# Adolescent-Friendly Pediatric Practice

# Adolescent-Friendly Pediatric Practice

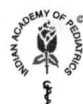 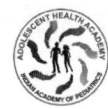 

### Editor-in-Chief
**Harish K Pemde** MD FIAP
Director–Professor and In-charge
Center for Adolescent Health
Department of Pediatrics
Lady Hardinge Medical College and
Kalawati Saran Children's Hospital
New Delhi, India
Vice President, International Association
of Adolescent Health
Chairman, IAP Adolescent Health
Academy (2022)

### Academic Editor
**TL Ratna Kumari** MD DCH FNNF
Former Professor of Neonatology
Madras Medical College, and
Institute of Child Health and
Hospital for Children, Chennai
Former Professor of Pediatrics and
Neonatology, ANIIMS, Port Blair
Editor-in-Chief, IJPP (2023–2025)
President
NNF, Tamil Nadu (2015–2016)

### Managing Editors
**Preeti M Galagali** MBBS MD PGDAP
Director and Consultant
Adolescent Health Specialist
Bengaluru Adolescent Care and
Counseling Centre
Bengaluru, Karnataka, India

**S Lakshmi Velmurugan** MD (Pediatrics)
Professor
Department of Pediatrics
Madras Medical College and Institute
of Child Health and Hospital for Children
Chennai, Tamil Nadu, India

### Admin Editor
**Harinder Singh** MBBS MD PGDAP FIAP PCC
(Adolescent Health, IMA-Sinha Institute)
Owner, Teen Clinic
Ludhiana, Punjab, India
Vice President, CIAP North Zone (2022)

### Associate Editors
Amitha Rao Aroor
Dhakshayani RV
J Shyamala
Jayashree K

S Kalpana
Shilpa Chandrashekhar
Sridevi A Naaraayan
Swati Ghate

### Forewords
S Thangavelu, Remesh Kumar R, Upendra S Kinjawadekar, Piyush Gupta, Vineet K Saxena, Swati Bhave, MKC Nair, CP Bansal, JS Tuteja, Sukanta Chatterjee, Geeta Patil, JC Garg, RN Sharma, Suhas Dhonde

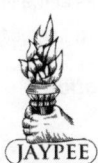

**JAYPEE BROTHERS MEDICAL PUBLISHERS**
*The Health Sciences Publisher*
New Delhi | London

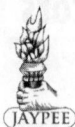 **Jaypee Brothers Medical Publishers (P) Ltd**

**Headquarters**
Jaypee Brothers Medical Publishers (P) Ltd
EMCA House, 23/23-B
Ansari Road, Daryaganj
New Delhi 110 002, India
Landline: +91-11-23272143, +91-11-23272703
+91-11-23282021, +91-11-23245672
Email: jaypee@jaypeebrothers.com

**Corporate Office**
Jaypee Brothers Medical Publishers (P) Ltd
4838/24, Ansari Road, Daryaganj
New Delhi 110 002, India
Phone: +91-11-43574357
Fax: +91-11-43574314
Email: jaypee@jaypeebrothers.com

**Overseas Office**
JP Medical Ltd
83 Victoria Street, London
SW1H 0HW (UK)
Phone: +44 20 3170 8910
Fax: +44 (0)20 3008 6180
Email: info@jpmedpub.com

Website: www.jaypeebrothers.com
Website: www.jaypeedigital.com

© 2024, Indian Academy of Pediatrics

The views and opinions expressed in this book are solely those of the original contributor(s)/author(s) and do not necessarily represent those of editor(s) or publisher of the book.

All rights reserved. No part of this publication may be reproduced, stored or transmitted in any form or by any means, electronic, mechanical, photocopying, recording or otherwise, without the prior permission in writing of the publishers.

All brand names and product names used in this book are trade names, service marks, trademarks or registered trademarks of their respective owners. The publisher is not associated with any product or vendor mentioned in this book.

Medical knowledge and practice change constantly. This book is designed to provide accurate, authoritative information about the subject matter in question. However, readers are advised to check the most current information available on procedures included and check information from the manufacturer of each product to be administered, to verify the recommended dose, formula, method and duration of administration, adverse effects and contraindications. It is the responsibility of the practitioner to take all appropriate safety precautions. Neither the publisher nor the author(s)/editor(s) assume any liability for any injury and/or damage to persons or property arising from or related to use of material in this book.

This book is sold on the understanding that the publisher is not engaged in providing professional medical services. If such advice or services are required, the services of a competent medical professional should be sought.

Every effort has been made where necessary to contact holders of copyright to obtain permission to reproduce copyright material. If any have been inadvertently overlooked, the publisher will be pleased to make the necessary arrangements at the first opportunity.

**Inquiries for bulk sales may be solicited at:** jaypee@jaypeebrothers.com

*Adolescent-Friendly Pediatric Practice*

*First Edition:* **2024**

ISBN: 978-93-5696-157-9

*Printed at* Rajkamal Electric Press, Kundli, Haryana.

# Contributors

**Amitha Rao Aroor** MBBS MD (Pediatrics)
Professor in Pediatrics and Adolescent Specialist
AJ Institute of Medical Sciences
Mangaluru, Karnataka, India

**Anuradha HS** MBBS DNB (Pediatrics)
PGDAP CPD Educator USA
Founder and Director
Tots 2 Teens Healthcare
Bengaluru, Karnataka, India

**Atul M Kanikar** MBBS DCH
Practicing Pediatrician and Adolescent Care Specialist
Nashik, Maharashtra, India

**B Lakshmi Shanthi** MBBS DCH PGDAP
Consultant Pediatrician and Adolescent Health Expert
Running Comprehensive Pediatrics and Adolescent Health Clinic
Medical Officer in Coimbatore Municipal Corporation
Coimbatore, Tamil Nadu, India

**Chandrika Rao** MBBS DCH MD (Pediatrics)
Post Graduate Diploma in Adolescent Medicine, Post Graduate Diploma in Medical Law and Ethics
Professor of Pediatrics and Adolescent Physician
MS Ramaiah Medical College and Hospital
Bengaluru, Karnataka, India

**Chitra Dinakar** MBBS DCH DNB (Pediatrics)
Pediatrician
Ashwini Clinic
Bengaluru, Karnataka, India

**CP Bansal** MBBS MD PGDAP FIAP FICMCH
Practising Pediatrician and Adolescent Care Specialist
Director
Shabd Pratap Hospital
Gwalior, Madhya Pradesh, India

**Dhakshayani RV** MD (Pediatrics)
Associate Professor
Department of Pediatrics
Government Medical College
Nagapattinam, Tamil Nadu, India

**Gowrishankar NC** MD DCH DNBPED FIAP
Head
Department of Pediatrics and Pediatric Pulmonologist
Mehta Multispecialty Hospital India Pvt Ltd
Chennai, Tamil Nadu, India

**Harinder Singh** MBBS MD PGDAP FIAP PCC
(Adolescent Health, IMA-Sinha Institute)
Owner, Teen Clinic
Ludhiana, Punjab, India
Vice President
CIAP North Zone (2022)

**Harish K Pemde** MD FIAP
Director–Professor and In-charge
Center for Adolescent Health
Department of Pediatrics
Lady Hardinge Medical College and Kalawati Saran Children's Hospital
New Delhi, India
Vice President, International Association of Adolescent Health
Chairman, IAP Adolescent Health Academy (2022)

**Hemchand K Prasad**
MD PDCC (Ped Endo) FPE FPD
Consultant
Department of Pediatric Endocrinology
Mehta Multispecialty Hospital India Pvt Ltd
Chennai, Tamil Nadu, India

**J Shyamala** MBBS DipNB (Pediatrics) DCH
Senior Consultant Pediatrician and Head
Department of Pediatrics
Apollo Children Hospitals
Chennai, Tamil Nadu, India

**Jayashree K** MBBS MD
Pediatrician and Adolescent Health Specialist
Associate Professor
Department of Pediatrics
Kasturba Medical College, Mangaluru
Manipal Academy of Higher Education
Manipal, Karnataka, India

**Kamal Kumar Singhal** DCH MD DM (Pediatrics Pulmonology)
Professor
Division of Pediatric Pulmonology
Department of Pediatrics
Lady Hardinge Medical College and
Kalawati Saran Children's Hospital
New Delhi, India

**Kritika Agarwal** MBBS MD (Pediatrics)
Consultant Pediatrician
Member of IAP, AHA
Manipal Hospital
Bengaluru, Karnataka, India

**Malathi Sathiyasekaran**
MD DCH DM MNAMS
Senior Consultant Pediatric Gastroenterologist
Rainbow Children's Hospital and MGM Hospital
Chennai, Tamil Nadu, India

**Mary Augustine**
MBBS MD (Dermatology)
Professor
Department of Dermatology
St John's Medical College Hospital
Bengaluru, Karnataka, India

**Megha Mahajan** MD DM
Child and Adolescent Psychiatrist
Consultant Child Psychiatrist
Fortis Hospital, Bengaluru
Aastha Children's Clinic
Bengaluru, Karnataka, India

**MKC Nair** DS
Director
NIMS-Spectrum-Child Development Research Centre (CDRC)
NIMS Medicity
Thiruvananthapuram, Kerala, India
Former Vice Chancellor, KUHS
Founder Director, CDC
Emeritus Professor in Child Adolescent and Behavioral Pediatrics, CDC

**Nedunchelian K** MD (Pediatrics) DCH
Senior Consultant Pediatrician
Head (Academics and Research)
Metha Multispecialty Hospitals India Pvt Ltd
Chennai, Tamil Nadu, India

**Newton Luiz** MD DCH DNB
Consultant Pediatrician
Dhanya Mission Hospital
Kerala, India

**Piyali Bhattacharya**
DCH MD (Ped) FIAP FRCP (London)
Consultant Pediatrician
Sanjay Gandhi Postgraduate Institute of Medical Sciences
Lucknow, Uttar Pradesh, India

**Poonam Bhatia**
MBBS DCH PGDAP DCMH (NIMHANS)
Director
Tots 2 Teens Child Guidance Clinic
Dewas, Madhya Pradesh, India

**Preeti M Galagali** MBBS MD PGDAP
Director and Consultant
Adolescent Health Specialist
Bengaluru Adolescent Care and Counseling Centre
Bengaluru, Karnataka, India

**Prerna Kukreti** MD (Psychiatry)
Associate Professor (Psychiatry)
Lady Hardinge Medical College and Associated Hospitals
New Delhi, India

# Contributors

**Rajiv Mohta** MBBS MD (Pediatrics) PGDAP
Adolescent Specialist and Pediatrician
Mohta Children and ENT Hospital
and Adolescent Counseling Centre
Nagpur, Maharashtra, India
Healthcare Consultant
Nelson Child Hospital
Member of IAP, AHA

**Ramaswamy Ganesh** MBBS DNB
MNAMS MRCPCH (UK) FRCPCH (UK) PhD
Senior Consultant Pediatrician
Rainbow Children's Hospital
Chennai, Tamil Nadu, India

**Riya Lukose** DCH DNB MRCPCH
IAP Fellowship in Developmental and
Behavioral Pediatrics
Pediatrician
Amala Institute of Medical Sciences
Thrissur, Kerala, India

**S Kalpana** MD (Pediatrics) European
Diplomate in Pediatric Respiratory Medicine
Associate Professor
Department of Pediatrics
Government Vellore Medical College
Adukamparai, Tamil Nadu, India

**S Lakshmi Velmurugan**
MRCPCH (UK) MBBS
Professor
Department of Pediatrics
Madras Medical College and Institute of
Child Health and Hospital for Children
Chennai, Tamil Nadu, India
Executive Editor
Indian Journal of Practical Pediatrics
President, IAP Chennai City Branch
(2023)

**Sangeeta Yadav** MD (Pediatrics)
Professor of Excellence
Former Head
Department of Pediatrics
Maulana Azad Medical College and
Associated
LN Hospital, University of Delhi
New Delhi, India

**Shashi Kiran** MD
Consultant Child Psychiatrist
Tees, Esk and Wear Valleys
NHS Foundation Trust
Durham, UK

**Sheila Balakrishnan** MD DNB
Additional Professor
Department of Obstetrics and Gynecology
The Government Medical College
Thiruvananthapuram, Kerala, India

**Shekhar Seshadri** MBBS MD (Psychiatry)
Senior Professor in Child and
Adolescent Psychiatry
The National Institute of Mental Health
and Neuro-Sciences
Bengaluru, Karnataka, India

**Shilpa Chandrashekhar**
MBBS MD (Pediatrics)
Assistant Professor
Department of Pediatrics
Karnataka Institute of Medical Sciences
Hubballi, Karnataka, India

**Shivangi Bora** MBBS MD (Pediatrics)
Senior Resident
Department of Pediatrics
St John's Medical College Hospital
Bengaluru, Karnataka, India

**Shoba Srinath** DPM MD
Consultant Child and Adolescent
Psychiatrist
Retired Senior Professor
Child and Adolescent Psychiatry
The National Institute of Mental Health
and Neuro-Sciences
Bengaluru, Karnataka, India

**Shruti Kalkekar** MBBS DCH PGPN PGDAP
Consultant Pediatrician and Adolescent
Health Expert
Running Comprehensive Pediatrics and
Adolescent Health Clinic
Director
Dr Kalkekar's Cura Advanced Child
Health Clinic
Navi Mumbai, Maharashtra, India

## Contributors

**Shyamal Kumar** MD PGPN PGDBM
Developmental Pediatrician
Rani Children Hospital
Ranchi, Bihar, India

**Sreyoshi Ghosh** MBBS MD DM
Consultant Child and Adolescent
Psychiatrist
Bengaluru, Karnataka, India

**Sridevi A Naaraayan** MD (Pediatrics)
Professor
Department of Pediatrics
Madras Medical College
Chennai, Tamil Nadu, India
Secretary, IAP CCB
Member, Editorial Board, IJPP

**Suresh Natarajan** MBBS DNB MNAMS
MRCPCH (UK) FRCPCH (UK) DAA PhD
Senior Consultant Pediatrician
Rainbow Children's Hospital
Chennai, Tamil Nadu, India

**Swati Ghate** DCH PGDAP MA
(Clinical Psychology)
Joint Director
Babylon's Newton Institute of Child
and Adolescent Development
Jaipur, Rajasthan, India

**Swati Y Bhave**
MD DCH FCPS FIAP FAAP (Hon)
Professor Emeritus
Dr DY Patil Medical College and
Research Center, Pimpri
Dr DY Patil Vidyapeeth, Pune
Visiting Consultant Pediatrician
(Adolescent)
Sassoon Hospital and Govt BJ Medical
College, Pune
Senior Consultant in Adolescent
Pediatrics and Head and In-charge
of Adolescent Wellness Clinic
Jehangir Hospital
Pune, Maharashtra, India
Executive Director, AACCI, Mumbai
(Association of Adolescent and Child
Care in India)

**Tejas Golhar** FRANZCP MBBS MD PDF
(CAP) Cert. Child and Adolescent Psychiatry
Consultant Child and Adolescent
Psychiatrist
Goulburn Valley Health, Australia
and Department of Psychiatry
University of Melbourne, Australia

**TL Ratna Kumari** MD DCH FNNF
Former Professor of Neonatology
Madras Medical College, and
Institute of Child Health and
Hospital for Children, Chennai
Former Professor of Pediatrics and
Neonatology, ANIIMS, Port Blair
Editor-in-Chief, IJPP (2023–2025)
President, NNF, Tamil Nadu (2015–2016)

**Utkarsh Bansal** MBBS MD (Pediatrics)
MAMS FACEE (Peds EM) Fellow Neonatal
Medicine (ISPT & Learn-ECMS, Australia)
Professor and Head (Pediatrics)
Hind Institute of Medical Sciences
Safedabad
Consultant Pediatrician
Neonatologist and Adolescent Physician
Om Child Care and Vaccination Clinic
Lucknow, Uttar Pradesh, India

**Utkarsh Sharma** MBBS MD
(Pediatrics and Neonatology)
Vice-Principal cum Professor and Head
Department of Pediatrics and
Neonatology
Shri Guru Ram Rai Institute of Medical
and Health Sciences
Dehradun, Uttarakhand, India

**V Poovazhagi** MD DCH PhD
Professor and Head
Pediatric Intensive Care Unit
Institute of Child Health and Hospital
for Children
Chennai, Tamil Nadu, India

**Varsha Bharti** MBBS
Medical Officer
Child Development Center
Thiruvananthapuram, Kerala, India

**Vijayarani M** DCH PGDAP
Pediatrician and Adolescent Physician
Sneham—Child and Adolescent Clinic
Vellore, Tamil Nadu, India

**Viji Thirugnanam**
DNB (Pediatrics Trainee)
Pediatrician
Mehta Multispecialty Hospitals India Pvt Ltd
Chennai, Tamil Nadu, India

**Vinayak Koparde**
MD (NIMHANS) DM (NIMHANS) Dip CAP (UK)
Associate Professor
Jawaharlal Nehru Medical College
Belagavi
Consulting Child and Adolescent Psychiatrist
Child Development Center
KLES Dr Prabhakar Kore Hospital and MRC, Belagavi
Springboard Child Health
Belagavi, Karnataka, India

**Yamuna S** MBBS DCH DNB (Pediatrics)
Pediatrician and Adolescent Physician
Child and Adolescent Clinic
Chennai, Tamil Nadu, India

# Foreword

With adolescent health issues receiving much-needed attention from both society and caregivers of late, this effort to compile a textbook dealing with adolescent issues is laudable. The editorial board and the authors have taken a stupendous effort to address all adolescent health issues in this book. I am sure that this book will serve as a guide to all stakeholders in adolescent health particularly pediatricians and family physicians. IJPP is always at the forefront of kindling the academic interest of pediatric postgraduates and practicing pediatricians.

IJPP-AHA is proud to be associated with this pathbreaking academic venture and hopes that it will inspire pediatricians to chart new paths in adolescent health care.

**S Thangavelu**
Senior Consultant (Pediatrics) and Director
Department of Pediatrics
Mehta Multispeciality Hospitals India Pvt Ltd
Chennai, Tamil Nadu, India
*Former* Reader in Pediatrics
Pediatric Intensive Care Unit
Institute of Child Health, Madras Medical College
Chennai, Tamil Nadu, India

# Foreword

It is well known that India has a rich demographic dividend in the form of 20% population being adolescents. They are destined to shape its future. Their health status and productivity shall directly reflect on the country's socioeconomic growth for decades to come.

IAP is well cognizant of this fact for a long and has been working hard incessantly for adolescents for over two decades. Adolescent Health Academy, IAP's vibrant subspecialty chapter has been instrumental in creating a palpable wave of adolescent health awareness across the country. IAP is also trying its best to get the adolescent age group officially and legally under the umbrella of pediatricians' care. We have proposed to the authorities to rename the pediatrics departments in all our medical colleges as *Department of Pediatrics and Adolescent Medicine*. This will also make them optimally functional in providing healthcare to adolescents and in training their students for the same.

Empowering pediatricians and budding doctors on Adolescent Health are big challenges of the day. It gives us great pleasure to see that IAP, AHA and IJPP have joined hands and come out with IAP's first textbook on Adolescent Health. *Adolescent-Friendly Pediatrics Practice* caters very systematically to almost all the important physical and mental health concerns encountered in adolescent office practice. This book presents the latest and lucid information to the readers in a simple and practically useful manner. The chapters of the book are painstakingly written by very eminent national and international experts and carry the flavor of their vast personal experience in the field. There are lots of flowcharts, figures and tables to make the contents attractive, crisp and reader friendly. We are sure, this book will fill the void of a comprehensive and practical textbook on adolescent health.

We extend our warm wishes to all the authors for their very concrete and sincere contributions. Dr Harish K Pemde and team have left no stone unturned to edit the book to its perfection. M/s Jaypee Brothers Medical Publishers (P) Ltd have always been with IAP in most of its academic publications. We are happy to see their usual perfection reflected in this book. This book will surely be a great help to us on our path of providing comprehensive care to children till they become adults.

**Remesh Kumar R**
President, IAP 2022
**Upendra S Kinjawadekar**
President, IAP 2023
**Piyush Gupta**
President, IAP 2021
**Vineet K Saxena**
HSG, IAP 2022-23

# Foreword

It is a pleasure to write the foreword for the book, *Adolescent-Friendly Pediatrics Practice*, the first IAP Book on adolescent medicine published jointly by the Adolescent Health Academy and the Indian Journal of Practical Pediatrics (IJPP).

It is pertinent to note that India has the largest youth population in the world, with one in every five individuals between 10 to 19 years of age. The demographic dividend opportunity in *our country is the longest in the world*, whose potential can be harnessed provided they are in their optimal physical and mental health.

It is well recognized that adolescent health has triple implications for the present generation as well as the generations to come. The period of Adolescence (10 to 19 years) is hence a critical period of substantial concern. Although many programs and services to cater to adolescent health and improve their quality-of-life have appeared in increasing numbers over the past few decades there is still a continuing pursuit for solutions to varied problems among adolescents, with this forethought in the background a comprehensive approach has been made to equip primary caretakers and adolescent physicians to deal effectively with the common adolescent health issues in office practice.

The book is an excellent amalgamation of updated articles covering all important aspects of adolescent clinical care, published in the last 2 decades. It is a handy desktop reference for practicing pediatricians, postgraduates and all health professionals interested in adolescent healthcare. We sincerely hope that this book reaches tens and thousands of healthcare professionals looking after adolescents.

**Swati Bhave**
Former President, IAP and Chairperson, AHA
**MKC Nair**
Former President, IAP and Chairperson, AHA
**CP Bansal**
Former President, IAP and Chairperson, AHA
**JS Tuteja**
Former Chairperson, AHA

# Foreword

We believe that while it may take a village to raise a child, it takes an army to mold an adolescent. Adolescent health care is an elaborate network that cannot be navigated solely by doctors or caregivers. In a world where adolescents have access to an extensive array of views and opinions, raising one is no longer a 'step-by-step plan'. Navigating this new and rapidly changing time had puzzled adolescent specialists for a really long time. Managing the physical and emotional health of an adolescent was a juggling act that was truly tough to balance. It becomes the ardent duty of healthcare professionals to help and guide adolescents and their parents through this tumultuous phase of life.

This book offers some insight into this quandary. It sheds light on various aspects of adolescent health care, keeping-in-mind the latest developments. It provides one with a general understanding of the period of adolescence and the changes that it brings, be they physical, emotional or social. It seamlessly moves on to an approach to adolescent health care, with a special focus on adolescent counseling. It then turns to common problems that may affect adolescents and a guide to their approach and treatment. Finally, it touches on chronic illnesses and the handling of these illnesses. With contributions by eminent adolescent specialists from India and abroad, along with selected articles from IJPP journal volumes over the past decade, this book compiles some of the greatest and most varied approaches to adolescent healthcare.

This book is of great significance, especially at a time when the world (and adolescents especially) is just beginning to heal from the effects of the COVID pandemic, which took great tolls, both physically and emotionally. With the world slowly moving towards the 'new normal' of living, this book seems to slowly nudge us into the 'new normal' of adolescent medicine.

Best of luck, today and always!

**Sukanta Chatterjee**
Chairperson, AHA (2023)
**Geeta Patil**
Chairperson, AHA (2024)
**JC Garg**
Chairperson, AHA (2021)
**RN Sharma**
Secretary, AHA (2022-23)
**Suhas Dhonde**
Treasurer, AHA (2022-23)

# Preface

Adolescents constitute 20% of India's population. It was slightly more than 2 decades ago when the Indian Academy of Pediatrics (IAP) declared that pediatricians can look after children up to 18 years of age. Since then, a lot has happened in this field in India. In addition to the annual conferences of Adolescent Health Academy (AHA), the Subspecialty Chapter of IAP, many training programs, continuing medical education (CMEs), and workshops have happened across the country. A large number of pediatricians have developed interest in Adolescent Health and Medicine and have started practicing this subspecialty. Several resources were created to support the pediatricians looking after children up to 18 years of age. These resources were in the form of resource book for IAP Presidents' Action Plan Programs, some training programs, conference proceedings, and, in 2020-2021, the Webinar videos and video symposiums.

IAP's journals Indian Journal of Practical Pediatrics (IJPP) and Indian Pediatrics have published a large number of articles on the topics related to adolescent health and medicine. IJPP published a large number of review articles on these topics over the last 2 decades. A large number of pediatricians have benefitted from them. IJPP, thus, helped in the development of the specialty of adolescent health and medicine in India. We, the AHA and IJPP, came together and decided to come out with a compendium of these articles earlier published in IJPP. Although some of the articles were quite old, the topics are still relevant. Out of the many articles published, we chose several of them. We also decided to publish these articles in the form of a book. We found that the topics were many, but some important topics were missing. We, then, decided to add few more chapters to make it a near complete book on the subject.

The Editorial Board (EB) further contacted the original authors with a request to update their articles in view of recent developments in science. We also added new authors for the additional chapters (that were not earlier published in IJPP). Simultaneously, we also requested IAP to approve this book as IAP book. We are grateful to IAP-EB 2022 to accept our request and approve this as IAP book and for referring this book to M/s Jaypee Brothers Medical Publishers (P) Ltd, New Delhi for publication. Thus, this book became the first IAP book on the subject of Adolescent Health and Medicine.

Rest is history as all the authors are senior pediatricians and Who's Who of the adolescent health experts and pioneers of the subject in India, and some young and enthusiastic pediatricians and other experts. All have worked hard to bring this book.

We are sure that this book will further add significantly to the resources on adolescent health and medicine in India. All those practicing adolescent health and medicine will find it useful in their routine practice and in managing adolescents and young adults having medical and mental health issues. We have planned to revise and update this book every 3 years, and your feedback, comments, and suggestions are welcome.

**Harish K Pemde**
**TL Ratna Kumari**
**Preeti M Galagali**
**S Lakshmi Velmurugan**
**Harinder Singh**

# Acknowledgments

## Names of the Office Bearers and the Members of the Executive Board of the Indian Academy of Pediatrics (2022)

**Remesh Kumar R**
President

**Upendra S Kinjawadekar**
President-Elect

**Piyush Gupta**
Immediate Past President

**Vineet K Saxena**
Secretary General

**K Radhakrishna**
Vice President-Central Zone

**Sudhir Mishra**
Vice President-East Zone

**Harinder Singh**
Vice President-North Zone

**Subramanya NK**
Vice President-South Zone

**Chetan B Shah**
Vice President-West Zone

**Samir Hasan Dalwai**
Treasurer

**Alok Bhandari**
Joint Secretary-Liaison

**Purna A Kurkure**
Jt. Secretary-Admin

**Devendra Mishra**
Editor-in-Chief, IP

**S Thangavelu**
Editor-in-Chief, IJPP

**Anthati S Kireeti**
Executive Board Member

**P Anil Kumar**
Executive Board Member

**R Ramakrishna Paramahamsa**
Executive Board Member

**Mritunjay Pao**
Executive Board Member

**Chandra Mohan Kumar**
Executive Board Member

**Sheo Bachan Singh**
Executive Board Member

**Arun Prasad**
Executive Board Member

**Sushil Kumar**
Executive Board Member

**Ajay Kumar Gupta**
Executive Board Member

**Lalan K Bharti**
Executive Board Member

**Manish Gupta**
Executive Board Member

**Virendra Sadanand Gaokar**
Executive Board Member

**Kanaksinh U Surma**
Executive Board Member

**Ramesh M Bajania**
Executive Board Member

**Samir R Shah**
Executive Board Member

**AVS Ravi**
Executive Board Member

**Mahaveer Prasad Jain**
Executive Board Member

**Ravinder K Gupta**
Executive Board Member

**Joy Bhaduri**
Executive Board Member

**Geeta Patil**
Executive Board Member

**Madhu S Pujar**
Executive Board Member

**SN Prashanth**
Executive Board Member

**Shiva Prakash Sosale C**
Executive Board Member

**Jose Ouseph**
Executive Board Member

**M Narayanan**
Executive Board Member

**MK Nandakumar**
Executive Board Member

**Riaz I**
Executive Board Member

**Kewal Kishore Arora**
Executive Board Member

**Mahesh Maheshwari**
Executive Board Member

**Narendra R Nanivadekar**
Executive Board Member

**Pramod M Kulkarni**
Executive Board Member

**Ramakant D Patil**
Executive Board Member

**Sanjay B Deshmukh**
Executive Board Member

**Bela Verma**
Executive Board Member

**Shyamkumar Laishram**
Executive Board Member

**Santanu Deb**
Executive Board Member

**Prasant Kumar Saboth**
Executive Board Member

**Susruta Das**
Executive Board Member

**Gurdeep Singh**
Executive Board Member

**Harpreet Singh**
Executive Board Member

**Anurag Tomar**
Executive Board Member

**Rameshwar L Suman**
Executive Board Member

**A Chenthil**
Executive Board Member

**A Somasundaram**
Executive Board Member

**J Balaji**
Executive Board Member

**R Somasekar**
Executive Board Member

**G Vijaya Kumar**
Executive Board Member

**Kottooru Srisailam**
Executive Board Member

**S Srikrishna**
Executive Board Member

**Dhiraj M Gupta**
Executive Board Member

**Om Shankar Chaurasiya**
Executive Board Member

**Kaustav Nayek**
Executive Board Member

**Rajeev Krashak**
Executive Board Member

**Sutapa Ganguly**
Executive Board Member

**Utkarsh Sharma**
Executive Board Member

**Sheila S Mathai**
Services

**Asok Kumar Datta**
Executive Board Member

## Adolescent Health Academy Executive Board (2022)

**Harish K Pemde**
Chairperson

**Prashant Saboth**
Executive Board Member (East Zone)

**JC Garg**
Past Chairperson

**Prashant Kariya**
Executive Board Member (West Zone)

**RN Sharma**
Secretary

**Ranjith P**
Executive Board Member (South Zone)

**Suhas Dhonde**
Treasurer

**Geeta Bansal**
Executive Board Member (North Zone)

**Piyali Bhattacharya**
Executive Board Member (Central Zone)

## Editorial Board of Indian Journal of Pediatric Practice (2022)

**S Thangavelu**
Editor-in-Chief

**S Shanti**
Associate Editor

**G Durai Arasan**
Managing Editor

**C Vijyabhaskar**
Associate Editor

**TL Ratna Kumari**
Executive Editor

**Dhakshayani RV**
Executive Member

**Annamalai Vijyaraghvan**
Associate Editor

**Elayarani Elavassan**
Executive Member

**S Lakshmi**
Associate Editor

**S Kalpana**
Executive Member

**V Poovazhagi**
Associate Editor

**K Senthil Ganesh**
Executive Member

**J Shyamala**
Executive Member

**A Somasundaram**
Executive Member

**Sridevi A Naaraayan**
Executive Member

**B Sumathi**
Executive Member

**Vineet K Saxena (Ex-Offico)**
Executive Member

The editors appreciate the contribution of M/s Jaypee Brothers Medical Publishers (P) Ltd, New Delhi, India. We thank Shri Jitendar P Vij (Group Chairman), Mr Ankit Vij (Managing Director), Mr MS Mani (Group President), Ms Chetna Malhotra (Senior Director—Professional Publishing, Marketing, and Business Development), Ms Pooja Bhandari (Director—Production) and Ms Kritika Dua (Senior Development Editor) for tireless follow-up and finishing the book within the timeline.

# Contents

## Section 1: Understanding Adolescence

1. **Normal Adolescent Growth and Development** .................... 3
   *Swati Y Bhave, Sangeeta Yadav*

2. **Body Image during Adolescence** ................... 18
   *Amitha Rao Aroor, Preeti M Galagali*

3. **Adolescent Sexuality** ....................... 30
   *Chandrika Rao*

4. **Parenting an Adolescent** ................. 43
   *Yamuna S, Vijayarani M*

5. **Media Usage in Adolescents** ....................... 50
   *Jayashree K, Preeti M Galagali*

## Section 2: Dealing with Adolescent Client

6. **Psychosocial Assessment of Adolescents Using HEEADSSS** ...... 61
   *B Lakshmi Shanthi, Shruti Kalkekar*

7. **Sexual and Reproductive Health Assessment of Adolescents** ................................ 73
   *Poonam Bhatia, Anuradha HS*

8. **Monitoring Physical Growth of Adolescents** ............... 85
   *Sridevi A Naaraayan, Nedunchelian K*

9. **Adolescent Counseling** ................. 98
   *Atul M Kanikar, CP Bansal*

10. **Motivational Interviewing** ....................... 106
    *Swati Ghate, Sreyoshi Ghosh*

11. **Making Pediatric Practice Adolescent Friendly** ..................... 116
    *Kritika Agarwal, Rajiv Mohta*

12. **Psychopharmacological Interventions in Children and Adolescents** ............................. 125
    *Tejas Golhar, Shashi Kiran, Shoba Srinath*

## Section 3: Common Medical Problems

13. **Adolescent Headache** .................................................. 139
    *Amitha Rao Aroor, Preeti M Galagali*

14. **Adolescent Sleep Problems** ........................................ 153
    *Jayashree K, Preeti M Galagali*

15. **Dermatological Issues in Adolescence** ..................... 162
    *Shivangi Bora, Mary Augustine*

16. **Irritable Bowel Syndrome in Children and Adolescents** .......... 175
    *Ramaswamy Ganesh, Suresh Natarajan, Malathi Sathiyasekaran*

17. **Adolescent Obesity** .................................................. 190
    *Viji Thirugnanam, Hemchand K Prasad*

18. **Adolescent Polycystic Ovary Syndrome** ................... 208
    *MKC Nair, Sheila Balakrishnan, Varsha Bharti*

19. **Coping Strategies in Adolescents: Developmental Issues** ........ 216
    *Shashi Kiran, Shekhar Seshadri*

20. **School Performance in Adolescence** ....................... 225
    *Preeti M Galagali, Newton Luiz*

21. **Adolescent Anxiety and Depression** ....................... 237
    *MKC Nair, Shyamal Kumar*

22. **Disruptive Behavior Disorders in Adolescents: Management** ... 247
    *Harish K Pemde, Prerna Kukreti*

23. **Management of Adolescent Suicidal Behavior in Office Practice** .......... 256
    *Preeti M Galagali, Amitha Rao Aroor*

24. **Anemia in Adolescents** ............................................. 268
    *Piyali Bhattacharya*

25. **Menstrual Disorders in Adolescence** ...................... 276
    *J Shyamala, Chitra Dinakar, Shilpa Chandrashekhar*

26. **Relationship Counseling** .......................................... 294
    *MKC Nair, Shyamal Kumar, Riya Lukose*

27. **Office Management of Substance Abuse** ................ 301
    *Jayashree K, Preeti M Galagali*

## Section 4: Chronic Diseases in Adolescents

28. **Tuberculosis in Adolescents** ......... 315
    *Utkarsh Bansal, Gowrishankar NC, Dhakshayani RV*

29. **Asthma in Adolescents** ......... 333
    *S Lakshmi Velmurugan, Utkarsh Sharma, S Kalpana*

30. **Pneumonia in Adolescents** ......... 343
    *V Poovazhagi, Kamal Kumar Singhal*

31. **Psychotic Disorders in Adolescents** ......... 349
    *Megha Mahajan, Vinayak Koparde*

*Index* ......... *361*

# SECTION 1

# Understanding Adolescence

1. **Normal Adolescent Growth and Development**
   *Swati Y Bhave, Sangeeta Yadav*
2. **Body Image during Adolescence**
   *Amitha Rao Aroor, Preeti M Galagali*
3. **Adolescent Sexuality**
   *Chandrika Rao*
4. **Parenting an Adolescent**
   *Yamuna S, Vijayarani M*
5. **Media Usage in Adolescents**
   *Jayashree K, Preeti M Galagali*

# CHAPTER 1

# Normal Adolescent Growth and Development

*Swati Y Bhave, Sangeeta Yadav*

## ■ INTRODUCTION

The World Health Organization (WHO) defines adolescence to be between the ages of 10 and 19 years. Adolescence is a very dynamic and important state of human development, as it is the transitional stage where a child matures to transform into an adult. This leads to many changes happening at the same time in the physical, psychological, emotional, and social domains.

## ■ NORMAL PHYSICAL GROWTH AND DEVELOPMENT

As pediatricians, we make parents of young children aware of the normal range of development of physical and mental milestones so that they do not have undue concerns or fears but at the same time are alert to the red flag signs for early intervention. Similarly, as adolescent physicians it is important to make both parents and adolescents themselves aware of the process of puberty and the normal variations seen in adolescents. This anticipatory guidance and preventive counseling will prevent a lot of concerns related with pubertal changes, especially the issues associated with *early bloomers and late bloomers*, which will prevent a lot of anguish and psychological problems, caused in the minds of both parents and adolescents.

### Puberty

This signifies the beginning of biological growth during adolescence and is a period of rapid growth and bodily changes involving changes caused by increased hormonal activity.

In childhood, the hypothalamic gonadotropin-releasing hormone (GnRH) pulse generation is kept under restrain. At puberty there is maturation of the central nervous system (CNS) centers that lessen the restraint. A certain level of general maturity must normally be reached before the CNS activates puberty. A pubertal level of maturation is also closely tied with body mass and nutrition. The bone age (or skeletal age) corresponds to pubertal maturation better than the chronological age.

The release of hypothalamic GnRH is regulated by a number of neurotransmitters and neuroendocrine hormones. These processes are magnified during pubertal development. The hormonal regulation of the growth spurt and the alterations in body composition depend on the release of the several hormones such as gonadotropins, leptin, sex steroids, and the growth hormone.

It is very likely that interactions among these hormonal axis are more important than their main effects, and that alteration in body composition and the regional distribution of body fat actually are signals to alter the neuroendocrine and peripheral hormone axes **(Fig. 1)**.

The biological changes that occur during puberty are development of primary sex characteristics (changes in the organs directly related to reproduction—gonadal maturation), sexual maturation making them capable of fertility, appearance of secondary sexual characteristics (bodily signs of sexual maturity that do not directly involve reproductive organs), increase in height and weight, i.e., adolescent growth spurt, completion of skeletal growth, increase in skeletal mass, and changes in body composition. During puberty, the succession of these events is consistent among adolescents. However, there are likely to be deviations in the age of onset, duration, and tempo of these events between and within individuals.

The onset of puberty corresponds to a skeletal age of approximately 10-11 years in girls and 13 years in boys. Girls complete each stage of puberty earlier than boys. Gonadal steroid hormones (primarily estradiol in both sexes) enhance bone mineral accrual and affect adult height by promoting epiphyseal fusion through direct effects on the growth plate. The pubertal

There is negative feedback as follows.
The gonadotropins inhibits GnRH from hypothalamus. Inhibin from the gonads secretion inhibits anterior pituitary release of FSH.
The estrogen and progesterone in females and testosterone in males inhibits anterior pituitary response to GnRH.

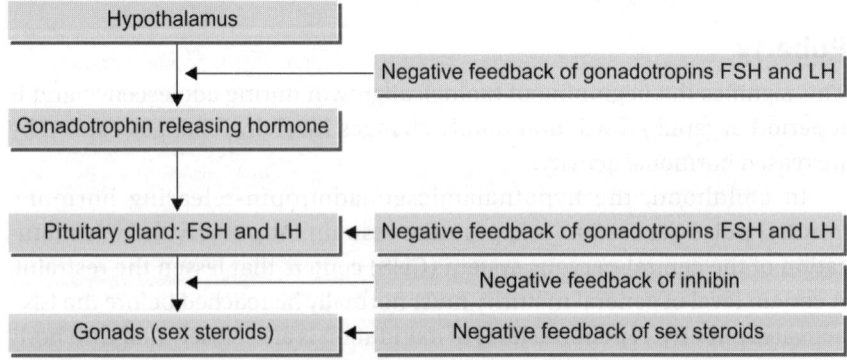

**Fig. 1:** Endocrine regulation related to puberty. (FSH: Follicle-stimulating hormone; GnRH: gonadotropin-releasing hormone: LH: luteinizing hormone)

growth consists of a phase of acceleration, followed by a phase of deceleration, and the eventual cessation of growth with the closure of epiphyses.

Certain diseases can cause puberty to occur early (precocious puberty) or late (delayed puberty). Physical changes represent just a fraction of the developmental processes that adolescents experience. Biological, psychosocial, and cognitive changes that begin during puberty, continue throughout adolescence and directly affect not only the physical status, but also influence their final personality as an adult in the society.

## Monitoring of Puberty in Office Practice

Parents are sometimes concerned that their child is going through puberty too early or too late. It is true that there are some medical causes of precocious or delayed puberty. Chances are that the child is going through puberty at the time that is right for him or her. The primary physician checks the child's physical growth. Monitoring is the key part of the child's medical care during the middle childhood to early teen years.

Clinicians need to evaluate the stages of puberty in their adolescent clients and the well accepted standard reference is use of sexual maturity rating (SMR), also known as Tanner staging **(Table 1)**. Sexual maturation correlates remarkably well with linear growth, changes in weight and body composition, and hormonal changes.

## Variations in Puberty

Adolescents are very keen to "fit-in" with peers. That is why they choose the same style of dressing, choice of music, hobbies and lifestyle choices, etc. Any adolescent who looks different or has different opinion is targeted for bullying or ostracization. Most children in a class go through the same stage of puberty. If an adolescent has early puberty (early bloomers) or late puberty (late bloomers), it results in significant variation in physical characteristics though they are still perfectly in the range of normalcy. Since they look different, they do not fit-in with the peers.

Unless they are taught about puberty and variations through school programs and also through parent and teacher programs these outliers face a lot of issues, that can not only lead to body image issues but also psychological problems. Such adolescents need to receive timely counseling before it escalates into a mental health issue. Anticipatory guidance on body changes and emotional changes eases the adolescents' anxiety in these issues.

Boys who are *early bloomers* are at an advantage as they are bigger and stronger than peers. They are more likely to be looked upon as natural leaders but if they have aggressive tendencies, they can have bullying behaviors. Boys who are *late bloomers* are perceived as tiny and physically inferior and can become victims of abuse, especially by older homosexual boys or men.

**TABLE 1:** Sexual maturity rating (SMR).

| Females | Males |
|---|---|
| *Breast development* | *Genital development* |
| **B1:** Prepubertal: Elevation of papilla only | **G1:** Preadolescent |
| **B2:** Breast buds with enlargement of areola | **G2:** Testis is >2.5 cm in longest diameter or 4 mL volume |
| **B3:** Further enlargement of breast tissue and areola, without separation of contours | **G3:** Growth of penis in width and length and testis enlarges |
| **B4:** Breast contour is separate from chest wall. Areola and papilla form a secondary mound | **G4:** Penis and testes are larger, scrotum darker and thicker |
| **B5:** Mature breast with projection of papilla | **G5:** Adult size and shape |
| *Pubic hair* | *Pubic hair* |
| **P1:** Prepubertal: No pubic hair | **P1:** Prepubertal: No pubic hair |
| **P2:** Sparse long, straight, slightly curly, minimally pigmented hair | **P2:** Sparse, slightly curly and pigmented hair at the base of penis |
| **P3:** Darker and coarser hair on mons pubis | **P3:** Thicker, curlier hair spreads laterally |
| **P4:** Adult type hair, not yet spreading to thighs | **P4:** Adult type hair, not yet spreading to thighs |
| **P5:** Adult type distribution of hair | **P5:** Adult type distribution of hair |

It can also lead to poor self-esteem due to negative body image, as girls do not think them sexually attractive. This also puts them at a higher risk of abuse of anabolic steroids, and harmful protein supplements for body building.

An early bloomer girl has a "woman's mature body with a child's innocent mind and emotional maturity". Such girls become targets of older boys and "sugar daddies" for sexual exploitation and abuse. She may also learn to use her body to her advantage, to get privileges. A late bloomer girl also develops poor body image and lowered self-esteem, as boys do not think them sexually attractive. This can lead to high-risk sexual behavior like sexual experimentation to attract attention.

Teachers in school also expect more maturity and responsibility from the early bloomers as they look bigger than peers, this is very unfair to them as they are likely to have the same emotional and cognitive maturity as their peers though they appear physically bigger.

## Body Image Issues Related to Puberty

Unless adolescents are primed to understand the process of puberty, some adolescents find it difficult to handle these physical changes. This leads to body image issues because they look gawky and awkward during the various stages of puberty and have constant pressure of media and peers to look cool and hep. Negative body image leads to low self-esteem that becomes a major factor for adolescent high-risk behavior.

## PARENTAL UNDERSTANDING OF NORMAL ADOLESCENT DEVELOPMENT

Most adults are not aware about the adolescent neurodevelopment and impact on adolescent behavior. They are also not aware about the psycho-emotional-social and sexual development of adolescence in various stages of early (10–13 years), middle (14–16 years), and late (17–19 years). Hence many parents and teachers have a lot of misunderstanding and misinterpretation of teen behavior that often leads to conflicts at home and school. Adolescent pediatricians need to educate teens themselves and parents and teachers through school and community programs.

Parents and teachers can help adolescents to transit into adulthood by the following:
- Formation of an identity with respect to self, future, and the world,
- Come out of the childhood dependence on parents and other adults and be empowered to become an adult capable of independent decision making and survival,
- They should be able to establish a new relationship, changing from *child-parent* to *adult-adult* as per the principles of transactional analysis, and
- Determination of goals in vocation, career and profession, family functioning and personal lifestyle and moral and ethical values.

Parents often feel neglected, unappreciated by teenagers or during their middle age crisis they become threatened by their offspring. Communication between parents and adolescents are distorted based on the above assumptions, which result in major conflicts.

## NORMAL PSYCHOSOCIAL DEVELOPMENT

Normal adolescent psychosocial development includes a variety of aspects. *Cognitive skills* that enhance their ability to reason and to think abstractly. *Emotional maturity and self-identity* develops a stronger recognition of their own personal identity, including recognition of a set of personal moral and ethical values, and greater perception of feelings of self-esteem or self-worth, establishing a new sense of who they are and who they want to become. *Social development* involves relating in new ways both to peers and adults and to experiment with new behaviors.

### Cognitive Development

Cognitive competence includes the ability to think, reason, plan, and solve problems. Ability to reflect on thinking is called metacognitive capacity which facilitates to understand thoughts, emotions, and feelings and thus show empathy toward others.

Children have "concrete thinking" which means understanding of immediate, that is the existential moment, i.e., here and now. They can relate to short-term consequences only. They cannot appreciate possibility of many solutions for a single problem. They lack ability to learn from previous experiences and apply the acquired knowledge in the context of a new experience. They cannot see the future as a continuum to the present.

According to Piaget, early adolescence is the period when the initial seeds of abstract thought processes are sown in a child who is a concrete thinker so long. By middle adolescence abstract thinking begins to emerge, which becomes more fine-tuned in late adolescence.

## Identity Crisis in Adolescents

Adults tend to treat adolescents sometimes as a child and sometimes as an adult. This leads to confusion and identity crisis in the mind of the teens and leads to career pressures. The developing brain with its limbic preponderance leads to reward seeking and experimentation which results in high-risk behavior compounded by peer pressure.

Biological and psychological changes of puberty are seen in all races and cultures, but psychosocial changes are culture specific and occur in the context of social environment. The tasks involved in social life move from dependence to independence, developing the self-identity and maturation in the peer relationships. Some are very aggressive; others are very submissive.

Every adolescent goes through a confused state of mind:
- Who am I?
- What is the goal of my life?
- Am I capable enough?
- How will I sail through life?

Their developing cognitive skills help to improve their abstract thinking and reasoning powers. Emotional development helps them to get a sense of personal identity. Social development helps them to relate to both peers and adults. They also develop greater sense of self awareness and their own set of moral values and ethics.

Most adolescents can go through the three phases of adolescence fairly smoothly, especially when they have a stable environment at home and school and adults give them positive psychosocial support.

### *Self-awareness and Self-esteem*

It is important for parents and teachers to help adolescents to develop positive self-esteem and a sense of identity. Because this is one of the important protective factors against high-risk behavior in adolescents such as eating disorders, substance abuse, and unsafe sexual experimentation.

## Adolescent Brain Development

It was presumed that the human brain matures by 18 years and hence the legal age permitting voting is 18 years in most countries as it was thought that by this age the brain is mature enough to take adult decisions. However, research over last two decades has shown that the human brain does not fully mature till 21–24 years of age. It has also been found that it develops from behind forward beginning from cerebellum, and the frontal cortex which has the executive functions matures last.

This means the adolescent brain is working through the hypothalamic limbic system which makes them vulnerable to amygdala hijack and the dopamine reward pathway.

This results in the high-risk experimentation seen in adolescents and vulnerability to all addictions that are dopamine dependent such as tobacco, alcohol, drugs, junk food, internet, social media, etc.

Due to immature frontal cortex the decisions which require mature thought and understanding of the future consequences of todays' action are not well developed making them impulsive and succumbing to negative peer pressure.

## Coping Skills in Adolescents

Due to intense academic competition, there is tremendous pressure in school and home for career choices and performance which increases the incidence of mental health issues such as anxiety, depression, and suicide.

The WHO life skills education programs help to enhance coping skills to deal with various stresses. Abstract thinking can be enhanced by learning life skills such as decision making and problem-solving skills. This can also be strengthened in the home and school setting by parents and teachers, helping adolescents to negotiate every roadblock in their life successfully.

## Emotional Development

Emotions in an adolescent play an important role in guiding behavior. This paves the path to lasting relationships with peer and family. Adolescents are always struggling to resolve major conflicts between internal pressures and social demands from society and family. In the absence of an understanding companionship, frustrations and disappointments are expressed as anger outbursts.

In early adolescence physical growth, preoccupation with body and interest in sexually explicit material are normal. Need for autonomy, demands for privacy, and increased argumentativeness are also normal. Emotional distancing from parents, waning peer group influence, and increasing conformity to an extraparental adult role model happens during middle adolescence. Establishment of intimate long-lasting relationships with friends and members of the opposite sex, achievement of complete emancipation, and initiation of realistic plans for future economic independence take place in late adolescence.

For a holistic personality development, it is very important to have emotional skills necessary to manage stress and be sensitive and effective in relating to other people. These skills have been called "emotional intelligence". This involves self-awareness, relationship skills, and the ability to get along well with other people and to make friends.

The most important skills that adolescents may develop as a part of their emotional development include recognizing and managing emotions, developing empathy, learning to resolve conflict constructively, and developing a cooperative spirit.

## Social Influences

Stable, protective, and nurturing environment at home, school, and community foster positive adolescent development and protects from high-risk behavior.

A close bond between parents and teens is shown by many researchers to be a protective factor against high-risk teen behavior. Some amount of conflict between adolescents and parents appears to be a way of learning how to become independent from parents and at the same time also wanting to be close to them. Care should be taken to remain connected and assure them of unconditional love even during conflict situations.

There is a symbolic movement of adolescents away from parents and family. Hence, involvement in family functions, weddings, etc., comes down to a minimum. There would be serious conflicts between parents and youngsters if anything is enforced against the will and cooperation of the adolescent. Parents should be aware of this movement away from home and ought to consider this as a step toward emancipation, which would enable the young adult to make relationships on their own. Parents should be made to understand that adolescents return to family environment during late adolescence, not for nurturance but to discuss issues on an adult-adult plane.

Society has its own demands on adolescents who are given confusing messages. At one point of time they are treated as mature individuals capable of viewing their future and taking appropriate steps toward acquisition of knowledge and choice of career. At another point of time they are looked down as immature dependents who need parental support and guidance in all facets including choice of educational stream, institution, place of work, choice of partner, timing of marriage, pregnancy, childbirth, etc.

## School and Peer Influence

Adolescents spend most of their time with the peer group in school and extracurricular activities. Parental neglect or abuse pushes adolescents into adverse peer influences. Parents are considered to be outdated and not objective enough to understand the needs and ideas of the youngsters. Parents have to understand and accept this and make special effort to keep positive relationship and communication with their adolescents, which protects adolescents from negative peer pressure.

Early adolescents have small same gender peer groups who have similar academic, social, and economic status. The peer group represents the code of normality and source of assurance and acceptance of social and moral code of ethics. Good peer group enhances their self-esteem and confidence. Individuals with many friends possess high self-esteem. Adolescents are attracted to peer groups who conform to their upbringing and concepts about future. Switching of peer groups happens if the youngsters do not feel comfortable in a particular group.

Peer group is very important for developing a sense of identity and learning social skills, especially during early adolescence. Being accepted and appreciated by peers is very rewarding for personality development. The influence of the peer group will depend on the stage of development. It also includes development of the "positive self", which is a very important aspect of adolescent identity development.

Adolescents are self-conscious and are worried about external appearances. They have a feeling that they are continuously "on stage" and everyone else is staring at them. Girls view themselves as overweight and are prone for eating disorders like anorexia nervosa. Boys and girls have their peer group decide the dress code and behavior during early and middle adolescence. Girls share a lot of confiding issues with their friends whereas boys form peer groups based on activities and leisure. Extraparental adult role model has a great influence on the adolescents' psychosocial development. During late adolescence, the youngsters introspect more and peer group influences decrease. Individual intimate friendships are formed which may remain as long-lasting relationships in future.

Adolescents spend a large part of their life in school and learn to develop social and cognitive skills with peers. It also provides safety and stability. If teachers show partiality or favoritism to students, it will have an adverse effect on the self-esteem of the student concerned and emotions of the peers. Good teachers should act as ideal adult role models. Negative behavior by teachers can lead to negative behavior of students.

## Moral and Value Development

This refers to the development of a sense of values and ethical behavior, moral reasoning, and prosocial behavior; and is very much dependent on the sociocultural and religious milieu of his or her upbringing. Moral values shape up human personality and decide how a person will behave in society and with other human beings.

Summary of all changes and adult support required at various stages **(Table 2)**.

### ■ POINTS TO REMEMBER

- Normal psychosocial development is affected by a variety of factors such as personality of the adolescent, the parenting style, the atmosphere at home, school, and community, peer influences, mentors, and role models available. For advocacy and awareness of adolescent holistic wellbeing, education and training of adolescent care takers is of supreme importance in adolescent health services.
- Adolescent pediatricians need to make both parents and adolescents aware of the normal physical and psychosocial development in the three stages of adolescence so that they do not misinterpret "normal adolescent behavior" as an abnormal wayward behavior.
- This can be done by doing programs in educational institutes and in the community for "out of school adolescents". This knowledge will help adolescents go through the transition in a healthy manner with good support from parents at home and teachers in schools.
- For adolescents to develop resilience create a positive environment to act as protective factor to reduce negative peer influence and risk taking behavior, a supportive environment in homes, community, and teaching institutions is vital.
- It is very important to monitor normal development of individual adolescent in the clinic setting and give appropriate anticipatory guidance and preventive counseling.
- Clinicians dealing with adolescents need to be aware of these phases, as this knowledge guides the approach to an adolescent patient. Health professionals should always give adequate time during the initial session to and adolescent for determining his/her degree of biological maturity and level of cognitive development. These characteristics should be used to determine the individual needs and the type of educational messages that shall have to be given while counseling the adolescent.
- All stake holders dealing with adolescents should train themselves in the WHO life skills education program and involve themselves in imparting this knowledge to empower the not only the adolescents but also teachers in schools and colleges and parents in community. Timely interventions provide help in developing coping skills.

**TABLE 2:** Summary of normal development in adolescents and adult support needed.

| | Early adolescence (10–13 years) | Middle adolescence (14–16 years) | Late adolescence (17–19 years) | Adult support |
|---|---|---|---|---|
| Pubertal staging | Tanner's stage 1–2 | Tanner's stage 3–5 | Tanner's stage 5 | • Ensure puberty monitoring |
| Physical changes | • Secondary sexual characteristics developing<br>• Peak height velocity (PHV)–peaks in girls<br>• Menarche in most<br>• Same age boys look smaller<br>• Boys may worry about delayed growth | • Secondary sexual characteristics well defined<br>• Most getting comfortable with body changes<br>• PHV declines in girls<br>• PHV peaks in boys<br>• Spermarche take place | • Final changes in secondary sexual characteristics<br>• Height stabilizes<br>• Boys gain muscle bulk and power<br>• Girls develop feminine curves | • Education about puberty at home and in school programs<br>• Help to understand puberty variations<br>• Help build positive body image |
| Psychological | • Awareness of sexual identity<br>• Reward orientation<br>• Self-concept: They are very conscious about self<br>• They feel they are on stage all the time and are the focus of attention of everyone around | • Wants to be left alone<br>• Want privacy<br>• Can put no-entry board on their doors<br>• Body image issues may still be seen in some especially with late bloomers<br>• Considers themselves invincible and more high-risk taking<br>• Verbal dexterity is increased<br>• Idolization (religious political)<br>• Period of heightened vulnerability to risk taking and problems in regulation of affect and behavior<br>• Rise late in the morning<br>• Untidiness issue of conflict with parents | • Again, start reconnecting with family<br>• Personal identity–start thinking about what sort of adult persona they want to be<br>• Thoughts about future, progress in education and employment career, and what sort of person they want to be<br>• Religious and political views start getting crystalized<br>• Want to start becoming financially independent | • Help build positive self-esteem and help to deal with body image issues.<br>• Understand that moving away from family is an important stage of development and not rejection of parents or family<br>• Positive relationship and close communication is a protective factor against high-risk behavior<br>• Avoid constant conflicts<br>• Choose battles |

*Contd...*

Contd...

|  | Early adolescence (10–13 years) | Middle adolescence (14–16 years) | Late adolescence (17–19 years) | Adult support |
|---|---|---|---|---|
| Emotional | Emotional lability, hot cognition | • Typical terrible teens<br>• Rejection and rebellion argumentative, rebellious, and anger outbursts are common<br>• Start developing understanding that a person's emotions are influenced by their previous experiences also | • Impulsiveness decreases with more mature cortical brain control over limbic system<br>• More composed and mature<br>• Empathy develops | • Understanding the brain development stages<br>• Responding to their *hot cognition* with mature adult *cold cognition*<br>• Help and teach emotional regulation |
| Cognitive development | • Concrete thinking predominant<br>• Cannot plan for future and cannot understand the future implications of current decisions and actions | • Abstract thinking emerges<br>• Future outcome of current acts are visualized during calm status<br>• But abstract thinking reverts to concrete thinking in times of emotional stress/crisis and can succumb to negative peer pressure | • Complex abstract thinking<br>• *Neer, Ksheer, Vivek* (Law and morality)<br>• Can think for themselves and resist peer group influence | • Abstract thinking can be enhanced by helping them to make their own decision and WHO life skill education program |
| Sexuality | • Exchange notes on normalcy of body changes with friends<br>• Same age same sex friends predominate<br>• Are curious about opposite sex but like to or may pretend to ignore opposite sex peers | • Sex thoughts, self-stimulation is at peak<br>• Experimentation starts<br>• Can lead to unwanted side effects<br>• Sexual orientation begins<br>• Attracted to opposite sex friends<br>• Transient phase–same sex attraction can occur<br>• Some girls may hate menstruation and require counseling for acceptance | • Sexual orientation more defined<br>• Can be aware that they have a different sexual orientation<br>• May need support and guidance as they may face discrimination | • Need to give awareness and education about all aspects of sexuality at home by parents and in school through professional programs |

Contd...

| | Early adolescence (10–13 years) | Middle adolescence (14–16 years) | Late adolescence (17–19 years) | Adult support |
|---|---|---|---|---|
| Social | • Peer identification begins<br>• Socially moves away from family<br>• Sensation seeking exploratory behavior, e.g., smoking<br>• Initiation of moral concepts | • Conflict over finances—feel parents are ATMs—want more than what parents can afford<br>• Fantasize about heroes and heroines<br>• Addiction to social networking<br>• Late night watching TV or internet<br>• Like to participate in lot of social and extracurricular activities like to learn new languages<br>• Planning for vocation | • Period of terrible teens is over for most<br>• Can understand parent's financial status<br>• Their views are mature, and outlooks are broader<br>• They do understand others' viewpoints and reason for the same<br>• They are aware of their rights and responsibilities<br>• Less of peer group more of intimate relations | Parental understanding about the normal social development and not start labeling the adolescent about not loving the family and going away from them. Understanding that they are not rejecting parents – but need peer group to develop their identity and personality |
| Family relationships | • As they emotionally mature, they want to become independent, and this may lead to their being somewhat detached from the family<br>• Symbolic movement away from family<br>• Do not like to participate in family functions | • Demonstrates needs for privacy and autonomy<br>• Struggles for independence in all activities<br>• Questions authority—at home, school, and community<br>• Moves away from the family<br>• Feels peers understand them better<br>• Late night sleeping and late getting up<br>• Major interpersonal conflicts with parents | • Returns to family norms with a broader outlook and perceives rights and responsibilities as an adult<br>• Better relationship with parents and other adults<br>• More composed and mature<br>• Emancipation completed in most<br>• Plans for future economic independence and viability | • Understand adolescents' opinions and values<br>• Do not constantly get angry about their *back answering*<br>• Inculcate healthy life style by role modeling and not nagging |

Contd...

Contd...

| | Early adolescence (10–13 years) | Middle adolescence (14–16 years) | Late adolescence (17–19 years) | Adult support |
|---|---|---|---|---|
| Peers | • Starts identifying with peer groups<br>• Their dressing sense, tattoos, hair styles, ear piercings, etc., follow peer group pattern | • Peers are respected more than parents<br>• Peer group approval considered as foremost | • Peer influence less prominent<br>• Individual intimate friendships evolve | • Making them understand about positive and negative peer pressure<br>• Get to know their peers and not keep castigating their friends |

*Source:* Adapted and modified from Agarkhedkar S, Bhave SY. Psychosocial and emotional development. In: Bhave SY (Ed). Bhave's Textbook of Adolescent Medicine, 2nd edition. New Delhi: Peepee Publishers; 2016. pp. 81-4.

## SUGGESTED READING

1. Agarkhedkar S, Bhave SY. Psychosocial and emotional development. In: Bhave SY (Ed). Bhave's Textbook of Adolescent Medicine, 2nd edition. New Delhi: Peepee Publishers; 2016. pp. 81-4.
2. American Psychological Association. Developing Adolescents: A Reference for Professionals. Washington, DC: American Psychological Association; 2002.
3. Arias-Carrión O, Stamelou M, Murillo-Rodríguez E, Menéndez-González M, Pöppel E. Dopaminergic reward system: a short integrative review. Int Arch Med. 2010;3:24.
4. Culbertson JL, Newman JE, Willis DJ. Childhood and Adolescent Psychological Development. Pediatr Clin North Am. 2003;50:741-64.
5. Erikson EH. Identity: Youth and Crisis. New York: WW Norton & Company; 1968.
6. Guy-Evans O. (2021). Amygdala Hijack and the Fight or Flight Response. [online] Available from www.simplypsychology.org/what-happens-during-an-amygdala-hijack.html. [Last accessed February, 2023].
7. Harris TA. I am Ok, You're OK: A Practical Guide to Transactional Analysis. New York: Harper & Row Publishers; 1969.
8. Hofman AD. Adolescent growth and development. In: Hofman AD, Greydanus DE (Eds). Adolescent Medicine, 3rd edition. Stamford, CT: Appleton & Lange Publisher; 1997. pp. 10-22.
9. Marshall WA, Tanner JM. Variations in pattern of pubertal changes in girls. Arch Dis Child. 1969;44(235):291-303.
10. Marshall WA, Tanner JM. Variations in the pattern of pubertal changes in boys. Arch Dis Child. 1970;45(239):13-23.
11. Rogol AD, Roemmich JN, Clark PA, Growth at Puberty. J Adolesc Health. 2002;31:192-200.
12. Spear LP, Silveri MM. Special Issue on the Adolescent Brain. Neurosci Biobehav Rev. 2016;70:1-3.
13. Sutherland P. Cognitive Development Today: Piaget and His Critics. California, United States: SAGE Publications; 1992.
14. Tanner JM, Whitehouse RH, Marshall WA, Carter BS. Prediction of adult height, bone age, and occurrence of menarche, at ages 4 to 16 with allowance for mid-parental height. Arch Dis Child. 1975;50:14-26.
15. World Health Organization. (1994). Life skills education for children and adolescents in schools. Pt. 1, Introduction to life skills for psychosocial competence. Pt. 2, Guidelines to facilitate the development and implementation of life skills programmes, 2nd rev. [online] Available from https://apps.who.int/iris/handle/10665/63552. [Last accessed February, 2023].
16. Yadav S, Jain TS. Adolescent Care. New Delhi: Cambridge Press; 2000.

# CHAPTER 2

# Body Image during Adolescence

*Amitha Rao Aroor, Preeti M Galagali*

## ■ INTRODUCTION

Body image is a crucial part of adolescent development and has an impact on overall health. The importance of body image increases during adolescence and can affect identity development. This review outlines the factors affecting body image development and approach to an adolescent with body image concerns.

## ■ DEFINITION

Body image is a dynamic concept and is defined as the internal representation of one's external appearance. It has four components, which include:
1. Perceptual (perception of size and shape of body and body parts)
2. Cognitive (thoughts and beliefs about the body)
3. Affective (feeling about the body)
4. Behavioral (actions taken to attain "ideal" body image).

It is a continuum of healthy perception of one's body (accurate and positive) to unhealthy perception (inaccurate and negative). Positive body image is having realistic perception of one's body and feeling good about it as it is. Negative body image is distorted perception of a person about his/her body with feeling of shame or anxiety and leads to low self-esteem. Various behaviors are adapted to attain ideal body image. These include dieting, laxative use, excessive physical activity, muscle building exercises, usage of steroids, and supplements. Behavioral manifestations also include checking (repeated monitoring of shape and weight), body avoidance (avoid exposure of viewing one's body, e.g., covering mirrors) and comparison (judgment about body size by examining others' bodies).

### Range of Body Image Disturbances

Body image disturbances can range from mild preference for various body characteristics to severe disturbance including eating disorders. It can be about the appearance of whole body or specific body parts. Body image disturbances can be either body image distortion (perceptual disturbance, i.e., failure to evaluate size) or dissatisfaction (conceptual disturbance, i.e., affective component and negative cognition).

## Impact of Negative Body Image

Negative body image is linked to various mental health issues such as low self-esteem, depression, anxiety, and substance use. Disturbance of body image is a core component of anorexia nervosa, bulimia, and body dysmorphic disorder. Body dissatisfaction is the single strongest predictor of eating disorders. Suicide has a positive correlation with negative body image.

## ■ BODY IMAGE DEVELOPMENT DURING ADOLESCENCE

Rapid and diverse pubertal changes occurring during adolescence along with emphasis on "ideal body" have led to an increase in body image issues. Early puberty in girls and late puberty in boys increases the risk. Neurodevelopmental immaturity makes them sensitive to body image issues, and poor coping skills lead to an excessive preoccupation and dissatisfaction with body image. Numerous biological, psychological, and sociocultural factors contribute to the development of body image in adolescents as shown in **Table 1**.

## Physical and Biological Factors

Dissatisfaction toward one's own body develops because the body features do not fit internalized beauty norms. During puberty there is a change in body proportions along with development of secondary sexual characteristics.

**TABLE 1:** Factors affecting body image.

| | |
|---|---|
| Physical and biological factors | • Body weight, body shape<br>• Pubertal changes<br>• Medical diseases |
| Peer factors | • Pressure to fit in<br>• Fat talk<br>• Bullying at school for body size |
| Familial factors | • Parent's concern about weight and appearance<br>• Obsession about exercise<br>• Negative comments about body from family members |
| Psychological factors | • Low self esteem<br>• Depression<br>• Perfectionist attitude<br>• Body comparison tendencies<br>• Athletics |
| Traditional and social media | • Seeing ideal body in media<br>• Public opinion, judgment, comparison<br>• Number of 'likes' on social media platforms |

Lack of explanation regarding pubertal changes may lead to misconceptions about these changes with feeling of guilt and shame.

## Sociocultural Factors

Include influence of parents, family, peers, societal norms, and media. An increased sense of social pressure to have an ideal body, comments by parents and family members, parental values, and quality of relationship contribute to the level of satisfaction with the body. Body talks with peers lead them to be self-conscious of their bodies and various behaviors to attain a perfect body. Peer teasing and bullying related to body weight, shape, and appearance influence teen's perceptions about their bodies. Media functions as a "super peer" and defines the look and body shape to attain via images with unrealistic and unattainable body measures. Girls are encouraged to lose weight and look beautiful while boys are encouraged to be strong and have bulky muscles. The tripartite influence model states that peers, family, and media are channels that propagate messages of body ideals and have a direct impact on body dissatisfaction.

## Psychological Factors

There has been documentation of a strong connection between body image and self-esteem. Perfectionism is a risk factor for poor body image as they set high standards for themselves.

**Flowchart 1** outlines key processes in the development of body image in adolescents. As shown in the **Flowchart 1**, body image development is

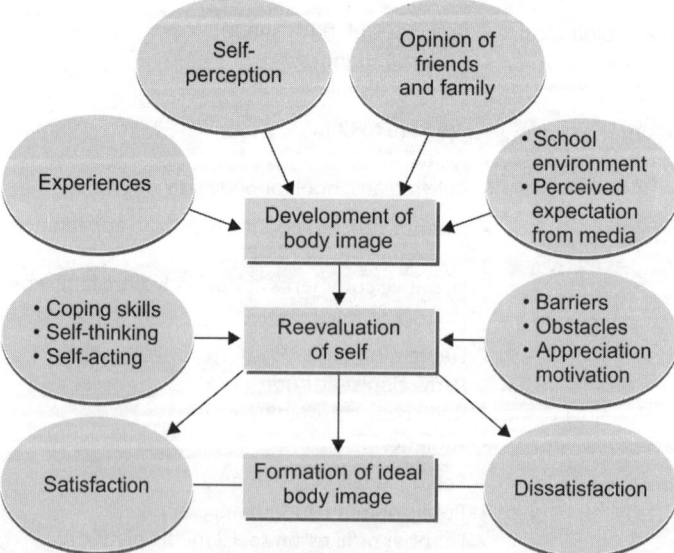

**Flowchart 1:** Development of adolescent body image.

a complex process. It is a response to the internal and external stimuli experienced by the adolescent. Reevaluation of oneself is a crucial element that influences the satisfaction level. Beliefs, emotions, and life skills reinforce this reevaluation. There are barriers, obstacles, and also positive appreciation for developing a healthy body image. An adolescent with strong self-efficacy and adaptive coping skills will have a positive appreciation of their body, even when it does not fit into ideal standards. Those who are dissatisfied with their bodies are prone to develop disordered eating.

## PREVALENCE OF BODY IMAGE ISSUES IN INDIAN ADOLESCENTS

Previously, body image concerns were thought to be a problem of the Western world. Recent literature, however, reveals a substantial prevalence in South East Asia and India. Depending on the study methodology, the prevalence of body image issues in Indian adolescents is reported to be ranging from 25 to 85%. Studies from various parts of India have shown prevalence of disordered eating behavior to be 10–30% among adolescent girls and young adults. The prevalence was higher among girls, those in urban areas, with high socioeconomic status and influenced by media usage.

## CLINICAL PRESENTATION

Adolescents with body image issues usually present to pediatricians with:
- Concerns about normal pubertal changes and growth spurt such as size of breasts and penis, gawkiness, physiological gynecomastia, and acne.
- Poor academic performance with intense desire and preoccupation to attain an ideal body image of "zero figure" for girls and "six packs" for boys, usually under the influence of peers and media.
- Disordered eating behavior like skipping meals, following fad diets (e.g., keto diet and intermittent fasting), caloric restriction, fat avoidance, and binge eating.
- Performing excessive physical exercise with the aim to lose weight.
- Conflicts between parents and adolescents regarding eating habits, lifestyle, unconventional appearance, and exercise patterns.
- Physical disorders such as anemia and osteoporosis.
- Mental disorders such as eating disorders, depression, anxiety, body dysmorphic disorder, problematic internet use, bullying, and suicidal behavior.
- Menstrual irregularity and amenorrhea.
- Use of drugs and food supplements, e.g., anabolic steroids to put on muscle mass.
- Medical emergency with electrolyte imbalance and hypotension as in eating disorders.

## HISTORY TAKING

History should be elicited from adolescents and their parents in a sensitive, nonjudgmental, and empathic manner offering privacy and confidentiality. The following should be explored while taking a HEEADSSS psychosocial history from an adolescent with body image concerns **(Table 2)**.

Asking an open-ended question such as, "How do you feel when you look at yourself in the mirror?" would encourage adolescents to share their body image concerns with clinicians. HEEADSSS evaluates strengths and problem areas in an adolescent's life related to body image. Warning signs of negative body image when present should be identified **(Box 1)**.

For early detection of eating disorders, the clinical history should focus on the adolescent's perception of self, history of past illness or admission, patterns of eating and drinking, caloric intake, purging, restricting, binging, laxative use, exercise patterns, and menstrual history. Comorbidities such as depression, anxiety, and obsessive-compulsive disorder should be looked

**TABLE 2:** HEEADSSS Psychosocial history in body image concerns.

| Item | Key points |
|---|---|
| **H**ome | Socio economic status, literacy level of family members, relationship with parents, type of parenting, abuse, mental, and eating disorders |
| **E**ducation | Recent change in school and in academic performance, peer group, bullying |
| **E**ating habits | Caloric and nutrient intake, details of body image concerns |
| **A**ctivities | Hobbies, type and duration of media usage and physical activity, time spent with peers and outdoors, quantity and quality of sleep, recent loss of interest in activities |
| **D**epression | Change in mood, behavior and interest, suicide ideation or attempt |
| **S**ubstance use | Attitude towards drug use, type and frequency of drug use |
| **S**exuality | Details regarding sexual health, menstruation, intimate partners, sexual encounters, sexual violence, abuse |
| **S**afety | Indulgence in violent acts |

**BOX 1:** Warning signs of negative body image.

- Feeling inadequate about or criticizing one's own body
- Constantly viewing themselves in comparison to others
- Not wanting to leave the house because of the way they look
- Overemphasis on certain body parts
- Obsessed about losing weight/sudden weight loss
- Skipping meals
- Frequent visit to bathroom after meals

for and diagnosed using The Diagnostic and Statistical Manual of Mental Disorders, Fifth Edition (DSM-5) criteria.

## ■ ASSESSMENT OF BODY IMAGE

A wide variety of valid and reliable scales and questionnaires have been recommended to screen for various components of body image. Choice of scale should be individualized depending on the age and sex of the child and should be appropriate to the level of maturity. If gross disturbances are noted, the adolescent needs to be evaluated for body dysmorphic disorder. Few of the scales recommended are as follows:

- *Figure rating scale (schematic drawings):* Consist of several gender specific silhouettes of the human body in multiple shapes and sizes. The child is asked to select the image representative of the current and the ideal selves. The difference between the two ratings gives the degree of body dissatisfaction.
- *Body Shape Questionnaire (BSQ):* Consists of questions regarding one's feelings about their appearance which are rated by 6-point Likert scale. Depending on the score obtained, severity is classified as no concern/mild/moderate/severe concern about body image. Original questionnaires have 34 items. Shortened 16 and 8 item scales have also been derived.
- *Adolescent body image satisfaction scale (ABISS):* 16 item scale has shown good validity to assess body image among adolescent males.
- *Body image questionnaire:* Evaluates affective and cognitive components. It assesses satisfaction with respect to the adolescent's overall body as well as specific parts.
- *Multidimensional body self relations questionnaire (MBSRQ):* Original form has a 69-item version (7 main subscales and 3 special multi-item scales). A shorter form with 34-item version MBSRQ-AS (MBSRQ-appearance scale) evaluates only the appearance-related component with 2 main subscales and 3 multi-item scales. It provides a 9-item body area satisfaction scale to measure satisfaction/dissatisfaction with specific area. It is recommended for adolescents >15 years of age.
- *Assessment of drive for muscularity:* Especially in males as they are most often dissatisfied with small body size and lack of tone and bulk of muscles. These scales include drive for muscularity scale, muscle appearance satisfaction scale, etc.
- Use of computer software to assess the perceptual disturbances in body image.
- *SCOFF questionnaire:* SCOFF screening questionnaire can be used to screen for eating disorders. SCOFF is an acronym standing for sick, control, one, fat, and food, respectively **(Box 2)**.

**BOX 2:** SCOFF Questionnaire.

- Do you make yourself sick because you are uncomfortably full?
- Do you worry that you have lost control over how much you eat?
- Have you lost more than one stone (14 lb) in last 3 months?
- Do you believe yourself to be fat when others say that you are too thin?
- Would you say that food dominates your life?

*Interpretation:* Each 'yes' scores 1 point and a score >2 is a pointer towards anorexia nervosa or bulimia

For those who test positive on SCOFF, Eating Attitudes Test with 26 questions (EAT 26) can be used to determine risk for eating disorders. An EAT score of >20 qualifies for a detailed assessment by a mental health professional. DSM-5 criteria are used to make the final diagnosis of eating disorders including anorexia nervosa and bulimia nervosa. In both these disorders, self-evaluation is deeply influenced by body shape and weight. Anorexia nervosa is characterized by a restriction in energy intake and an intense fear of gaining weight while bulimia nervosa is characterized by episodes of binge eating followed by compensatory behavior like diuretic use and laxatives.

## ■ EXAMINATION

Important points to be noted in examination include:
- Skin, eyes, teeth, and hair for issues of acne, hirsutism, dandruff, atopy, malocclusion, caries, myopia, texture, color, body piercing, tattoo, and cosmetic usage.
- Tanner staging and secondary sexual characteristics for concerns regarding pubertal changes, size of breasts and genitalia, and gynecomastia.
- Body mass index, height and weight for issues of stature, and weight and muscular frame.
- Detailed systemic and musculoskeletal assessment would be required for those with physical disabilities and chronic medical disorders.
- Clinical pointers toward eating disorders if present should be identified **(Box 3)**.

## ■ INDICATIONS FOR REFERRAL

Indications for referral to mental health professionals are:
- EAT score >20
- Poor response to counseling even after regular sessions for 4–6 weeks
- Severe substance use disorder, severe depression, suicidal ideation, and behavior
- Adolescents fulfilling DSM-5 criteria for diagnosis of eating disorders.

**BOX 3:** Clinical pointers towards presence of eating disorders.

- Under nutrition, loss of fat
- Bradycardia, hypotension, orthostatic pulse, poor capillary refill, distant heart sounds
- Hypothermia
- Dental erosion on molars
- Sialadenosis
- Facial petechiae
- Subconjunctival hemorrhage
- Bruises on metacarpophalangeal joints
- Carotenemia
- Edema
- Xerosis

## ■ MANAGEMENT

Management of body image dissatisfaction depends on its severity and associated comorbidity. Minor concerns regarding body image can be managed by counseling parents and adolescents. A multidisciplinary hospital-based team including psychiatrist, psychologist, nutritionist, adolescent health specialist, and intensivist is needed to manage eating disorders and its complications.

The following should be addressed while managing body image concerns and providing anticipatory guidance during annual well adolescent visits **(Table 3)**.

### Normative Pubertal Changes

The adolescents and their parents should be reassured regarding changes in physique as puberty sets in such as widened shoulders for boys and broadening of hips for girls.

**TABLE 3:** Educating adolescent and parents and promotion of healthy body image.

| Adolescent | Parents |
| --- | --- |
| • Educate about the normal pubertal changes<br>• To focus on the positive features, rather than on the negative ones<br>• Think about positive traits not related to appearance<br>• To critically analyze images of models in media<br>• Not to compare self with others/celebrities<br>• Surround with people who have healthy body image<br>• Keep realistic goals about losing weight and to aim for gradual change<br>• Healthy diet and exercise | • Follow healthy life style. Be a good role model<br>• Praise the teen for achievements<br>• Express unconditional love<br>• Do not criticize appearance, but support instead<br>• Make their teens aware of tricks of beauty industry and teach realistic expectations |

## Body Mass Index

Age-appropriate charts should be used to diagnose overnutrition, undernutrition, and short stature. These charts are useful as follow-up tools to assess anthropometry when the adolescent is on treatment.

## Healthy Lifestyle

Adolescents are encouraged to adopt a healthy diet approach that involves eating from all food groups, avoiding a diet with high fat, salt, and sugar, ensuring moderate to intense physical activity for 1 hour every day and 8–9 hours of sleep. Meditation, yoga, involvement in hobbies, restricting screen time, and learning stress management techniques are helpful in managing anxiety regarding body image concerns.

## Self-esteem

Importance of developing an all-round personality and a nurturing, stimulating, and safe environment at home is discussed with parents and adolescents. This urges the adolescent to look beyond "outer/external" beauty as the only determinant of self-worth and highlights the importance of "inner" beauty characterized by grit, resilience, will power, and psychosocial competence. Parents are advised to spend quality time with their children and adopt an authoritative parenting style using assertive communication.

## Media Education

Media usage, online activities, and their effect on body image concerns are assessed in detail. Adolescents and parents are guided toward healthy media usage, media literacy, and online etiquette. Media literacy focuses on interpreting media messages appropriately and not getting influenced by media stereotypes. Screening is also done for social media addiction and problematic internet use.

## Life Skills

Life skill education enables adolescents to make healthy lifestyle choices and enhance self-esteem.

## Education of Parents

Parents should be role models for their children by following a healthy diet and exercise pattern, focus on nonappearance related positive traits and avoid harsh criticism, and comparisons regarding body image.

## Therapies

The therapeutic counseling is by using a combination of approaches which include developing acceptance, challenging sociocultural messages of "thin ideal" and targeting selective attention to disliked body parts as well as importance given to another's approval. Psychological therapies include cognitive behavioral therapy (CBT), acceptance and commitment therapy (ACT), virtual reality exposure therapy, and mindfulness-based therapy. CBT targets all the three components, i.e., size perception (overestimation of size), cognitive affective component (negative thoughts, overvalued beliefs, emotions, and idealization of thin ideal), and behavioral component (body checking, avoidance, and comparison). Yoga may be recommended as an adjunct to improve mind-body awareness.

## CONCLUSION

Adolescents are vulnerable to body image dissatisfaction. Adolescence is also an age of opportunity where a health professional can counsel them to develop a positive body image and love their body in spite of flaws and imperfections. This would enhance their self-esteem and prevent onset of serious mental disorders such as eating disorders, depression, and suicidal behavior.

## POINTS TO REMEMBER

- Body image is the dynamic perception of one's body and is determined strongly by self-evaluation.
- Development of body image follows biopsychosocial model and body image disturbance may be associated with negative health outcomes.
- Adolescents needed to be screened for body image concerns during routine visits with detailed history, HEEADSSS assessment, and examination. Body dissatisfaction may be assessed using appropriately selected questionnaires. If indicated, timely referral to a mental health specialist should be made.
- Promotion of healthy body image must be included as a part of the anticipatory guidance in all adolescents. It includes the explanation of normal pubertal changes, encouragement to follow a healthy lifestyle, media education, and mastering life skills.

## SUGGESTED READING

1. American Psychiatric Association. Diagnostic and statistical manual of Mental disorders, Fifth edition. Arlington, VA: American Psychiatric Association; 2013.
2. Dixit S, Agarwal GG, Singh JV, Kant S, Singh N. A study on consciousness of adolescent girls about their body image. Indian J Community Med. 2011;36(3):197-202.
3. Gaddad P, Pemde HK, Basu S, Dhankar M, Rajendran S. Relationship of physical activity with body image, self-esteem sedentary lifestyle, body mass index and eating attitude in adolescents: a cross-sectional observational study. J Family Med Prim Care. 2018;7:775-9.

4. Galagali P, Luiz N. Poor School Performance in Adolescence. Ind J Pract Pediatr. 2015;17:116-22.
5. Ganesan S, Ravishankar SL, Ramalingam S. Are Body Image Issues Affecting Our Adolescents? A Cross-sectional Study among College Going Adolescent Girls. Indian J Community Med. 2018;43(Suppl 1):S42-6.
6. Greco LA, Barnett ER, Blomquist KK, Gevers A. Acceptance, body image, and health in adolescence. In: Greco LA, Hayes SC (Eds). Acceptance and Mindfulness Treatments for Children and Adolescents: A Practitioner's Guide. California, United States: New Harbinger Publications; 2008. pp. 187-214.
7. Hartman-Munick SM, Gordon AR, Guss C. Adolescent body image: influencing factors and the clinician's role. Curr Opin Pediatr. 2020;32(4):455-60.
8. Kartha GK, Navya CJ, Aswathy MG, Joshy VM. Body Image Perception among Adolescent students in a private School in Thrissur, Kerala. Int J Public Health Res. 2019;6(2):68-75.
9. Klein DA, Goldenring JM, Adelman WP. HEEADSSS 3.0: The psychosocial interview for adolescents updated for a new century fueled by media. Contemp Pediatr. 2014;31(1):16-28.
10. Morgan JF, Reid F, Lacey JH. The SCOFF questionnaire: assessment of a new screening tool for eating disorders. BMJ. 1999;319(7223):1467-8.
11. Mountford VA, Koskina A. Body image. In: Wade T (Ed). Encyclopedia of Feeding and Eating Disorders. Singapore: Springer; 2015.
12. Nivedita N, Sreenivasa G, Sathyanarayana Rao TS, Malini SS. Eating disorders: Prevalence in the student population of Mysore, South India. Indian J Psychiatry. 2018;60:433-7.
13. Phillips KA, Rogers J. Cognitive-behavioural therapy for youth with body dysmorphic disorder: current status and future directions. Child Adolesc Psychiatr Clin N Am. 2011;20(2):287-304.
14. Riva G, Gaudio S, Serino S, Dakanalis A, Ferrer-García M, Gutiérrez-Maldonado J. Virtual reality for the treatment of body image disturbances in eating and weight disorders: a guide to assessment, treatment, and prevention. In: Cuzzolaro M, Fassino S (Eds). Body Image, Eating, and Weight. Berlin, Germany: Springer; 2018. pp. 333-51.
15. Shashank KJ, Gowda P, Chethan TK. A Cross sectional Study to assess the eating disorder among female medical students in a Rural Medical College of Karnataka State. Natl J Community Med. 2016;7(6):524-7.
16. Shroff H, Thompson JK. Body image and eating disturbance in India: media and interpersonal influences. Int J Eat Disord. 2004;35(2):198-203.
17. Soohinda G, Mishra D, Sampath H, Dutta S. Body dissatisfaction and its relation to Big Five personality factors and self-esteem in young adult college women in India. Indian J Psychiatry. 2019;61:400-4.
18. Tort-Nasarre G, Pollina Pocallet M, Artigues-Barberà E. The Meaning and Factors That Influence the Concept of Body Image: Systematic Review and Meta-Ethnography from the Perspectives of Adolescents. Int J Environ Res. Public Health. 2021;18:1140.
19. Upadhyah AA, Misra R, Parchwani DN, Maheria PB. Prevalence and risk factors for eating disorders in Indian adolescent females. Natl J Physiol Pharm Pharmacol. 2014;4:153-7.

20. Voelker DK, Reel JJ, Greenleaf C. Weight status and body image perceptions in adolescents: current perspectives. Adolesc Health Med Ther. 2015;6:149-58.
21. Yadav VP. Understanding the body image of adolescents: a psychological perspective. Int J Appl Res. 2017;3(6):588-94.
22. Yanover T, Thompson JK. Assessment of body image in children and adolescents. In: Smolak L, Thompson JK (Eds). Body Image, Eating Disorders, and Obesity in Youth: Assessment, Prevention, and Treatment. Washington, DC: American Psychological Association; 2009. pp. 177-92.

# CHAPTER 3

# Adolescent Sexuality

*Chandrika Rao*

## ■ INTRODUCTION

Sexuality is a complex topic from the time of Aristotle's ideas to Sigmund Freud's era and more so in the modern era. The adolescent development and formation of their identity is a transition phase for the adolescents, parents, and society. In the 21st century, adolescent sexual behavior is being discussed openly, emphasizing the importance of sexuality, sexual behaviors, and relationships with its risks.

The World Health Organization, international health agencies, and Indian Academy of Pediatrics also identify adolescent-friendly health services as a worldwide priority, with 70% of more than one billion youth (10–19 years) living in developing countries. The important role that the health providers play in ensuring a positive sexual attitude is being recognized and stressed on now.

## ■ DEFINITION

Sexuality is often considered only as the act of sex and often the discussion is limited by that concept. However, human sexuality is more than the act of sex and involves the person's concept of his or her own body image, sexual identity, role at home and society, personal feelings, and self-esteem. Some of the terminologies commonly used are as follows:

*Anatomic sex:* This refers to the anatomic sexual reproductive organs. Anatomic sex is only one component of sexuality.

*Gender identity:* This refers to the feeling within the person as being either masculine or feminine. Gender identity and anatomic sex sometimes do not match. For example, a person can be born as a boy but feels and behaves like a girl. This is sometimes referred to as transgender.

*Sexual orientation:* This refers to the sexual attraction one feels toward another person. One may be attracted to people of the opposite sex (heterosexual or straight), the same sex (homosexual, gay, or lesbian), or both (bisexual). Sexual orientation is influenced by many factors, including anatomic sex, gender identity, and the society. It is common for adolescents to feel confused about their sexual orientation, which is normal. These feelings may change as the person matures or may persist. It is important for adolescents and adults to be comfortable with all aspects of sexuality (anatomic sex, gender identity, and sexual orientation).

## ADOLESCENT SEXUAL DEVELOPMENT

There are many theories regarding adolescent sexuality. The popular ones are listed here.

- Freud's psychoanalytic theory states that the stages of psychosexual development are genetically determined. Sigmund Freud had proposed his theory of psychosexual development, where he described about oral phase, anal phase, phallic phase, latency phase, and genital phase as the landmark steps of psychosexual development **(Table 1)**.

  He opined that physiological changes are affected by emotional changes, and negative emotions like anxiety, depression, and tension have greater impact. He also stressed on the role of self-image in the development of sexuality.

- *Anna Freud's theory:* She emphasized on id, the ego, and the superego. She opined that adolescent conflicts arise due to poor formation of id and ego of the individual.
- *Erikson's theory:* He opined that the sense of personal identity is more important than sexuality. Individual efforts, peer relationships, and value system contribute to a stable identity. The adolescent should form his own identity and not mimic an elder's or peer's identity as it will lead to confusion and dissatisfaction in adult life.
- According to Piaget, cognitive development through adolescence involves movement from concrete to abstract thinking and a decrease in egocentric thought.
- The social constructionist perspective examines the role of power and culture in the development of adolescent sexuality. In a practical sense, this explains why some girls may believe that sex is necessary to maintain relationships.
- *Developmental feminist perspective:* Gender norms in society influence gender identity formation. Adolescent girls may learn to consider

**TABLE 1:** Phases of psychosexual development.

| Phases | Lifetime |
| --- | --- |
| Oral phase | Birth to 18 months |
| Anal phase | 18 months to 3 years |
| Phallic (oedipal) phase | 3–5 years |
| Latency phase | 5 years to puberty |
| Genital phase | Puberty to till end of life |

themselves as objects of desire and focus on what others expect out of them than being assertive about what they need. Society having double standards in viewing the same male and female sexual behavior differently indicates that premarital sex also influences adolescent sexual development. Adolescents are often judged for their sexual behavior by their gender. Elder siblings also influence sexual attitudes as per this theory.

- *Social learning and the sexual self-concept:* Peer pressure plays an important role. The sexual experiences in childhood and adolescence, family roles, and media are responsible for forming a self-concept and learning. Research has shown boys to experience lower sexual self-esteem and higher sexual anxiety. They also experience ambivalent feelings as society expects them to be dominant. Girls in age group of 14–17 years demonstrate high self-esteem and decreased anxiety. Researchers state that these behaviors are not impulsive but have been affected by self-concept and experiences.
- *Biopsychosocial model:* Biological factors, psychological factors, and social factors have equal importance in determining the sexuality in adolescents. Biological factors are the genetic factors and neuroendocrine factors, which determine the biological sex. During adolescence the gonadal hormones, cortisol, and many other hormones play a role in causing the onset of puberty. Individual's personality or temperament is the psychological factor that decides the attitude toward sexuality. Introvert adolescents may face difficulty in responding sexually. The attitude of the parents toward sexuality, parenting style, peer relationship, and cultural influences are the social factors which decide the sexual attitude of the adolescent.
- *Other:* Media, political, legal, philosophical, spiritual, ethical, and moral values significantly influence the sexuality development.

## ADOLESCENT SEXUAL DEVELOPMENT

Adolescent sexuality development can be seen of as a long-term shift that is self-regulated, qualitative, and progressive rather than simply induced by the environment.

Early adolescence in age groups of 10–13 years show increased interest in opposite sex, excess interest in sexual feelings, and may masturbate. Girls achieve menarche and males experience nocturnal emissions. In middle adolescence in age groups of 14–16 years old, puberty is often completed. They explore relationships with other gender and like to spend more time with same or opposite gender friends. In late adolescence (approximately 17–19 years old), goals are established. Adolescents begin to understand consequences of sexual behavior; begin to understand pregnancy and sexually transmitted diseases (STDs). They explore relationships and

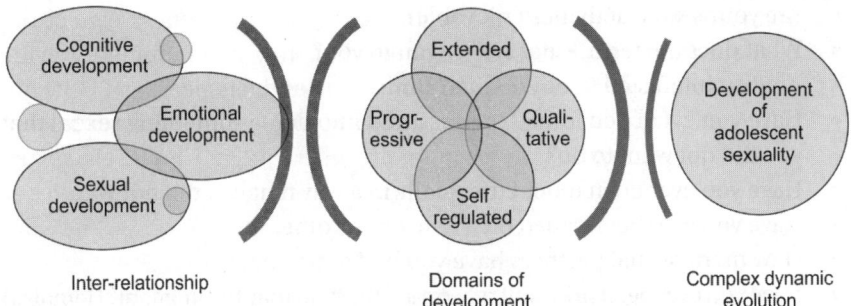

**Fig. 1:** Long term shift towards adolescent sexuality development.

understand their own sexual orientation. Adolescents may be sexually active and begin long-term relationships. They understand the role of media.

The oedipal complex (a child's attraction to the parent of the opposite sex) is common during the adolescent years. Parents can acknowledge the adolescent's physical changes and gradually lay down ground rules to not cross parent-child boundaries.

Sexual orientation begins during puberty. Sexual orientation and gender identity are not a choice and appear to be established by early childhood. Feelings of homosexuality or lesbianism, transgender may emerge to discontinue later or may continue. These are influenced by both biological and environmental influences.

The fifth edition of the Diagnostic and Statistical Manual of Mental Disorders (DSM-5) defines gender dysphoria (GD) as a condition in which a person has marked incongruence between the expressed or experienced gender and the biological sex at birth. Adolescents with GD experience a strong desire to be treated as the other gender and want to have the characteristics of that gender. The previous diagnostic term, gender identity disorder, was rejected in the DSM-5 to avoid pathologizing identity.

## ■ ADOLESCENT ASSESSMENT

The HEADDSSS questionnaire by Cohen et al. is usually used to assess adolescent sexual behavior and obtaining a comprehensive, confidential, and developmentally appropriate adolescent psychosocial history allows for the discovery of strengths and assets as well as risks. Nonjudgmental attitude, privacy, and confidentiality should be ensured. Resource material and reading material should be freely available.

The HEADDSS assessment has outlined the following questions under sexuality.
- Have you ever been in a romantic relationship?
- Tell me about the people that you have dated or tell me about your sex life.
- Have any of your relationships ever been sexual relationships?

- Are your sexual activities enjoyable?
- What does the term "safer sex" mean to you?
- Are you interested in boys? Girls? Both?
- Have you ever been forced or pressured into doing something sexual that you did not want to do?
- Have you ever been touched sexually in a way that you did not want?
- Have you ever been raped on a date or any other time?
- How many sexual partners have you had altogether?
- Have you ever been pregnant or worried that you may be pregnant? (females)
- Have you ever gotten someone pregnant or worried that that might have happened? (males)
- What are you using for birth control? Are you satisfied with your method?
- Do you use condoms every time you have intercourse?
- Does anything ever get in the way of always using a condom?
- Have you ever had a STD or worried that you had an STD?

## ROLE OF A PEDIATRICIAN

Pediatricians should have offices which are adolescent friendly and welcoming to youth. This includes having supportive office staff members who do not discriminate and do not behave differently with sexual minorities. They should encourage parents to talk to their teen about sexual behavior in a nonjudgmental way. Parents should be counseled that the adolescent interest in one's own body may be natural. It does not indicate that their child is involved in sexual activity. It is necessary to discuss abstinence, contraception, consent, and substance abuse with the adolescent and life skill training to adolescent to say "no". During communication, use inclusive words as gay, lesbian, bisexual, or transgender. This opens avenues for adolescent to communicate. For transgender youth, pediatricians should provide the opportunity to acknowledge and affirm their feelings of GD. Adolescent physicians should refer transgender youth to a qualified mental health professional who will assist with the dysphoria, educate them, and help them in their transition. The impact of sexuality in adolescence, i.e., (1) pregnancy, (2) contraception, (3) STDs, (4) dating violence, and (5) sexual abuse should be discussed with the adolescent. These are discussed here.

### Adolescent Pregnancy

Every year, an estimated 21 million girls aged 15–19 years in developing regions become pregnant and approximately 12 million of them give birth. In India, adolescent pregnancy is high in rural areas due to early marriage. Data shows that teen pregnancy in India is 62 out of every 1,000 women. Although they are married, pregnancy is usually not a choice but occurs due to inadequate knowledge about contraception, societal pressure to bear children once married, and very often rights violation. The age of the mother is determined by the verified date when the pregnancy ends, not by the estimated date of conception. Adolescent pregnancy is harmful for both mother and baby. Adolescent pregnancy may result in problems such as postpartum hemorrhage, anemia, hypertension, depression, premature and low birth weight babies, and increased number of neonatal complications.

The pediatrician plays an important role along with the obstetrician in antenatal care of an adolescent pregnant girl and can educate and counsel the teen and the parents and ensure good outcome of mother and child. Counseling on complete antenatal care, psychological support to family, immunization, diet, supplementation of iron and folic acid tablets, advice to abstain from drugs and alcohol, ensuring delivery in hospital, and care of newborn are the necessary things which a pediatrician has to do.

## Contraception

The various methods which can be recommended are as follows:
- *Natural methods:* Abstinence during fertile phase and withdrawal (coitus interruptus). Periodic abstinence may not be reliable for adolescents to follow as impulsive behavior dominates in this period.
- *Barrier contraceptives:* Male condoms, spermicidal agents, use of diaphragm or cervical cap in the vagina, use of hormones which alter the cervical mucus and prevent entry of sperm into the cervical canal (today sponge with spermicidal cream). Barrier methods are best for adolescents while condoms prevent pregnancy and infection.
- *Intrauterine contraceptive devices (IUCDs):* Copper T may not be suitable in nulliparous women. However it is a long term, coital independent method which a sexually active adolescent may choose if no contraindications are present.
- *Suppression of spermatogenesis:* Gossypol is the drug of choice.
- *Suppression of ovulation with hormones:* Estrogen and progesterone pills can be prescribed in adolescents. Third-generation combined oral contraceptives (COCs) pills have few side effects. Ultra-low-dose COCs pill with 15 µg ethinylestradiol have fewer side effects. Some may prefer three monthly injection of Depo-Provera at dose of 150 µg IM, implants, or skin patches.
- *Interceptive agents (postcoital contraception):* I-pill, two tablets as soon as possible within 48–72 hours.

## Sexually Transmitted Infections

Infections can spread through sexual intercourse, anal sex, oral sex, and using fingers, other body parts, or sex toys that have come in contact with another person's genitals or body fluids. Abstinence is the only 100% effective method to prevent STDs. Adolescents who have early sexual intercourse, multiple sexual partners, unprotected sex, homosexuality, poverty, drugs, or high risk sex behavior are at greater risk of getting STD.

Some of the most important causes of sexually transmitted infections (STIs) are chlamydia, gonorrhea, human papillomavirus (HPV), and herpes simplex virus, and the treatment is given in the **Table 2**.

### Human Papillomavirus

This may be a silent infection. HPV 6 and 11 can cause condylomata acuminata. This can be treated with local application of podophyllin 25% in alcohol for 6 hours daily or 25% trichloroacetic acid plus fluorouracil to cause sloughing in 3–7 days and can be repeated weekly but contraindicated if adolescent is pregnant. Diathermy, laser ablation, and surgical excisions are other available treatment options. HPV causes cervical cancer in women, penile cancer in men, and anal or oropharyngeal cancer in either sex and can be prevented by vaccine. Children ages 11–12 years should get two doses of HPV vaccine, given 6–12 months apart. Children who start the HPV vaccine series on or after their 15th birthday need three doses, given over 6 months.

### Human Immunodeficiency Virus

Recommendations are that human immunodeficiency virus (HIV) screening should be routinely done in sexually active adolescents. Posters and pamphlets are useful in dissemination of information in the pediatrician's clinic.

## Dating Violence

Girls under age 18 are twice more likely to be beaten by their child's father than women over age of 18. 10–30% of teenagers have experienced violence in a dating relationship in different populations studied.

## Sexual Abuse

The topic of sexuality is a taboo and sex education in schools is not prevalent in India. There must be better education in this area, from an early age and without taboos (Castro and Santos-Iglesias, 2016). The focus should be on the importance of prevention and promotion of sexual health, teaching from early ages how to identify possible situations or intentions of abuse, educating in gender equality, and promoting healthy sexuality. This will help prevent sexual abuse. The Protection of Children from Sexual Offences (POCSO) Act in India has helped to have a legal structure for diagnosis and management. Pediatricians must be aware and manage sexual abuse cases.

**TABLE 2:** Sexually transmitted infections (STIs) and treatment.

| Syndrome | Organisms/diagnoses | Treatment[a] |
|---|---|---|
| Urethritis and cervicitis | • *Neisseria gonorrhoeae* and *Chlamydia trachomatis*<br>• Other causes: *Mycoplasma genitalium, Ureaplasma urealyticum, Trichomonas vaginalis,* and herpes simplex virus (HSV) | • Ceftriaxone, 250 mg, IM, in a single dose[b]<br>Or<br>• Cefixime, 400 mg, orally, in a single dose[b] plus either<br>• Azithromycin, 1 g, orally, in a single dose<br>Or<br>• Doxycycline, 100 mg, orally, twice a day for 7 days |
| | HSV—primary infection | • Acyclovir, 400 mg, orally, three times/day for 7–10 days<br>Or<br>• Acyclovir, 200 mg, orally, five times/day for 7–10 days<br>Or<br>• Famciclovir 250 mg, orally, three times/day for 7–10 days<br>Or<br>• Valacyclovir 1 g, orally, twice daily for 7–10 days |
| Adolescent vulvovaginitis | *T. vaginalis* | • Metronidazole, 2 g, orally, in a single dose<br>Or<br>• Tinidazole, 2 g, orally, in a single dose |
| | Bacterial vaginosis | • Metronidazole, 500 mg, orally, twice daily for 7 days<br>Or<br>• Metronidazole gel 0.75%, 1 full applicator (5 g), intravaginally, once a day for 5 days<br>Or<br>• Clindamycin cream 2%, 1 full applicator (5 g), intravaginally at bedtime, for 7 days |
| | *Candida* species | • Ketoconazole (400 mg/day)<br>Or<br>• Itraconazole (50–100 mg/day)<br>Or<br>• Fluconazole (100 mg/week) for 6 weeks, and clotrimazole (500 mg vaginal suppositories once per week) |

*Contd...*

*Contd...*

| Syndrome | Organisms/diagnoses | Treatment^a |
|---|---|---|
| | HSV—primary infection | • Acyclovir, 400 mg, orally, three times/day for 7–10 days<br>*Or*<br>• Famciclovir, 250 mg, orally, three times/day for 7–10 days<br>*Or*<br>• Valaciclovir, 1 g, orally twice/day for 7–10 days |
| Pelvic inflammatory disease (PID) | *Neisseria gonorrhoeae, Chlamydia trachomatis*, anaerobes, coliform bacteria, and *Streptococcus* species | • *Mild:* Ceftriaxone 250 mg IM in a single dose<br>*Plus*<br>• Doxycycline 100 mg orally twice a day for 14 days with or without metronidazole 500 mg orally twice a day for 14 days<br>• *Severe:* Cefotetan 2 g IV every 12 hours<br>*Or*<br>• Cefoxitin 2 g IV every 6 hours<br>*Plus*<br>• Doxycycline 100 mg orally or IV every 12 hours |
| Syphilis | *Treponema pallidum* | • Preferred therapy: Benzathine penicillin G 2.4 million units IM for one dose<br>• Alternative therapy (for penicillin-allergic patients):<br>  – Doxycycline 100 mg PO BID for 14 days, or<br>  – Ceftriaxone 1 g IM or IV daily for 10–14 days, or<br>  – Azithromycin 2 g PO for one dose |
| Genital ulcer disease | *T. pallidum* | Same as for syphilis |
| | HSV—primary infection | See prepubertal vulvovaginitis |
| | *Haemophilus ducreyi* (chancroid) | • Azithromycin, 1 g, orally, in a single dose or ceftriaxone, 250 mg, IM, in a single dose<br>*Or*<br>• Ciprofloxacin, 500 mg, orally, twice daily for 3 days^c<br>*Or*<br>• Erythromycin base, 500 mg, orally, three times/day for 7 days |
| | *Klebsiella granulomatis* [granuloma inguinale (Donovanosis)]^d | • Doxycycline, 100 mg, orally, twice a day for at least 3 weeks and until all lesions have healed completely<br>*Or* |

*Contd...*

*Contd...*

| Syndrome | Organisms/diagnoses | Treatment[a] |
|---|---|---|
| | | • Azithromycin, 1 g, orally, once/week for at least 3 weeks and until all lesions have healed completely<br>Or<br>• Ciprofloxacin, 750 mg, orally, twice a day for at least 3 weeks and until all lesions have healed completely<br>Or<br>• Erythromycin base, 500 mg, orally, four times/day for at least 3 weeks and until all lesions have healed completely<br>Or<br>• Trimethoprim-sulfamethoxazole, 1 double-strength (160 g/800 mg) tablet, orally, twice a day for at least 3 weeks and until all lesions have healed completely |
| Sexually acquired epididymitis | *C. trachomatis*, *N. gonorrhoeae* | • Ceftriaxone, 250 mg, IM, in a single dose<br>Plus<br>• Doxycycline, 100 mg, orally, twice daily for 10 days |
| | Enteric organisms (for patients allergic to cephalosporins and/or tetracycline) | • Levofloxacin, 500 mg, orally, once daily for 10 days<br>Or<br>• Ofloxacin, 300 mg, orally, twice a day for 10 days |
| Gonococcal infections of the pharynx | *N. gonorrhoeae* | Ceftriaxone, 250 mg, IM, in a single dose |
| Anogenital warts | Human papillomavirus | Patient-applied:<br>• Podofilox 0.5% solution or gel or imiquimod 5% cream<br>Or<br>• Sinecatechins 15% ointment<br>Provider-administered:<br>• Cryotherapy<br>Or<br>• Podophyllin resin 10–25%<br>Or<br>• Trichloroacetic acid<br>Or<br>• Bichloroacetic acid<br>Or<br>• Surgical removal |

*Contd...*

*Contd...*

| Syndrome | Organisms/diagnoses | Treatment[a] |
|---|---|---|
| Vulvovaginal candidiasis | | Intravaginal agents:<br>• Butoconazole, 2% cream, 5 g, intravaginally, for 3 days[a,b]<br>Or<br>• Butoconazole, 2% cream (sustained release), 5 g, single dose intravaginal application for 1 day<br>Or<br>• Clotrimazole, 1% cream, 5 g, intravaginally, for 7–14 days[a,b]<br>Or<br>• Clotrimazole 2% cream, 5 g, intravaginally, for 3 days[a,b]<br>Or<br>• Miconazole, 2% cream, 5 g, intravaginally, for 7days[a,b]<br>Or<br>• Miconazole, 4% cream, 5 g, intravaginally, for 3 days[a,b]<br>Or<br>• Miconazole, 100, mg vaginal suppository, 1 suppository for 7 days[a,b]<br>Or<br>• Miconazole, 200 mg vaginal suppository, 1 suppository for 3 days[a,b]<br>Or<br>• Miconazole, 1,200 mg vaginal suppository, 1 suppository for 1 day[a,b]<br>Or<br>• Nystatin, 100,000-U vaginal tablet, 1 tablet for 14 days<br>Or<br>• Tioconazole, 6.5% ointment, 5 g, intravaginally, in a single application[a,b]<br>Or<br>• Terconazole, 0.4% cream, 5 g, intravaginally, for 7 days[a]<br>Or<br>• Terconazole, 0.8% cream, 5 g, intravaginally, for 3 days[a]<br>Or<br>• Terconazole, 80 mg vaginal suppository, 1 suppository for 3 days[a]<br>Oral agent:<br>• Fluconazole, 150 mg oral tablet, 1 tablet in single dose |

## LEGAL ASPECTS

In India, legal age for consensual sex is 18 years under the Criminal Law (Amendment) Act, 2013. Marriage of a female <18 years of age or a male of <21 years of age is illegal. Marriage is voidable and not void. Marriage will become valid if no steps are taken by such "child" seeking declaration of marriage as void, (Hindu Marriage Act, 1955). The Medical Termination of Pregnancy (MTP) Act of India clearly states the conditions under which a pregnancy can be ended or aborted, the persons who are qualified to conduct the abortion, and the place of implementation. One of the qualifications is abortion in unmarried girls under the age of 18 years is to be conducted with the consent of a guardian. (Medical Termination of Pregnancy, 1971).

Legal instruments alone cannot solve complex social issues unless accompanied comprehensive sexuality education, autonomy and empowerment of girls, access to reproductive health services, gender-sensitive and efficient law enforcement, and social support for adolescent girls when they are in conflict with their families.

## KEY RECOMMENDATIONS

- To have a team of pediatricians, psychologists, counselors, and teachers for sexuality education.
- Schools can facilitate platforms for open discussion about sexuality with parents and adolescents.
- Train volunteers to support peer-led culturally sensitive interventions.

## POINTS TO REMEMBER

- Sexuality is influenced by adolescents over body language, sexual identify, role at home and society, personal feeling, and self-esteem.
- Feelings of homosexuality, transgender may emerge to discontinue later or may continue.
- HEADDSSS questionnaire is usually used to assess the adolescent behaviors.
- Pediatricians should have an adolescent friendly clinic to address to sexuality and related assess such as adolescent pregnancy, STDs, and sexual abuse.

## SUGGESTED READING

1. American Psychiatric Association. Diagnostic and Statistical Manual of Mental Disorders, Fifth edition. Washington, DC, US: American Psychiatric Association; 2000.
2. American Psychiatric Association. Diagnostic and Statistical Manual of Mental Disorders, Fifth edition. Washington, DC: American Psychiatric Press; 2013.

3. American Psychological Association. Guidelines for psychological practice with lesbians, Gay and Bisexual clients. Am Psychol. 2012;67(1):10-42.
4. Braverman PK. HPV Vaccine in Adolescents. Pediatr Ann. 2019;48(2):e71-7.
5. Cohen E, MacKenzie RG, Yates GL. HEADSS, a psychosocial risk assessment instrument: Implications for designing effective intervention programs for runaway youth. J Adolesc Health. 1991;12(7):539-44.
6. Galagali PM, Rao C, Dinakar C, Gupta P, Shah D, Chandrashekaraiah S, et al. Indian Academy of Pediatrics Consensus Guidelines for Adolescent Friendly Health Services. Indian Pediatr. 2022;59(6):477-84.
7. Gee H. The oedipal Complex in adolescence. J Analytical Psychol. 1991;32(2):193-210.
8. Hegde A, Chandran S, Pattnaik JI. Understanding Adolescent Sexuality: A Developmental Perspective. J Psychosexual Health. 2022;4(4):237-42.
9. Kumar A, Singh T, Basu S, Pandey S, Bhargava V. Outcome of the teenage pregnancy. Indian J Pediatr. 2007;74:927-31.
10. Levine DA; Committee On Adolescence. Office-based care for lesbian, gay, bisexual, transgender, and questioning youth. Pediatrics. 2013;132:e297-313.
11. Mbizvo MT, Zaidi S. Addressing critical gaps in achieving universal access to sexual and reproductive health (SRH): the case for improving adolescent SRH, preventing unsafe abortion, and enhancing linkages between SRH and HIV interventions. Int J Gynaecol Obstet. 2010;110 Suppl:S3-6.
12. Ministry of Health and Family Welfare. The Medical Termination of Pregnancy Act, 1971. [online] Available from https://main.mohfw.gov.in/acts-rules-and-standards-health-sector/acts/mtp-act-1971. [Last accessed January, 2023].
13. Saewyc EM, Magee LL, Pettingell SE. Teenage pregnancy and associated risk behaviours among sexually abused adolescents. Perspect Sex Reprod Health. 2004;36:98-105.
14. StudyMode. (2012). The developmental theories of Jean Piaget, Sigmund Freud, and Erik Erikson. [online] Available from http://www.studymode.com/essays/The Developmental Theories of Jean Piaget-866031.html. [Last accessed January, 2023].
15. Sully EA, Biddlecom A, Daroch J, Riley T, Ashford L, Lince-Deroche N, et al. Adding It Up: Investing in Sexual and Reproductive Health 2019. New York: Guttmacher Institute; 2020.
16. Treffers PE. Teenage pregnancy, a worldwide problem. Ned Tijdschr Geneesk. 2003;147:2320-5.
17. UNFPA. Generation of Change: Young People and Culture, Youth Supplement: State of World Population 2008. New York: UNFPA; 2008.
18. Wertsch JV, Sohmer R. Vygotsky on learning and development. Hum Dev. 1995;38:332-7.
19. Workowski KA, Berman S; Centers for Disease Control and Prevention (CDC). Sexually transmitted diseases treatment guidelines, 2010. MMWR Recomm Rep. 2010;59:1-110.

# CHAPTER 4

# Parenting an Adolescent

*Yamuna S, Vijayarani M*

## ■ INTRODUCTION

Parents are defined to encompass "all those who provide significant and/or primary care for adolescents, over a significant period of the adolescent's life, without being paid as an employee", including biological parents, foster parents, adoptive parents, grandparents, other relatives, and fictive kin such as godparents.

Indian adolescents live with their parents until they move out either for education or for employment. In spite of physically staying away from the parental shelter most adolescents are being in touch with their parents in a regular manner. How and for what the parents interact with their adolescents determine the connection between them.

Psychosocially, an adolescent is in the process of searching for his identity keeping in mind the expectations of his parents, other family members, and school and the social setting in which he lives. The parents are in the process of admitting the fact that their adolescent may not need their inputs soon in all aspects of life. It is easy for the parents to rejoice and accept independent walking by their toddler as an important milestone; but is very difficult to acknowledge the independent decision making skills by their adolescent as a significant appreciable milestone. Not only does it cause concern in the parents but also makes them realize that they have to let go of their role as parents soon.

The World Health Organization (WHO) has gathered and analyzed significant information from existing research and experience obtained from various intervention programs conducted in many countries to help parents recognize their role in preventing adolescents from indulging in high-risk health behaviors. In 1997, WHO, United Nations Population Fund (UNFPA), and United Nations Children's Fund (UNICEF) jointly issued a technical report on "programming for adolescent health and development" where the following five areas were proposed as major themes of intervention that could be carried out to promote healthy development of this population **(Box 1)**.

**BOX 1:** Major theme of intervention.

- Creating a safe and supportive environment
- Providing accurate information
- Building skills
- Providing counsel
- Improving health services

Thus, the home comprising the family members including parents is central to program interventions to prevent adolescent ill health. Family and parents provide support and love, promote moral development and a sense of responsibility, provide role models and education about culture, set expectations, negotiate for services and opportunities, and filter out or counteract harmful or inconsistent impact from the social environment.

## ■ FAMILY CONNECTION AS A PROTECTIVE FACTOR

By definition, factors are called "protective" if they discourage one or more behaviors that might lead to negative health outcomes (e.g., having sex with many partners) or encourage behaviors that might prevent a negative health outcome (e.g., using condoms and contraception). Factors that are associated with increasing the likelihood of negative consequences of behavior are called risk factors. Family connectedness, school connectedness, presence of a trustworthy adult, and spirituality are the major protective factors in the lives of adolescents. Thus, parents play a key role in three of the four protective factors and contribute to a large extent in enjoying the fourth protective factor.

Literature reveals that parents are the most significant adults in the life of adolescents. Information to create awareness on aspects such as growing up, mood variations, substance use, and sexuality are better received if offered by parents during early adolescence. Boys and girls between 10 and 14 years are called "very young adolescents" who are connected with the parents and are still receptive as they are in the process of understanding themselves. As adolescents of this group learn to think about their identity they begin to question their parents about the relevance of each instruction given by their parents. Though this perturbs the parents, it gives them an opportunity to place the facts and explain the consequences of the various actions that could be performed by the emotionally charged adolescent.

The five dimensions of parenting which have influence on adolescents are as follows:

1. *Connection:* A positive and stable emotional bond between the parent and the adolescent established over the entire lifespan of the child conveys love, affection, compassion, and warmth. Early childhood attachment helps in forming secure relationships.

2. *Behavior control:* Structured approach to supervise, monitor, limit, and regulate the behavior of adolescents with negotiation and guidance to promote health in the adolescents; conveying that the wellbeing of their children is of foremost importance, helps in regulating behavior.
3. *Respect for individuality:* Allowing the adolescent to search for his or her identity resulting in self-worth and self-concept, e.g., seeking information about substances and then taking a decision to stay away from using them is a healthier way. This takes time but with guidance the process can be augmented.
4. *Modeling of appropriate behavior:* Children and adolescents imbibe values, ethics, and etiquette practiced by their parents and significant adults. Appropriate role modeling promotes healthy behaviors in adolescents.
5. *Provision and protection:* Parents may not have resources to provide all material comforts and information to their adolescent, but they can promote access to resources by empowering their children. Protection cannot be offered all through but skills to protect oneself from harm can be imparted by the parents, e.g., empowering with skills to say "no" to sexual exploitation.

Parents should be given information about adolescent health and development and should be provided opportunities to equip themselves with communication skills to transform the knowledge to enlighten the adolescents in a useful manner.

## ▪ STYLES OF PARENTING

Depending on the parental expectations and responsiveness to their children, Diana Baumrind classified parenting styles into four types, i.e., (1) Authoritarian: Highly demanding and less responsive, (2) Permissive/indulgent: Highly responsive and not demanding, but over indulging, (3) Authoritative: Highly demanding and highly responsive with role modeling, and (4) Neglectful: Not demanding and not responsive and not available. **Table 1** highlights the additional characteristics of each of the parenting style. Each parenting style promotes specific psychosocial developmental aspects in the child. Highly responsive parent will create an immense sense of wellbeing and trust in the child. Promoting higher responsiveness in parents is being currently thought to improve treatment outcomes by enhancing adherence.

## ▪ POSITIVE PARENTING AND ADOLESCENT BEHAVIOR

Numerous studies have made us understand that adolescents who have parents who practice authoritative style of parenting evolve as well-adjusted, well-informed, and capable adolescents who seem to have the skills to

**TABLE 1:** Characteristic feature of the four parenting styles.

| Feature/parenting style | Authoritarian | Permissive/indulgent | Authoritative | Neglectful |
|---|---|---|---|---|
| Demandingness/expectations | High | Nil | High | Nil |
| Responsiveness | Less | High | High | Nil |
| Style of communication | Aggressive | Passive/submissive | Assertive | Poor/limited to few words |
| Expression of love | Care is considered as love | Well expressed | Well expressed | Rarely expressed |
| Demonstrative love | Not expressed | Well expressed | Well expressed | Nil |
| Time spent with children | Less | High | High | Minimal |
| Value inculcation | Through instruction, "Do as I say, and not do as I do" | Left to child as, "Whatever you do is right for you"! | "We are value-loaded and follow what we practice" explanations are provided for each expectation | No attempt at value inculcation is made |
| Insistence on discipline | High with psychological control like black mailing, name calling, and sometimes physical abuse | Nil | Firm and high with explanation and negotiation and differential reinforcement like encouragement for positive behaviors and ignoring negative behaviors | Nil |
| Role modeling | Minimal | Nil, entire household is child centered | Very high | Nil |
| Compassion | Nil | High | Very high | Nil |
| Freedom of speech and expression | Nil | Total freedom, child will not know how to make use of the freedom, and gets confused and anxious | • Freedom of expression is given, with lot of inputs from parents on the right and the wrong<br>• Guidance on modification is offered with compassion | As there is not much of contact, expression is determined by the children who feel not guided |
| Moralistic | Highly moralistic | Willing to relax all moral values to see happiness in children | High, but not judgmental. Guidance is offered always | Not applicable |

*Contd...*

Contd...

| Feature/parenting style | Authoritarian | Permissive/indulgent | Authoritative | Neglectful |
|---|---|---|---|---|
| Opinionated | Yes | Nil | Not opinionated but explains possible opinions that can be formed by certain behaviors | Not applicable |
| Care of children | Care is complete, all acts of service done in a methodical manner but in an impersonal manner. Attempt to self-care is not encouraged. Dependency is seen as obedience and subordination. | Very good with personal attention to begin with; later with scare that the child might scold the parents for lapses | Very good with personal attention, involving children in inculcation of habits of self-care very early in life, generation of independence and preparation of the children to survive without the support of parents is practiced | Care is not adequate and children usually fend for themselves with breach in self-care and hygiene |
| Appreciation and encouragement | Rarely offered | Offered more than necessary as the parents are scared at consequences if not offered | Offered in right doses at right occasions | Not offered as the parents are rarely aware of accomplishments |
| Criticism | Liberal and frequent | Nil | Yes, but with explanations and ways to rectify | Rarely take note of deviance in behaviors or actions |
| Outcome in children | • Submissive or rebellious, lack of self-control, self-esteem, and self-confidence as they have been controlled always<br>• Performance anxiety is high and accomplishments are less | Self-driven, anxious at outcomes as they have not been exposed to challenges appropriately with guidance from parents; self-esteem low with reduced confidence at new activities | Self-motivated, self-disciplined, and self-confident children with high self-esteem and frequent success in many tasks | Feel that they lack direction or may latch on to people to receive direction which may be right or wrong |
| Children's perception about the parents | Strict, controlling parents who gave no space for growth | Ineffective parents who offered no guidance and direction | Excellent parents who were available always but at the same time encouraged independence; offered help whenever necessary | Nonavailable parents who were totally away in mind, body, and actions |

handle challenges independently using effective problem-solving skills. Parental willingness to provide autonomy since early childhood for handling age-appropriate challenges with an assurance of guidance in the event of necessity promotes emancipation in the adolescent. Parental responsiveness like being available to share strong emotions that emerge within the family setting or outside contribute to the acquisition of emotional regulation skills in the adolescents. Availability of an active listener, especially the parent enhances expression of emotions with a resultant reduction in issues such as depression, suicidal ideation, violence, use of weapons, delinquency, school dropout, substance use, and drunken driving. Thus, positive reinforcement of an accepted behavior with inputs to understand the negative consequences of a behavior that cannot be accepted paves the way to better activities during adolescence.

Adolescents feel less burdened and relieved when they are able to share their emotions and experiences with their parents; especially if the parents are capable of appropriate empathy and compassion. Adolescents do not look for readymade solutions but regard parents as a source of major support in the events of crises.

## PARENTING AND SEXUALITY

In most parts of the world, sex is considered a taboo subject and rarely do parents give information to their children. Open communication by parents about matters relating to sex, especially when an adolescent shows curiosity to know more about marriage, relationships, child birth and related issues, have been found to delay sexual debut, are related to an increased use of contraception and promote more stable relationships with reduction in promiscuity. Equipping parents to handle this challenge using an effective communication style is the major agenda for healthcare professionals.

## PARENTING AND LIFESTYLE IN ADOLESCENTS

Lifestyle factors such as physical activity, nutritional intake, sleep routine, hygiene, and hobbies are influenced by the parents' inputs either as suggestions or as role models. Parents who observe authoritarian style insist on certain practices with firmness amounting to aggression. Few adolescents might perceive this as an intrusion into their privacy and might rebel actively by arguing with the parents or passively by noncooperation. Parents who are permissive would allow the adolescent to take decisions and thus indirectly promote ill health. Authoritative parents establish a routine with appropriate explanation and negotiation.

## ROLE OF HEALTHCARE PROFESSIONALS

Healthcare professionals can play a major role in the following ways:
- Making parents comfortable with the growth and development during adolescence

- Equipping the parents with the aspects of the psychosocial developmental stage in which the adolescents are expected to evolve
- Enriching the parents with strategies to assist in the exploration of identity by their adolescent son or daughter
- Enabling the parents to allow space for the adolescent to develop autonomy and permit individualization
- Empowering the parents with essential communication tools to establish effective connection with their adolescents
- Enhancing the existing monitoring and guidance principles practiced by the parents that would help in early detection of deviations in behavior
- Expanding the horizon of the parents by including the peer group of their adolescents in a nonjudgmental manner
- Exposing the parents to the benefits of sharing information on sexuality with their adolescents and thus ascertaining the value of open parent-adolescent communication on delicate topics as a successful method to prevent high risk health behaviors in the next generation.

## POINTS TO REMEMBER

- Educate the parents on adolescent growth and development.
- Empower parents on effective communication skills.
- Enlighten the parents to include taboo subjects such as sexuality and substance use in their discussions with adolescents.
- Ensure the inculcation of authoritative parenting style by all parents since the first meeting.

## SUGGESTED READING

1. Blum RW. Risk and protective factors affecting adolescent reproductive health in developing countries: an analysis of adolescent sexual and reproductive health literature from around the world: summary. Geneva, Switzerland: World Health Organization; 2005.
2. Darling N. Parenting Style and its Correlates. [online] Available from http://ecap.crc.illinois.edu/eecearchive/digests/1999/darlin99.pdf. [Last accessed February, 2023].
3. Eshel N, Daelmans B, de Mello MC, Martines J. Responsive parenting: interventions and outcomes. Bull World Health Organ. 2006;84:991-8.
4. World Health Organization. Helping Parents in Developing Countries Improve Adolescents' Health. Geneva, Switzerland: World Health Organization; 2007.
5. Yamuna S. Art of parenting. In: Parthasarathy A, Menon PSN, Gupta P, Nair MKC (Eds). IAP Textbook of Pediatrics, 5th edition. New Delhi. Jaypee Brothers Medical Publishers (P) Ltd.; 2013. pp. 1062-6.

# CHAPTER 5

# Media Usage in Adolescents

*Jayashree K, Preeti M Galagali*

## ■ INTRODUCTION

In this technology-driven era, millennials are using digital media more than anyone could imagine. Adolescents normatively have immature self-control, self-regulation, and cognition as compared to adults and are most vulnerable to ill effects of media.

Using media, adolescents are able to easily access information and entertainment and stay connected with friends and family. Popular social media of 2019 in India are listed in **Table 1** along with the percentage of individuals who use them.

Current scientific evidence has linked increased media use to decreased outdoor and physical activities, decline in academic performance, problematic internet use, difficulty in making and maintaining social relations, sleep disturbance, issues surrounding online safety, compromised privacy, and cyberbullying.

Digital citizenship is defined as appropriate and responsible behavior while using technology. Education about digital citizenship is important and encompasses learning to respect others and to protect oneself and others online.

The growth in interactive media platforms and their rapid adoption by young people is an indication of the compelling nature of social media tools,

**TABLE 1:** Social media usage in India 2022.

| | |
|---|---|
| Instagram | 76.50% |
| Facebook | 74.70% |
| Twitter | 44.90% |
| LinkedIn | 37.20% |
| Pinterest | 34.90% |
| MX TakaTak | 23.40% |
| Moj | 23.00% |
| Skype | 23.00% |

such as Instagram and Snapchat. Adolescents, who are highly attuned to peer relationships, find the social component of many of these platforms very rewarding. About 76% of teen-aged respondents in a recent Pew Research Center (a nonpartisan American think tank based in Washington, DC) survey reported that they use social media.

In 2018, three online platforms other than Facebook including YouTube, Instagram, and Snapchat were used by majority of the adolescents. Overall, 84% of teens revealed that they currently have access to a game console at home and 90% said that they play video games of any kind (whether on a computer, game console, or cell phone). Teenage girls are slightly more likely to say it would be hard to give up social media than teen boys (58% vs. 49%) and 35% of teens who say they use at least one of the five platforms this survey covered—YouTube, TikTok, Instagram, Snapchat, or Facebook—almost constantly. Over a period of time, the pattern to access media has changed with mobile phone screens replacing TV screens for entertainment. Technology addictions are more common among adolescents having single parent and lesser in nuclear and joint families. Psychiatric distress was seen more in mobile phone users as compared to those with internet addiction.

## ■ CORONAVIRUS DISEASE AND MEDIA

The coronavirus disease-2019 (COVID-19) physical distancing measures had a detrimental effect on adolescents' mental health. Adolescents worldwide alleviated the negative experiences of social distancing by spending more time on digital devices. A general increment in the use of digital technologies has been reported, especially of social media, with applications such as TikTok, Pinterest, Reddit, Facebook, Snapchat, Instagram, LinkedIn, and Twitter showing growth in active users ranging from 8 to 38%. Internet was filled with information about the COVID-19 pandemic, which helped a few adolescents gain knowledge about it. Few used social media due to fear of missing out (FOMO), which led to an obsessive cycle of social media usage. During the pandemic when schools were shut, most countries around the world resorted to online mode of teaching which kept many adolescents occupied with their academics. But at the same time, they got access to the internet which leads to video gaming problems and various other adverse effects of problematic internet use.

## ■ EFFECTS OF MEDIA ON ADOLESCENT HEALTH

Digital media usage has both advantages and disadvantages.

### Adverse Effects of Media

Social media use is associated with experiences of online harassment, short sleep hours, delay in time to fall asleep, sleep disruption, and body image

**BOX 1:** Health hazards of media use.

- Behavioral problems
- Obesity and postural problems
- Poor sleep hygiene
- Body image issues
- Academic underachievement
- Online dating, relationship issues, and trafficking
- Internet addiction
- Substance abuse
- Sexting and cyberbullying
- Depression and suicide
- Fear of missing out (FOMO)
- Nomophobia

issues among girls and boys. Adolescents, being constantly online, have sleep patterns affected, negatively impacting their mood. Anger due to peer rejection in early adolescence but not in young adults leads to increased viewing of antisocial media content. Adolescent victims of bullying who regulated their anger through maladaptive strategies (e.g., other-blame and rumination) showed higher levels of cyberbullying themselves. Traditional media as an information source was not significantly associated with sexual risk behavior outcomes, suggesting that social media platforms may offer special avenues for influencing sexual health behaviors (and potentially other health outcomes) not offered by traditional media sources. The adverse effects of media usage in adolescence are listed in **Box 1**.

A few important terms associated with digital hazards are explained here.

## Cyberbullying

When the internet, cell phones, or other devices are used to send or post text or images intended to hurt or embarrass another person, it is termed cyberbullying. It is a form of online harassment where derogatory remarks spread quickly and are known to become "viral". It is the most common online risk for all teens and could be devastating. It may result in severe psychological trauma. Several victims of cyberbullying are driven to suicide. Cyberbullying is a punishable offence under the Information Technology (IT) Act 2000 and the Indian Penal Code. Victims can complain regarding cyberbullying on the government's helpline number 112.

## Pornography

It refers to books, magazines, and films that are designed to cause sexual excitement by showing or describing sexual acts. Due to early exposure to media, children/adolescents are at risk of developing pornography addiction. Like any other addiction, the same dopamine neurotransmitter pathway is involved in this. By viewing sexually pornographic material, adolescents may face potential emotional, psychological, social, and physiological disorders and issues. As per "Protection of Children from Sexual Offences (POCSO) Act" criminalizes watching or collection of pornographic content involving children also. Sections 292 and 293 of the Indian Penal Code, 1860 make it illegal to sell, distribute, and exhibit or circulate obscene objects.

## Sexting

Sending, receiving, or forwarding sexually explicit messages, photographs, or images is termed sexting. It is very dangerous as adolescents can be blackmailed into recording videos showing pornography, and even sex trafficking. Sexting is a crime under POCSO Act.

## Internet Gaming Disorder

It is the excessive or uncontrolled internet gaming activity, leading to negative consequences in the psychosocial functioning of an individual. As internet gaming disorder (IGD) has been considered to be a significant public health issue, the Diagnostic and Statistical Manual (DSM) has stated that it is akin to an alcohol use disorder. There are nine criteria for IGD proposed in DSM-5, which are as follows:

1. Preoccupation
2. Withdrawal symptoms
3. Tolerance
4. Unsuccessful control
5. Impaired decision-making
6. Rewarding deficit
7. Escape
8. Deceit about internet gaming
9. Impaired function.

Similar criteria are used to define other addictive behaviors such as substance use disorder or gambling disorder.

## Focusing on Likes

It is the need to gain "likes" on social media. This can cause teens to make choices they would otherwise not make, including altering their appearance, engaging in negative behaviors, and accepting risky social media challenges.

*Fear of missing out:* It is a pervasive apprehension that others might be having rewarding experiences from which one is absent. This social anxiety is characterized by a desire to stay continually connected with what others are doing.

**BOX 2:** Benefits of digital media.

- Access to knowledge
- Emotional support and connectedness
- Strengthening relationships
- Self-identity
- Awareness regarding health-related issues
- Self-expression
- Community building and participation
- Mobile health, e.g., vaccination reminder apps, fitness apps, and suicide helpline

*Nomophobia:* It is a psychological condition where people fear of being without a mobile phone or being unable to use the phone for some reason, such as the absence of a signal or running out of battery power.

*Phantom vibration syndrome:* It is the perception that one's mobile phone is vibrating or ringing when it is not ringing. In a study done on medical students, it was found that 60% felt phantom vibrations and 42% felt phantom ringing.

## Benefits of Media

There are numerous advantages of media, if it is used in moderation. These are listed in **Box 2**.

Teens who struggle with social skills and social anxiety or who do not have easy access to face-to-face socializing might benefit from connecting with other teens through social media. Teens in marginalized groups—lesbian, gay, bisexual, transgender, transsexual, queer (LGBTQ) teens, and teens struggling with mental health issues—can find support and friendship through the use of social media. When teens connect with small groups of supportive teens via social media, those connections can be the difference between living in isolation and finding support.

## ■ ROLE OF PEDIATRICIAN

Anticipatory guidance should be provided during a clinical encounter with an adolescent. Details of eliciting media history are listed in **Table 2**. If there are issues with overuse of social media or mobile phones, then parents and the adolescent should be counseled for setting up digital boundaries and thereby decrease time spent on media. A few practical tips are enumerated in **Table 3**. The screening tool for internet addiction is young's internet addiction test and for IGD is problematic online gaming questionnaire. Psychotherapeutic interventions for media addiction include cognitive behavioral therapy (CBT) and motivational enhancement therapy. Whenever there are features of associated mental disorders such as depression and attention deficit hyperactivity disorder (ADHD), appropriate screening,

**TABLE 2:** Basic guide for eliciting media-related history from parents.

| | |
|---|---|
| Television/mobile screen | Time spent watching/watching with or without family member/discussion about the shows/TV installed in bedroom/TV watching rules/demands to buy products seen in advertisements |
| Movies/videos | Type of movies or videos being watched/any restrictions/nightmares or trouble after watching movies |
| Music | Type of music/discuss about the lyrics that parent object/any restriction on certain type of music |
| Video games | Familiarity with type of video games played/check on game's rating before buying/permission for downloading violent games/restriction on time spent playing video games |
| Internet | Access to individual computer/talking about the best use of the internet/aware of different websites visited/using any software to block visiting inappropriate/pornographic web sites |
| Books | Time spent reading books/providing variety of reading materials/discussing about the books read |
| Any other concerns | Use of tobacco or alcohol/body image or sexuality/display of aggressive behavior or foul language |

**TABLE 3:** Practical tips on setting digital boundaries.

| Digital apps/procedures | Advantages |
|---|---|
| Apps that show the time spent online | Gives accurate time spent on each app on daily basis |
| Apps that restrict access to social media sites | To restrict the time spent online, these apps which prevent accessing social media sites after usage for a fixed duration. Also, notification can be set up which pops up after certain amount of time is spent online |
| Use silent mode | Whenever working on something very important or during academic work this mode is used so that attention is not diverted and thereby time is well utilized |
| Turn off notifications | Helps indirectly in designating particular time to look at each app. Eagerness to check in to apps during notifications is controlled |
| Curating digital timelines | Follows accounts that make the teens feel good and unfollow any accounts that fill them with guilt or dread whenever they pop up. Mutes the posts if they cannot unfollow |
| Privacy settings | Determine those who might be able to see and share the messages that one posts |
| Hiding phone | Taking phone out of the pocket and off the coffee table or study table or hiding it in the bag, or even in a drawer, can stop teens from reaching for their phones without intention |

*Contd...*

*Contd...*

| Digital apps/ procedures | Advantages |
|---|---|
| Use a watch | To check the time, use a watch there by the pull to use mobile to check time is reduced. This helps reducing mindless scrolling |
| Set time aside | Setting time aside to scroll through apps and to respond helps teens to limit use of media devices |
| Set expectations | Letting friends and family know that teen is reducing screen time and might not reply as quickly as before will ensure their cooperation and encourage them to reduce screen time |
| Turn off devices before bedtime | To get a sound sleep, to turn phone off 1 hour before going to bed and to leave it outside the bedroom |

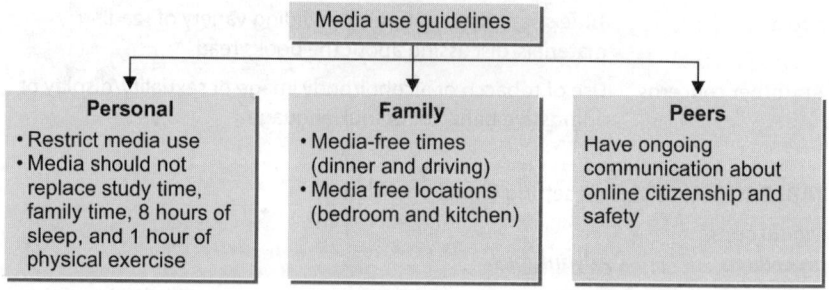

**Flowchart 1:** Media use guidelines.

therapy, and/or referral to psychiatrist should be advised. Parents should be encouraged to talk about using media appropriately early in childhood and build a relationship of trust surrounding social media. This would improve communication between parents and adolescents regarding issues of media usage. Adolescents should be made aware of the safe use of media in schools, colleges, and community centers and through radio, TV talks, and articles in print media. General media use guidelines are outlined in **Flowchart 1**. The Indian Academy of Pediatrics has set guidelines for parents regarding screen time which is provided in **Box 3**.

## ■ CONCLUSION

Adolescents of today are known as digital natives as they are born in a world full of digital devices and media messages. Healthy media use in adolescence promotes socioemotional well-being and enhances knowledge. Excessive and unmonitored media usage can result in poor physical and mental health. Pediatricians should give anticipatory guidance and screen for media-related health issues during adolescent health visits. Timely counseling and therapy will promote digital citizenship and prevent adverse health consequences.

**BOX 3:** The Indian Academy of Pediatrics (IAP) screen time and digital wellness guidelines for adolescents.

- Parents to ensure a warm, nurturing, supportive, fun-filled, secure home environment, stay updated with technology, use "teachable moments" while viewing media to convey family values, and to role model healthy media use
- Formulate media use rules and a family media plan before giving a device to the child/adolescent
- Balance screen time with essential daily activities (1 hour of physical activity, 8–9 hours of sleep, schoolwork, meals, hobbies, and peer and family interaction). If these are compromised, then the screen time is excessive and should be reduced
- Maximize educational and health promoting screen time and minimize recreational. Discourage multitasking
- Monitor digital content viewed. Avoid exposure to violent, age-inappropriate material, and online interaction with strangers/unknown people
- Mark digital free zones (bedroom, dining table, kitchen, bathroom, and motorized vehicles) and periodic digital fasting time
- Maintain correct posture while using digital devices and follow 20-20-20 rule
- Discuss media literacy to deconstruct digital messaging, online etiquette to ensure socially appropriate behavior, digital safety, and infodemic and permanence of digital footprint
- Share with trustworthy adults, report (to https://www.cybercrime.gov.in), block (sender) and save disturbing media messages to counter cyberbullying, sexting, and online sexual solicitation

## POINTS TO REMEMBER

- Adolescent media usage has become an integral part of present-day lifestyle.
- Awareness regarding benefits versus ill effects (cyberbullying and sexting) is the need of the hour.
- Education about staying safe in the digital world.
- Pediatricians should give anticipatory guidance.
- Parents need to talk regarding healthy media use to their adolescents.

## SUGGESTED READING

1. American Psychiatric Association (APA), Diagnostic and Statistical Manual of Mental Disorders, 5th edition (DSM-5). Arlington, VA: American Psychiatric Publication; 2013.
2. Balhara YPS, Verma K, Bhargava R. Screen time and screen addiction: beyond gaming, social media and pornography–a case report. Asian J Psychiatr. 2018;35:77-8.
3. Den Hamer AH, Konijn EA. Adolescents' media exposure may increase their cyberbullying behavior: a longitudinal study. J Adolesc Health. 2015;56:203-8.
4. Gupta P, Shah D, Bedi N, Galagali P, Dalwai S, Agrawal S, et al. Indian Academy of Pediatrics Guidelines on Screen Time and Digital Wellness in Infants, Children and Adolescents. Indian Pediatr. 2022;59(3):235-44.

5. Lemola S, Perkinson-Gloor N, Brand S, Dewald-Kaufmann JF, Grob A. Adolescents' electronic media use at night, sleep disturbance, and depressive symptoms in the smartphone age. J Youth Adolesc. 2015;44:405-18.
7. Lenhart A. (2015). Teens, Social Media & Technology Overview 2015. [online] Available from https://www.pewresearch.org/internet/2015/04/09/teens-social-media-technology-2015/. [Last accessed February, 2023].
7. Mangot AG, Murthy VS, Kshirsagar SV, Deshmukh AH, Tembe DV. Prevalence and pattern of Phantom ringing and Phantom Vibration among medical Interns and their relationship with smart phone use and perceived stress. Indian J Psychol Med. 2018;40:440-5.
8. MediaBriefAdmin. (2020). KalaGato Report: COVID 19 Digital Impact: A Boon for Social Media. [online] Available from https://mediabrief.com/kalagato-vocid-19-digital-impact-report-part-1/. (Last accessed February, 2023].
9. Nikken P, Schols M. How and Why parents guide the media use of young children. J Child Fam Stud. 2015;24(11):3423-35.
10. Sharma MK, Rao GN, Benegal V, Thennarasu K, Thomas D. Technology addiction survey: An emerging concern for raising awareness and promotion of healthy use of technology. Indian J Psychol Med. 2017;39:495-9.
11. Sherman LE, Payton AA, Hernandez LM, Greenfield PM, Dapretto M. The Power of the Like in Adolescence: Effects of Peer Influence on Neural and Behavioral Responses to Social Media. Psychol Sci. 2016;27:1027-35.
12. Smith A, Anderson M. (2018). Social Media Use in 2018. [online] Available from http://www.pewinternet.org/2018/03/01/social-media-use-in-2018/. [Last accessed February, 2023].
13. Statista. (2021). Growth of monthly active users of selected social media platforms worldwide from 2019 to 2021. [online] Available from https://www.statista.com/statistics/1219318/social-media-platforms-growth-of-mau-worldwide/. [Last accessed February, 2023].
14. The Global Statistics. (2023). India Social Media Statistics 2022. [online] Available from https://www.theglobalstatistics.com/india-social-media-statistics/. [Last accessed February, 2023].
15. Vogels EA, Gelles-Watnick R, Massara N. (2022). Teens, Social Media and Technology 2022. [online] Available from https://www.pewresearch.org/internet/2022/08/10/teens-social-media-and-technology-2022/#fn-28469-1. [Last accessed February, 2023].
16. Wieland DM. Computer Addiction: Implications for nursing psychotherapy practice. Perspect Psychiatr Care. 2005;41(4):153-61.
17. Young KS. Internet addiction: symptoms, evaluation, and treatment. In: Vande Creek L, Jackson T (Eds). Innovations in Clinical Practice: A Source Book. Florida: Professional Resource Press; 1999. pp. 19-31.

# SECTION 2

# Dealing with Adolescent Client

6. **Psychosocial Assessment of Adolescents Using HEEADSSS**
   *B Lakshmi Shanthi, Shruti Kalkekar*
7. **Sexual and Reproductive Health Assessment of Adolescents**
   *Poonam Bhatia, Anuradha HS*
8. **Monitoring Physical Growth of Adolescents**
   *Sridevi A Naaraayan, Nedunchelian K*
9. **Adolescent Counseling**
   *Atul M Kanikar, CP Bansal*
10. **Motivational Interviewing**
    *Swati Ghate, Sreyoshi Ghosh*
11. **Making Pediatric Practice Adolescent Friendly**
    *Kritika Agarwal, Rajiv Mohta*
12. **Psychopharmacological Interventions in Children and Adolescents**
    *Tejas Golhar, Shashi Kiran, Shoba Srinath*

# CHAPTER 6

# Psychosocial Assessment of Adolescents Using HEEADSSS

*B Lakshmi Shanthi, Shruti Kalkekar*

## ■ INTRODUCTION AND BACKGROUND

Issues related to psychosocial, behavioral, and lifestyle problems are very common in the adolescent age group. These in turn lead to risky behavior, unintentional injuries, substance abuse, unwanted pregnancy, sexually transmitted illness, and suicidal ideation which are the major causes of mortality and morbidity in adolescents. Unfortunately, very few adolescents seek professional help for such issues. Hence, psychosocial assessment during every contact of the adolescent with the pediatrician/family physician plays a key role.

In 1972, Dr Henry Berman described an approach for routine psychosocial history taking in adolescents using the HEEADSSS framework which was later refined by Dr Eric Cohen to integrate additional areas of importance. The HEEADSSS screening tool is a structured framework for conducting a comprehensive biopsychosocial assessment of the young person. It provides information about the young person's functioning in key areas of their life. The acronym HEEADSSS stands for Home, Education/Employment, Eating/Exercise, Activities, Drugs, Sexuality, Suicide/Depression, and Safety. Recently, questions on media usage have been added in the HEEADSSS 3.0 update.

Before starting the HEEADSSS assessment reassurance of confidentiality with the youth is a must. The beauty of HEEADSSS approach is it begins from the least personal questions to the most intimate questions. It provides an ideal format for a preventive health check-up. By exploring beyond presenting complaint of the adolescent, the healthcare provider can assess the psychosocial background and detect underlying health concerns and risk factors for timely intervention and preventive education.

The HEEADSSS screening should be performed by trained adolescent healthcare providers who have adequate knowledge about normal adolescent development and related health concerns. Undisturbed attention and empathetic listening with a nonjudgmental attitude set a good tone.

This is only a guide and not a diagnostic tool and can be catered as per need. The assessment should be reviewed at regular intervals.

## ■ CONFIDENTIALITY AND DOCUMENTATION

Privacy and confidentiality are two essential prerequisites of the assessment and parents of the adolescents should be informed of the same. After establishing a rapport with the adolescent, explain the purpose of the assessment, and obtain informed consent if the adolescent is above 18 years and assent for 12–18-year-olds. The healthcare provider's knowledge and expertise will determine the standard of healthcare to the adolescents. Explain confidentiality including the safety exceptions (harming self, others, or if somebody is harming them, sexual abuse).

## ■ HOME

Explore home situation, family life, relationships, and stability.

The questions need to be open ended and can be based as per the acronym for ease and comfort of history taking; however, the approach needs to be modified based on the clues from history. For instance the home environment may not be congenial for a particular adolescent and hence postponing this history would be ideal. Rather start by asking "where do you live?" "who lives with you?" **(Box 1)**. Most teenage problems are connected, in part, to relationships at home. The style of parenting also has an important role in adolescents' life. Authoritative parenting is a protective factor against high-risk behavior.

*A Guide to Using HEEADSSS*

## ■ EDUCATION/EMPLOYMENT

Find out the teen's connectedness to school and education, which is a good predictor of risk-taking behavior. Higher the connectedness lowers the risk-taking behavior. Ask specifically about the academic performance and any problems associated with it. Ask about bullying and pressures related to peer group. Older teens should be enquired about their employment, work hours, work satisfaction, and work pressure **(Box 2)**.

**BOX 1:** Home (sample questions).

- Where do you live? Who lives with you?
- What language is spoken at home?
- Explain your relationships at home.
- With whom do you feel comfortable to confide to?
- What are the cultural practices like?
- Has anyone joined or left your family of late?
- Have you moved out of your home recently?
- How often do you argue at home and what is the most common dispute?

**BOX 2:** Education/employment (sample questions).

- What are you good at/not good at?
- Have there been any changes at school/work?
- Have you changed schools recently?
- What is your future plan/ambition?
- Who are your friends at school?
- Do you feel safe at school? If not why?
- Have you ever been rusticated?
- Have you ever absented uninformed?

**BOX 3:** Eating and exercise (sample questions).

- Tell me about your routine food habits.
- Do you overeat or undereat to beat away mood swings?
- Any recent changes in body weight? Do you constantly brood over it?
- What do you like and not like about your body?
- Do you exercise regularly?
- What in your view constitutes a healthy diet?
- Do you overeat?
- Have you ever feigned illness or self-medicated to lose weight?

## ■ EATING AND EXERCISE

Explore how they look after themselves; eating, exercise, and sleeping patterns. Unhealthy eating habit is very common in adolescent age group which is a precursor for obesity and lifestyle diseases. Eating disorders are also common and cannot be unraveled without asking leading questions **(Box 3)**. Detailed history about the dietary patterns, physical activity, body image issues, crash dieting, sugary drinks, and JUNCS should be taken and anticipatory guidance given. Positive reinforcement should be given to adolescents who follow healthy lifestyle.

## ■ PEER-RELATED ACTIVITIES

Ask about their friendships, relationships, and how often do they indulge in risk taking or adventurous activities.

Start by asking "what do you do with friends?" **(Box 4)**. Take note when an adolescent says he does not have friends or feels bored all the time. The identity and self-esteem of adolescents is mostly related to their peer group.

## ■ DRUGS

Asking about drugs is a very sensitive discussion and should be dealt with caution. In early adolescents start by asking "do your friends use drugs/alcohol?" and then build up on the conversation. Older adolescents might open up on drugs-related questions if they develop the trust. Include

**BOX 4:** Peer-related activities (sample questions).

- What do you and your friends do for fun?
- Do you participate in sports/extracurricular activities?
- What are your hobbies?
- Do you read books?
- Do you listen to music or play instruments?
- Do you participate in any organized activities?
- What are the things you like about yourself?
- Do you enjoy playing online gaming with friends?

**BOX 5:** CRAFFT screening questionnaire.

- **C**—Have you ever traveled in a CAR driven by someone under the influence of drugs/alcohol?
- **R**—Do you ever use drugs/alcohol to RELAX, feel better or fit in?
- **A**—Do you ever use drugs/alcohol when you are ALONE?
- **F**—Do you FORGET things you did whilst using drugs/alcohol?
- **F**—Do your family or FRIENDS ever tell you to cut down drinking/drug use?
- **T**—Have you ever gotten into TROUBLE using drugs/alcohol?

**BOX 6:** Sexuality (sample questions).

- Have you ever fallen in love?
- Number of people you have dated?
- What is the level of intimacy in your relationship?
- Have you ever felt attracted to a person of the same sex?
- Do you masturbate, if so, how often?
- Have you ever missed your periods or on learning to be pregnant sought abortion services?
- What is your idea about contraception and prevention of sexually transmitted infection (STI)?
- Have you ever been forced to have sex or abused sexually?
- Do you indulge in sexting or watching porn? If so, how often?
- If you have been sexually active, are you comfortable/enjoy the act?

questions on caffeinated drinks, anabolic steroids, synthetic cannabinoids, and prescription drugs. Keep abreast of the latest trends of substance use in the teen's neighborhood. The "CRAFFT" screening tool is an easy to use screening test to assess the substance using teenager **(Box 5)**.

## ■ SEXUALITY

Explore their knowledge, understanding, experience, sexual orientation, and sexual practices. Look for risk taking behavior/abuse. This is the most sensitive part of the interview. It may be beneficial to seek permission before proceeding—"do you mind if I ask you a few more personal questions to learn how I can help you" **(Box 6)** or even say, "I know this is embarrassing, but I ask these questions to all my teen patients to have a better idea".

## ■ SUICIDE

Explore risk of mental health problems and strategies for coping and available support. Adolescents should be screened for depression whenever possible to ensure early diagnosis, appropriate therapy, and follow-up. Many teens admit to being stressed than to overt depression. The following questions can be asked to know about their mental status **(Box 7)**.

While screening for depression or suicide a quick patient health questionnaire-2 (PHQ-2) screening tool would be of immense help **(Table 1)**.

A score of 3 or higher has good sensitivity and specificity for diagnosing major depression in adolescents.

## ■ SAFETY

Injuries, suicide, and homicide are some of the major reasons for morbidity and mortality in adolescents; hence questions on safety are very important. Contributing factors such as bullying, violence in school, gang formation, sexual violence, and possessing weapons must be identified in the psychosocial history. Questions pertaining to online safety such as posting messages that may spread hatred/communal violence and sexting should be included **(Box 8)**.

In addition to the routine HEEADSSS interview two more S's can be added according to the present scenario. S for spirituality and S for social media or screen time.

**BOX 7:** Suicide (sample questions).

- How often do you feel bored?
- Have you ever felt hopeless/helpless?
- Do you have difficulty in sleep/appetite?
- Have you ever felt low/attempted suicide/counseling in the past?
- How often do you have emotional/aggressive outbursts?
- Have you ever engaged in self-harm/highly impulsive behavior?
- Do any of your family members suffer from depression or have attempted suicide?
- Have you ever suffered recurrent headache, gastric symptoms, and fatiguability?

**TABLE 1:** Screening for depression or suicide: Patient health questionnaire-2 (PHQ-2) screening tool.

| Over the past 2 weeks how often have you been bothered by any of the following? | Not at all | Several days | More than half the days | Nearly everyday |
|---|---|---|---|---|
| Little interest or pleasure in doing things | 0 | 1 | 2 | 3 |
| Feeling down, depressed, or hopeless | 0 | 1 | 2 | 3 |

**BOX 8:** Safety (sample questions).

- Do you feel safe at home?
- Do you feel threatened at school?
- Have you ever driven with a friend who was drunk?
- Have you driven a vehicle without following rules?
- Have you ever carried a weapon?
- Have you ever felt unsafe during your online activities?
- Do you feel vaccinations help you to prevent diseases?

**BOX 9:** Spirituality (sample questions).

- Do you believe in supreme power?
- Do you go to temple as a ritual or when you feel worried?
- Have you thought about the meaning of your life?
- Where do you find peace when in trouble?
- Have you tried meditation/yoga to calm down?

**BOX 10:** Social media/screen time (sample questions).

- What is the time spent on social media?
- Do you indulge in gaming, if so, time spent everyday?
- What do you think about media literacy?
- Have you ever been bullied online or have you bullied others?
- Have you ever indulged in binge watching?
- Have you ever watched porn, if so, how frequently?

## ■ SPIRITUALITY

Inculcation of spiritual beliefs and religious practices has shown to prevent high-risk behaviors in adolescents. At the same time teens with atheist/agnostic attitudes should not be judged and ridiculed. They should be encouraged to establish their own identity **(Box 9)**.

## ■ SOCIAL MEDIA/SCREEN TIME

Increased screen time has become an indispensable part of today's adolescents. The coronavirus disease (COVID) pandemic has added to the screen time by online classes, in addition to this, teens indulged in social media and gaming to beat the boredom which led to increased cases of problematic internet use (PIU). Presently media contributes 10–20% of any specific health problem. At the same time improved media access can lead to positive outcomes such as empathy, broad mindedness, social group acceptability, and respect for the elderly. Begin by asking preliminary question as presented in **Box 10**.

Standard scales like Young's Internet Addiction Test or Problematic and Risky Internet Use Screening Scale (PRIUSS) for screening PIU can be used

**TABLE 2:** Resilient teenager's characteristics.

| | |
|---|---|
| Home | • Empathetic parents<br>• Self-responsibility<br>• Involvement in daily chores<br>• Connected to siblings/relatives |
| Education and employment | • Satisfactory school performance<br>• Involvement in school<br>• Work contentment<br>• Participation in extracurricular activities and sports |
| Eating | • Eating balanced diet and avoiding JUNCS |
| Activities | • Leadership among peers<br>• Religious affiliation |
| Drugs | • Taking a vow to abstain<br>• Refusal skills |
| Sexuality | • Vowing to say "no"<br>• Refusal skills<br>• Healthy attitude toward sex |
| Suicidality | • No history of suicidal antecedents<br>• No family history of suicide<br>• Access to a soulmate<br>• Resilient coping skills<br>• Strong emotional quotient |
| Safety | • Seat belt/helmet use<br>• Problem solving skills<br>• Say "no" to substance<br>• Refusal to accompany an intoxicated driver |

depending on the response to the questions asked in **Box 10**. The prevalence rate of PIU in adolescents is 1–24.2%. Characteristics of resilient adolescents according to the HEEADSSS tool can be summarised as in **Table 2**.

# ALTERNATIVE TO HEEADSSS FOR YOUNG PEOPLE WITH INTELLECTUAL DISABILITY

The HEEADSSS may not be useful in adolescents with an intellectual disability. The Clinical Outcomes in Routine Evaluation–Outcome Measure (CORE-OM) measures psychosocial wellbeing and health in four domains: wellbeing, symptoms, functioning, and risk. It takes 5–10 minutes to complete. Adaptations include:
- *Young Person's CORE (YP-CORE):* It is a 10-item measure derived from the CORE-OM and designed for use with adolescents in the 11–16 years age. It is structurally similar to the CORE-OM but items have been rephrased to be more easily understood by the target age group.
- *CORE–Learning Disabilities (CORE-LD):* It is a variation being developed in Scotland and England for use in adolescents with learning difficulty.

## A Strength-based Approach—SSHADESS

The SSHADESS screening is a modified HEEADSSS screening, the reasons behind the modification include:
- It begins with strengths
- School is addressed before home
- A wider range of emotions are screened for

The SSHADESS has been designed for direct questioning of an adolescent in a private setting. It can also be used when a parent/caregiver brings an older child or younger adolescent who does not feel comfortable with a private interview. In such a situation, the general topics related to strengths, school, and activities are addressed and high-risk behaviors should not be addressed. Rather use this as an opportunity to offer anticipatory guidance and counseling for the parent to approach sensitive topics.

## Digital Survey e-HEEADSSS

The e-HEEADSSS is a better screening tool for in-patient setting in which significant increase in uptake rate with high disclosure rate. Digital survey provided a time-efficient self-administered, psychosocial screening tool introduced by nontrained staff, and had a consistent record of responses.

## THRxEADS for Teens with Chronic Disease

Chadia, Amari, and Kaufman discovered this clinical tool which serves as a complementary to HEEADSSS to explore key issues in teens with chronic disease, such as diabetes or cystic fibrosis (CF).

*THRxEADS:* T for transition, H for home, Rx for treatment, E for education/eating, A for activities/affect, D for drugs, and S for sexuality.

## The Headspace Modification

The headspace psychosocial guiding tool is used to assess areas of difficulty that may be indicative of psychosocial problems (anxiety, psychosis, and mania). It includes a wrap-up summary of positive interview of both the patient's strengths and goals (predisposing factors, precipitating factors, perpetuating factors, and protective factors).

## ■ PREVISIT PSYCHOSOCIAL ASSESSMENT

Post COVID teleconsultations have become common; hence, well-developed "back-end" computer systems to support psychosocial assessment even before the visit have been developed. They promote efficiency of use, validity of assessment, and ease of scoring. For example, Youth CHAT—this tool is used to explore the development in multidomains either through face-to-face visits or through teleconsultations.

## ■ TIPS FOR A SUCCESSFUL PSYCHOSOCIAL INTERVIEW

- The interview should proceed from basic, less intimate topics to those more personal.
- Identify strengths early so that they can be "built on" when motivating the patient to change or when encouraging positive behavior. Do not express shock, dismay, or be judgmental to the responses, this may disrupt the disclosure of the full history.
- Be careful not to ask closed questions for two reasons. First, they limit the magnitude of the responses. Second, when you ask a sensitive question and the patient does not yet fully confide in you, he/she may lie, and feel embarrassed to disclose honestly later.
- Look for real life problems that your patient has successfully overcome—the ability to face and overcome adversity known as resilience which is a highly protective factor in various circumstances.
- Praise—when it is needed as many vulnerable adolescents never hear any praise.
- Use active listening and paraphrasing—this allows the adolescent time to confirm and expand on his or her thoughts.
- Create a comfortable, trustworthy, and nonjudgmental setting—the adolescent should feel connected to you, for telling what is going on in their life.
- Share your concerns—it is ok to gently challenge your patient by saying, e.g., "I am worried that your smoking habit may be a barrier to your goal of serving in the military".
- Do not assume an adolescent who offers full and rapid disclosure is not at risk—sometimes vulnerable adolescents may disclose personal information very rapidly in an effort to bond with you.
- After the interview, ask permission to solve a problem identified—if you do not ask teens whether they want your advice; they may be less likely to listen to it.

## ■ WRAPPING IT UP

- Document the adolescent's developmental stage—whether early, middle, or late.
- Identify culture-specific needs.
- Summarize the assessment findings with the adolescent. Check with them which adults they trust and reinforce your role as a support.
- Ascertain whenever referrals may be needed and discuss it with them.

- Send and document appropriate referrals.
- Document a formulation of the assessment and subsequent plan in the record.

## DISCLOSURE IS NOT YOUR GOAL

There are two setbacks to performing a psychosocial interview. First, it can contextualize personal trauma through a prism of interrogation. Second, it might trigger unpleasant memories. For this reason, it is imperative that you clearly state a few points:
- Questions should be asked only once the rapport is established.
- The goal is to get the most pertinent history, not the thorough one.
- Your aim must be to initiate and sustain a workable relationship.
- Make sure to know what the teen wants out of the relationship.

## POINTS TO REMEMBER

- Psychosocial assessment is a key skill for healthcare providers who are dealing with teenagers. It must be performed by trained and skilled clinician who has adequate knowledge about normal adolescent development and related health concerns.
- A respectful, confidential, nonjudgmental, and empathetic interactive conversation will help to elicit the psychosocial information from adolescents. Clinician's positive attitude and genuine liking for youth will add on success.
- HEEADSSS is a standardized screening tool which provides systematic framework for psychosocial assessment. It helps in guiding health conversations, building on strength, providing helpful scientific facts, to detect underlying health concerns screening for risk factors, timely intervention, partnership for agreed plan of action, and preventive education. Involvement of parent in certain cases keeping confidentiality intact is must.
- Initial focus must be on rapport building to ease the conversation. Privacy and confidentiality are a key element for successful interviewing. Brief notes and documentation will help focused care for underlying health problem.
- Many modifications in HEEADSSS help to conduct psychosocial assessment in adolescents who are differently abled/especially challenged/with chronic illness.

## ACKNOWLEDGMENT

I would like to express my gratitude to Dr Preeti Galagali who gave me this golden opportunity to write an article on a very important topic "Psychosocial Assessment of Adolescents Using HEEADSSS". It also helped me in doing a lot of research and came to know about so many new things. Secondly, I am also grateful to Dr Anant Patil for scrutinizing the manuscript. I am also thankful to my family and friends who supported me to complete this in limited time frame.

## ■ SUGGESTED READING

1. Anand N, Sharma MK, Marimuthu P. Problematic internet use and its association with psychological stress among adolescents. Indian J Soc Psychiatry. 2021;37:269-74.
2. Brooks FM, Magnusson J, Spencer N, Morgan A. Adolescent multiple risk behaviour: an asset approach to the role of family, school and community. J Public Health (Oxf). 2012;34 (suppl 1):i48-56.
3. Butler PW, Middleman AB. Protecting adolescent confidentiality: a response to one state's "Parents' Bill of Rights". J Adolesc Health. 2018;63(3):357-9.
4. Chadi N, Amaria K, Kaufman M. Expand your HEADS, follow the THRxEADS! Paediatr Child Health. 2017;22(1):23-5.
5. Corry DA, Leavey G. Adolescent trust and primary care: Help-seeking for emotional and psychological difficulties. J Adolesc. 2017;54:1-8.
6. Ginsburg KR. The SSHADESS Screening: A strength based psychosocial Assessment. [online]. Available from: https://www.aap.org/contentassets/0e45de0366d54ec38fbfcb72382a0c6c/rt2e_ch32_sahm.pdf. [Last accessed January, 2023].
7. Goldenring J, Rosen D. Getting into adolescent heads: an essential update. Contemp Pediatr. 2004;21:64-79.
8. Hatala A, McGavock J, Michaelson V, Pickett W. Low risks for spiritual highs: risk-taking behaviours and the protective benefits of spiritual health among Saskatchewan adolescents. Paediatr Child Health. 2021;26(2):e121-8.
9. Ho J, Fong CK, Iskander A, Towns S, Steinbeck K. Digital psychosocial assessment: an efficient and effective screening tool. J Paediatr Child Health. 2020;56(4):521-31.
10. Klein D, Goldenring J, Adelman W. HEEADSSS 3.0—the psychosocial interview for adolescents updated for a new century fueled by media. Contemp Pediatr. 2014;31:16-28.
11. Liu L, Villavicencio F, Yeung D, Perin J, Lopez G, Strong KL, et al. National, regional and global causes of mortality in 5-19-year-olds from 2000 to 2019: a systematic analysis. Lancet Glob Health. 2022;10:e337-47.
12. Lora P, James D, Patel S. The HEEADSSS app: a service evaluation of the psychosocial screening app in young people. Arch Dis Child. 2022;107:A8.
13. Lorentzen V, Handegård BH, Moen CM, Solem K, Lillevoll K, Skre I. CORE-OM as a routine outcome measure for adolescents with emotional disorders: factor structure and psychometric properties. BMC Psychology. 2020;8:86.
14. Parker AG, Hetrick SE, Purcell R. Assessment of mental health and substance use disorders in young people: refining and evaluating a youth-friendly assessment interview. Aust Fam Physician. 2010;39:585-8.
15. Piko BF, Balázs MS. Authoritative parenting style and adolescent smoking and drinking. Addict Behav. 2012;37(3):353-6.

16. Rathi N, Riddell L, Worsley A. What influences urban Indian secondary school students' food consumption?—A qualitative study. Appetite. 2016;105:790-7.
17. Saw C, Smit A, Silva D, Bulsara MK, Tran Nguyen ET. Service evaluation and retrospective audit of electronic HEEADSSS (e-HEEADSSS) screening device in paediatric inpatient service in Western Australia. Int J Adolesc Med Health. 2020;34(6):401-9.
18. Sawyer SM. Psychosocial Assessments After COVID-19. J Adolesc Health. 2021;68(3):429-30.
19. Spaeth M, Weichold K, Silbereisen RK. The development of leisure boredom in early adolescence: predictors and longitudinal associations with delinquency and depression. Dev Psychol. 2015;51(10):1380-94.
20. Starship. (2022). Adolescent Consultation and the HEEADSSS assessment. [online] Available from: https://starship.org.nz/guidelines/adolescent-consultation/. [Last accessed January, 2022].
21. Weybright EH, Schulenberg J, Caldwell LL. More bored today than yesterday? National trends in adolescent boredom from 2008 to 2017. J Adolesc Health. 2020;66(3):360-5.

# CHAPTER 7

# Sexual and Reproductive Health Assessment of Adolescents

*Poonam Bhatia, Anuradha HS*

## ■ INTRODUCTION

Sexual and reproductive health is defined as a state of physical, emotional, mental, and social wellbeing in relation to sexuality; it is not merely the absence of disease, dysfunction, or infirmity. Sexual health requires a positive and respectful approach to sexuality and sexual relationships, as well as the possibility of having pleasurable and safe sexual experiences, free of coercion, discrimination, and violence.

Investment in adolescent reproductive and sexual health (ARSH) has a positive influence on overall health and economy of nation by reducing maternal mortality rate, infant mortality rate, incidence of teenage pregnancy, and sexually transmitted infections (STIs) including proportion of human immunodeficiency virus (HIV) positive cases.

The health assessment of every adolescent starts with psychosocial history taking by a screening tool HEEADSSS which covers every aspect of adolescent's life i.e., home, eating habits, education/employment, activities, drug use, sexuality, self harm, and safety. This basic yet essential assessment is part of history taking on any adolescent who visits our clinic. This art of history taking builds a rapport which not only helps clinician to understand the adolescent, but also gives, adolescent an opportunity to communicate their concerns related to sex and sexuality in an open and honest environment. The first S of pneumonic HEEADSSS represents sexuality history.

Every clinician needs to ask all adolescent patients aged 11 and older some essential sexual health questions related to puberty, gender identity, sexual attraction/orientation, and sexual activity. The additional questions explore sexual satisfaction, functioning, concerns, and support for one's gender identity and sexual orientation.

Objectives of sexuality history are to:
- Take complete sexual history including menstrual history in case of female adolescent client

- Discuss with and reassure adolescent boys about erections, ejaculation, masturbations as normative developmental process
- Discuss and clarify various myths/concerns related to masturbation in both genders
- Identify sexual behavior and classify their behavior as low-, moderate-, and high-risk behavior
- Perform targeted screening based on earlier mentioned history
- Identify teens at risk for sexually transmitted disease (STD) and counsel them on making healthy choices about their sexual activities
- Prevent teen pregnancy and support pregnant adolescents
- Identify teens who are suffering from sexual abuse
- Counsel adolescents on safe sexual practices, prevention of STD, and contraception
- Identifying and addressing various myths regarding sexuality and reproduction
- Assess and provide knowledge related to their sexual rights in light of current Indian laws.

## PREREQUISITES FOR TAKING SEXUALITY HISTORY

### Step 1

Psychosocial interviewing through HEEADSSS.

### Step 2

- Explain the concept of consent and confidentiality to parents and teens also when confidentiality needs to be broken.
- Interview parents and teens jointly and then separately also, set expectations.
- End the interview after explaining the screening tests, thanking the client and ensuring support.

### Step 3

Follow the Centers for Disease Control and Prevention (CDC) six Ps approaches as shown in **Figure 1**.

### *Partners*

Sexual activity that is informed, consensual, along with protection from STDs and unwanted pregnancy is said to be safe. Being sexually responsible means communicating openly and respecting the needs of partner, taking precautions against STIs, unplanned pregnancy, and with no element of abuse in relationship. Safe sex is an essential element of physical, mental, social, and economic health of partners.

# CHAPTER 7: Sexual and Reproductive Health Assessment of Adolescents

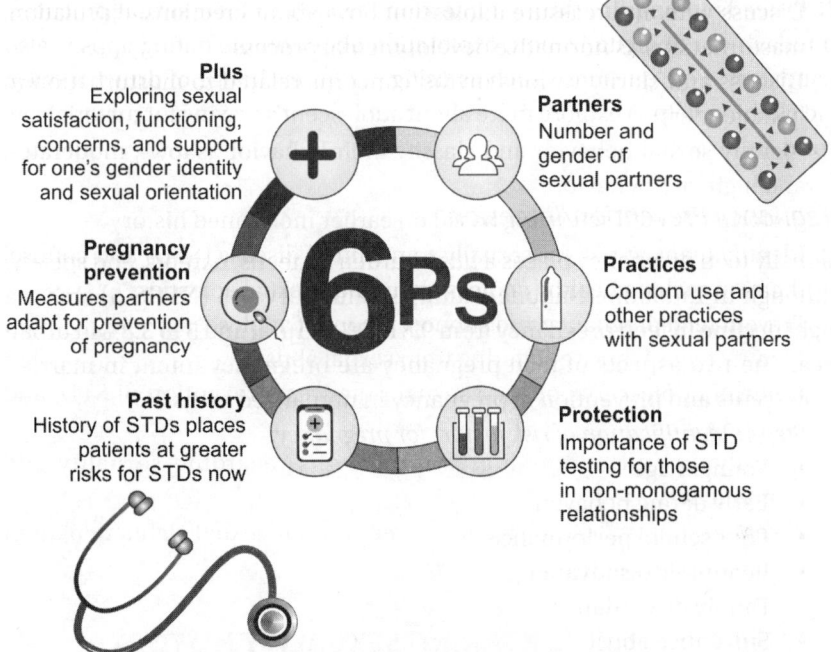

**Fig. 1:** The six Ps of sexual and reproductive health assessment.
*Source:* https://tinyurl.com/apoorvBhatia6PsDesign.

While taking sexual history ask open-ended questions in a nonjudgmental manner. Special attention should be paid to use gender neutral and inclusive terms like, "partner". To identify risk factors in a sexually active adolescent enquire the following: number of lifetime partners, number of partners in the past year, and gender of those partners. Such interrogation will help to frame preventive services and to plan for future counseling process for that particular adolescent.

Partner services are an important way of expanding clinical care to partners. The aim of partner services is to prevent transmission and reinfection with STI. The first step is the clinical evaluation of the sexually active adolescent patient, counseling for STI screening, and treatment followed by identifying their sex and needle sharing partners and providing treatment to them. Another way of notifying partners is to use digital media such as apps, emails, and social media. Every healthcare provider (HCP) should try their best to identify the primary partner and treat them and also encourage the patient to do so.

## Practices

To assess, the adolescent's risk of sexual diseases, to know, the anatomical sites of sampling, and to plan strategies for management and risk reduction

HCP, needs to enquire through questions related to their sexual practices. In today's era of digitalization, exploration about online dating apps is also mandatory. Few questions such as using sex for exchange of drugs, money, and clothing help to explore more about adolescent's craving for materialistic world.

### Pregnancy Prevention/Intension

Globally teen pregnancy places a huge burden on teens, parents, and society. Although in India, the National Family Health Survey-5 (NFHS-5) shows a slight decline in teen pregnancy from 9.8 to 8% in rural and 5 to 3.8% in urban area. The two aspects of teen pregnancy are pregnancy intent in married adolescents and prevention of pregnancy in unmarried teens.

- *Step 1: Identification of risk factors for pregnancy:*
  - Younger age
  - Early dating behavior
  - Poor school performance
  - Economic disadvantage
  - Family discordance
  - Substance abuse
  - Peer pressure
  - Sexual abuse
  - Mental health issues like depression
  - Media influence
- *Step 2: History:*
  - Menstrual history which includes LMP, duration, flow, etc.
  - Psychosocial history
- *Step 3:* Once the HCP understands the intent of an adolescent who is either sexually active or intends making a sexual debut, the advice is tailored accordingly.

To protect their bodies, avoid unintended pregnancies and unsafe abortions HCPs should guide every adolescent girl visiting clinic. This is done through nonjudgmental contraceptive counseling, providing complete information on modern methods of contraception, correct guidance on what is the right option for them, and the potential side effects. All HCPs should be adequately trained to provide unbiased care to adolescents irrespective of gender or marital status. Unmarried adolescents should have access to information about pregnancy prevention on social media and other digital channels.

### Protection from Sexually Transmitted Infection

According to the CDC, adolescents aged 15–24 years account for 50% of all new STD infections; hence, assessment of STI risk is a crucial part of adolescent reproductive and sexual health (ARSH).

**CHAPTER 7:** Sexual and Reproductive Health Assessment of Adolescents

**TABLE 1:** Risk stratification for contracting STIs based on sexual activities.

| | |
|---|---|
| No risk | Hand holding, massaging, hugging and rubbing against each other with clothes on, sharing fantasies, and self-masturbation are few of non risky activities that can be shared by partners |
| Low risk | Some examples of safe sexual activities are using a condom for every act of sexual intercourse, masturbating your partner, or masturbating together as long as males do not ejaculate near any opening or broken skin on their partners |
| Medium risk | These sexual activities carry some risk, such as introducing an injured finger into the vagina and sexual intercourse with improper use of a condom which carries a risk of HIV/STI transmission |
| High risk | Unprotected sexual intercourse is a highly risky sexual activity as it exposes both partners to body fluids which can be infected with HIV |

(HIV: human immunodeficiency virus; STI: sexually transmitted infection)

**BOX 1:** Protective factors to prevent early sexual debut in adolescents.

- Responsive parenting style, family connectedness, parental monitoring
- School connectedness, safe space and involvement in activities
- Positive peer influence and peers engaged in sports and other activities
- Good communication with sexual health partner and respectful sexual attitude
- High self-esteem and positive attitude toward sexual health and future
- Spiritual and religious affiliation
- Access to sexual health education and contraception
- Cohesive and trusted neighborhood offering after school programs

The first and foremost need is to identify risk factors that put adolescents at risk. The risk stratification for contracting STIs based on sexual activities is shown in **Table 1**. Various factors that make adolescents vulnerable to STI such as unsafe sexual practices, multiple partners, immature prefrontal cortex leading to risk taking behavior, immature vaginal and cervical epithelium of adolescent girls, lack of access to appropriate health services, poor reproductive hygiene practices, unsafe delivery and abortion. Other risk factors include sex with commercial sex workers; teens engaged in survival sex, i.e., sex for money, drugs, food, and housing; and early sexual debut. Increased vulnerability to STIs is observed when there are multiple sex partners, having sequential sex partnerships of limited duration or concurrent partnerships, failing to use barrier protection consistently and correctly, having lower socioeconomic status, and when access to healthcare is difficult for adolescent. Various factors through which sexual health risk of adolescents can be assessed are shown in **Figure 2**. After risk assessment adolescent's safety plan against STIs has be evaluated. **Box 1** shows various protective factors which prevent early sexual debut in adolescents.

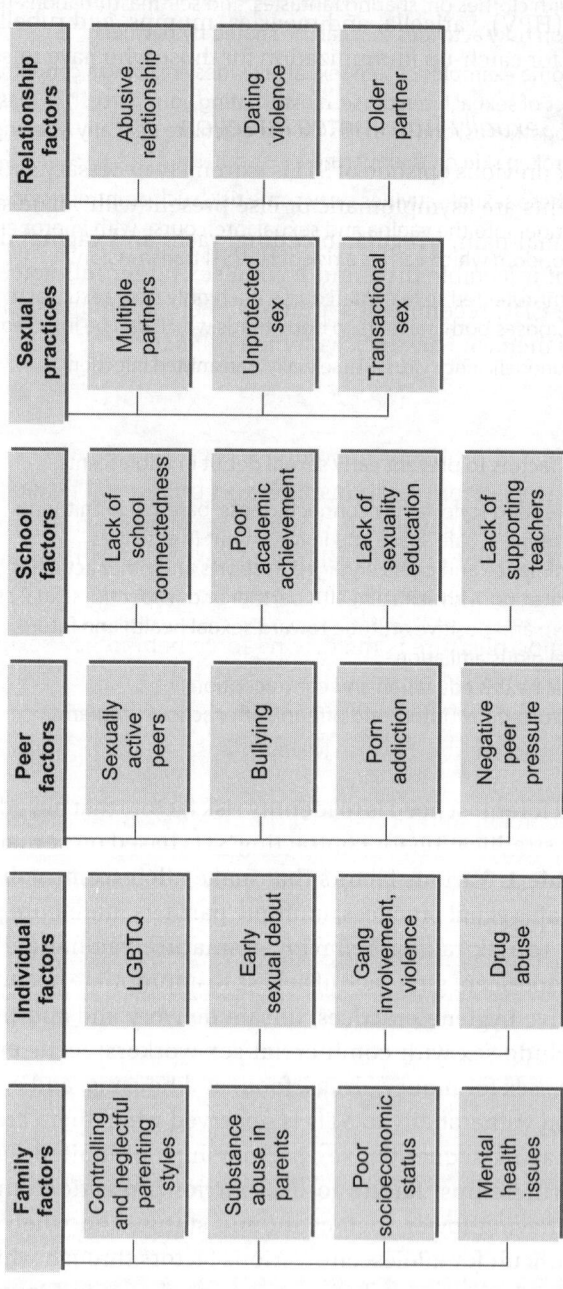

**Fig. 2:** Factors to identify adolescents with sexual health risk. (LGBTQ: lesbian, gay, bisexual, transgender, and questioning)

## CHAPTER 7: Sexual and Reproductive Health Assessment of Adolescents

The sexual attitudes and actions of adolescent's are guided by various myths which must be busted by HCP.

Enquire about their vaccination status for hepatitis A and B, human papillomavirus (HPV), varicella, and measles, mumps, and rubella (MMR) and guide them for catch-up immunization for those who have missed.

### Past History of Sexually Transmitted Infection

Interrogating for previous episode of STI is extremely necessary as 90% of the STIs in adolescents are asymptomatic or else present with vague symptoms such as abdominal pain, irregular bleeding, rash, and vaginal discharge. History of use of injectable drug and having sex under influence of drugs is essential. The CDC recommends annual screening for all sexually active adolescents and men who have sex with men (MSM).

### Plus

Sexual health-related problems encompass sexual orientation and gender identity, sexual expression, relationships, and pleasure. The sixth P—Plus includes pleasure, problems, and pride. It explores sexual functioning, satisfaction, and any other issue related to sexual health. Additionally it supports a person's gender identity and sexual orientation.

*Pleasure:* Obtaining pleasure is the driving force behind any sexual activity be it solo or with partner. The important fact about pleasure is that it begins in mind. The connection between thoughts, feelings, and behaviors has been established beyond doubt. So our thoughts affect our sexual experience of pleasure. The quality of intimacy between partners, previous history of sexual abuse, societal, and pressure of family are among the few factors which influence sexual pleasure. With the sexual act a blend of hormones are released which boosts immunity, induces sleep, elevates mood, and overall acting as a real stress buster.

Therefore asking questions related to sexual satisfaction is essential otherwise one can miss physical as well as emotional problems of teenagers. Researches prove that people with satisfactory sexual life do better in most of the fields of life.

*Problems:* This section brings out issues related to safety and consent. Boundaries and safety are interconnected to each other. Adolescents with high self-esteem feel empowered and normally do not surrender to partners demand. Adolescents should be able to set boundaries and communicate (through verbal and nonverbal) their desires, values, and choices to their partner.

Once the adolescent is comfortable, provider can discuss and resolve their queries related to their gender identity, dating violence, gender-based

**TABLE 2:** Myths and facts about sexuality.

| Myths | Facts |
| --- | --- |
| Oral sex is safe sex | Oral sex can lead to STI with exchange of body fluids |
| Pulling out before ejaculation helps avoid pregnancy | Pre-ejaculate can also lead to pregnancy |
| Is easy to tell if someone has STI | Most STIs are asymptomatic |
| You can get STI from a toilet seat | It is nearly impossible to contract an STI from a toilet seat |
| Only gay teens get HIV | Anyone who is sexually active can get HIV |
| Masturbation causes sexual dysfunction and infertility | Masturbation is normal |
| You cannot get pregnant when you have sex for the first time | Pregnancy is possible even after the first intercourse |

(HIV: human immunodeficiency virus; STI: sexually transmitted infection)

violence, etc. Globally, approximately 30% of girls suffer from physical and/or sexual violence in their lifetime. The sexual attitudes and actions of adolescents are guided by various myths which must be busted by HCP as shown in **Table 2**.

Use of substances such as alcohol, cannabis, and marijuana has been associated with high-risk sexual behavior (HRSB). Few examples of HRSB are involvement with multiple sexual partners, forgetting to use a condom or simply using it in an incorrect manner, having sex with sex workers, paid sex, or casual sex.

*Pride:* Body image is how we feel about our bodies and hence is essential part of sexuality. Sexual identity and relationships affect body image. Discussing about body image issues is essential as, those with poor body image might take sexually unhealthy decisions. Apart from struggling with their identities they also face societal discrimination, rejection from family and peers, and feel marginalized.

Healthcare provider must acknowledge that people can have varied sexual orientation, gender identity, or expression and when needed should take open stance for them. The queries of these teenagers should be resolved without any discrimination. In fact, sometimes clinician might be the only person on whom they can rely and share their concerns.

To promote positive attitude toward sex, equal opportunity should be given to every adolescent. This will empower them to take appropriate decisions related to their sexual and reproductive health and rights.

For better utilization of resources all adolescent friendly pediatricians should clearly display various health services **(Box 2)** that their clinic provides.

**BOX 2:** List of services available at healthcare facility.

- Information and counseling on sexual and reproductive health issues
- Promotion of healthy sexual behaviors
- Family planning information, counseling, and methods of contraception (including emergency contraceptive methods)
- Condom promotion and provision
- Testing and counseling services for pregnancy, human immunodeficiency virus (HIV), and other sexually transmitted infections (STIs)
- Management of STIs
- Antenatal care (ANC), delivery services, and postnatal care (PNC)
- Safe legal abortion and postabortion care
- Appropriate referral linkage between health facilities at different levels
- The right to information and education about sexual and reproductive health (SRH) services. Various rights are:
  - The right to decide freely and responsibly on all aspects of one's sexual behavior
  - The right to own, control, and protect one's own body
  - The right to be free of discrimination, coercion, and violence in one's sexual decisions and sexual life
  - The right to expect and demand equality, full consent, and mutual respect in sexual relationships
  - The right to the full range of accessible and affordable SRH services regardless of sex, creed, belief, marital status, or location

To probe deeper about sexuality additional questions can be asked which are given in **Table 3**.

## ■ CONCLUSION

As India caters to one of the largest youth populations in the world hence, it is the duty of the nation to protect and support the health of adolescents. By enhancing sexual education pediatricians can mitigate negative sexual health outcomes of adolescents. Pediatricians also have a great responsibility being the primary caregivers with an added advantage of a long-term relationship built from childhood. Apart from providing sex education they should also help teenagers to build life skills such as communication, assertiveness, and negotiating skills for development of responsible sexual behaviors.

It has been frequently experienced and proved that clinicians need special training in order to make these services accessible to youngsters.

Owing to taboo associated with sex, adolescents and even adults, hesitate to approach HCP for issues related to sexuality hence, in majority of countries sexual and reproductive health services do not reach the beneficiaries. Strengthening of preventive services is needed to protect sexual and reproductive health of adolescents.

**TABLE 3:** Additional sexual health questions for adolescents and adults (including those who are transgender).

| | |
|---|---|
| **Partners** | • Could you tell me about your current relationships (e.g., no partner, one partner, multiple partners)? |
| | • In the past 3 months, have you had sex with someone you didn't know or had just met? |
| | • Have you ever been forced or coerced to have sex/sexual activity against your will as a child or an adult?*<br>• *If yes*, does that experience affect your current sex life or sexual relationships? (Probe: In what ways?)<br>• *If yes*, does that make seeing a health care provider or having a physical exam difficult or uncomfortable? |
| | • Are you having any difficulties with your sexual relationships? |
| | • Do you or your partners have problems with sexual functioning (see "Problems" below)? |
| **Practices** | • In the past 3 months, what types of sex have you had? Anal? Vaginal? Oral? (Also, ask whether they give or receive each type of sexual activity.) |
| | • Have you or any of your partners used alcohol or drugs when you had sex? |
| | • Have you ever exchanged sex for drugs or money? |
| **Past history of STI(s)** | • Have you ever had a sexually transmitted infection (or disease)? *If yes*, which STI(s)? Where on your body were the infections? When did you have it? Were your partners tested and treated too? |
| | • Have you ever been tested for HIV? *If yes*, how long ago was that test? What was the result? |
| **Protection** | • What do you do to protect yourself from STIs, including HIV? |
| | • When do you use this protection? With which partners? |
| | • Have you been vaccinated against HPV? Hepatitis A? Hepatitis B? |
| **Pregnancy** | • Do you have any desire to have (more) children?<br>• *If yes*, how many children would you like to have? When would you like to have a child? What are you and your partners doing to prevent pregnancy until that time?<br>• *If no*, are you doing anything to prevent pregnancy? How important is it to you to prevent pregnancy? Would you like to talk about birth control options? |
| **Plus** — **Pleasure** | Start the conversation with, "It is part of my routine to ask about sexual health, including sexual functioning and pleasure, as part of your visit".<br>• How is your sex life going? What concerns do you have about your sex life?<br>　– Are you currently involved in any sexual relationships?<br>　– Is the sex you're having pleasurable for you? *If no*, why not? |

*Contd...*

## CHAPTER 7: Sexual and Reproductive Health Assessment of Adolescents

*Contd...*

| | | |
|---|---|---|
| | **Pleasure** | – Are you and your partners on the same page about what's pleasurable?<br>– Do you and your partners talk openly about sexual desires and boundaries? Are you able to advocate for sexual pleasure in your relationships?<br>• If not sexually active:<br>– Would you like to have a sexual relationship or a better sex life?<br>– Is there anything holding you back or getting in your way? [This could lead to a discussion of problems (see "Problems" below) and of other issues such as sexual assault and porn use.] |
| | **Problems** | • Are you having any difficulties when you have sex (e.g., pain, discomfort, vaginal dryness, lack of arousal, lack of orgasm, lack of erection)?<br>• Are you concerned about your sex drive or the sex drive of your partners (e.g., low or high level of interest in having sex, mismatched sex drives)? |
| | **Pride\*\*** | • What support, if any, do you have from your family and friends about your gender identity?<br>• What support, if any, do you have from your family and friends about your sexual orientation?<br>• Are you experiencing any harassment or violence–at home, at work, at school, or in your community–due to your sexual orientation or gender identity? |

(CDC: Centers for Disease Control and Prevention; HIV: human immunodeficiency virus; HPV: human papillomavirus; LGBT: lesbian, gay, bisexual, and transgender; STI: sexually transmitted infection)
*This could include, forced anal, vaginal, or oral sex; drug facilitated sexual assault; sexual harassment; stalking; groping; and/or birth control sabotage. Patient resources and a 24/7 hotline: The National Sexual Assault Online Hotline.
\*\*CDC, other government agencies, and community organization materials: Lesbian, Gay, Bisexual, and Transgender Health and LGBT Youth Resources.

## ■ ACKNOWLEDGMENT

We acknowledge that we are the authors of this article and our article is based on the guidelines given by CDC USA, WHO, and the Canadian Pediatric Society.

## ■ POINTS TO REMEMBER

- Ignorance and lack of information exposes adolescents to risky situations which might negatively impact their health.
- Informed and consensual sexual activities are the essential prerequisite of safe sex and the concept of safe sex should be discussed with every adolescent.

- People of varied sexual orientation, gender identity, or expression should be given equal opportunity which will motivate them to talk without any hesitation.
- Every adolescent should learn life skills such as communication skills, assertiveness, and negotiating skills for safe sexual behaviors.
- Investment in ARSH has a positive influence on overall health and economy of nation.

## SUGGESTED READING

1. Altarum Institute. Sexual Health and Your Patients: A Provider's Guide. Washington, DC: Altarum Institute; 2022.
2. Centers for Disease Control and Prevention. (2021). Partner Services. [online] Available from https://www.cdc.gov/std/treatment-guidelines/clinical-partnerServices.htm. [Last accessed February, 2023].
3. Centers for Disease Control and Prevention. A Guide to Taking a Sexual History. [online] Available from https://www.cdc.gov/std/treatment/SexualHistory.pdf. [Last accessed February, 2023].
4. Glasier A, Gülmezoglu AM, Schmid GP, Moreno CG, Van Look PF. Sexual and reproductive health: a matter of life and death. Lancet. 2006;368(9547):1595-607.
5. Healthline. (2021). 5 Reasons to Talk About Sexual Health with Your Doctor. [online] Available from https://www.healthline.com/health/hiv-aids/hiv-prevention/talk-about-sexual-health. [Last accessed February, 2023].
6. Johnson N. Comprehensive sexual health assessments for adolescents. Paediatr Child Health. 2020;25(8):551-2.
7. Leslie KM, Canadian Paediatric Society, Adolescent Health Committee. Adolescent pregnancy. Paediatr Child Health. 2006;11(4): 243-6.
8. Miller AS, Aisenbrey S, Kimmel DM. Awareness and Performance of Testicular Self-Examinations: An Analysis of Social and Cultural Barriers to Cancer Screenings in a US Orthodox Jewish Community. J Relig Health. 2022;61(6):4398-419.
9. Murro R, Chawla R, Pyne S, Venkatesh S, Sully EA. (2021). Adding It Up: Investing in the Sexual and Reproductive Health of Adolescents in India. [online] Available from https://www.guttmacher.org/report/adding-it-up-investing-in-sexual-reproductive-health-adolescents-india. [Last accessed February, 2023].
10. National Coalition for Sexual Health. Asking Essential Sexual Health Questions. [online] Available from https://nationalcoalitionforsexualhealth.org/tools/for-healthcare-providers/asset/AskingEssentialSexualHealthQuestions_2021.pdf. [Last accessed February, 2023].
11. Options for Sexual Health. (2022). Pleasure. [online] Available from https://www.optionsforsexualhealth.org/facts/pleasure/. [Last accessed February, 2023].
12. Options for Sexual Health. (2022). Safer Sex Tips. [online] Available from https://www.optionsforsexualhealth.org/facts/sti/safer-sex-tips. [Last accessed February, 2023].
13. World Health Organization. Defining Sexual Health. [online] Available from https://www.who.int/teams/sexual-and-reproductive-health-and-research/key-areas-of-work/sexual-health/defining-sexual-health. [Last accessed February, 2023].

# CHAPTER 8

# Monitoring Physical Growth of Adolescents

*Sridevi A Naaraayan, Nedunchelian K*

## ■ INTRODUCTION

Growth and development are the two inherent characteristics of the pediatric age group including adolescents, which differentiate them from the adults. As we all know they should progress hand in hand together in any normal individual. This chapter deals with the monitoring of *physical growth* of adolescents.

## ■ PHYSICAL GROWTH

*Physical growth* refers to an increase in body size (length/height and weight) and in the size of organs. Growth, a continuous process faces three spurts from the conception to adult stage, namely intrauterine period, infancy, and puberty. From birth to around age 1 or 2 years, children grow rapidly. Children tend to grow in at a steady growth velocity each year until the next major growth spurt occurs and the pubertal changes starts during early adolescence. Puberty is accompanied by rapid changes in body size, shape, and composition, which represent just a fraction of the developmental processes that adolescents experience. Pubertal growth proceeds with acceleration, followed by deceleration and completion of growth which is heralded by closure of epiphyses.

### Adolescence and Physical Growth

*Adolescence* is the period between 10 and 19 years of the age. With reference to physical growth, early adolescence (10–13 years) is accompanied by growth spurt and the beginning of sexual maturation, in midadolescence (14–15 years), the physical changes are complete and during late adolescence (16–19 years) along with physical growth, sexual maturity also gets completed.

Age of start growth of spurt in adolescence is found to be highly variable and depends on gender. Mean age is approximately 11 years in boys and 9 years in girls, and peak growth rate occurs in the second half of puberty (Tanner 3 and beyond) in both boys and girls at a mean age of 13.5 and

11.5 years respectively. Pubertal growth contributes to final height by 30-31 cm in boys (17-18% of the final height) and 27.5-29 cm in girls (17% of final height). Adolescence contributes to 20% of total growth in stature and up to 40-50% of body weight as somatic growth. The spurt in somatic growth which is initiated by the sex hormones is accompanied by sexual development.

Beyond the growth spurts, other physical changes that happen in both males and females during adolescence include body odor, acne, and more body hair. Many of the physical changes in adolescence are related to fertility.

## ■ GROWTH MONITORING

*Growth monitoring* can be considered as a process of tracking the growth by regularly measuring and comparing a person's growth, i.e., height, weight, BMI, etc. to a standard and assess growth adequacy. If inadequacy is encountered and a particular anthropometric index is abnormal remedial actions are undertaken. It is essential that we monitor the growth to ensure the adolescents are growing on par with the norms for the race and region. It must be done at regular intervals. For growth monitoring, it is the change in weight over a period of time which is more important, rather than the weight itself. The main purpose of growth monitoring is to assess growth adequacy and identify faltering at early stages before the adolescent reaches a substandard status with reference to ultimate adult stature and nutrition.

Monitoring of physical growth in adolescents can be considered under two main headings:
1. Monitoring the changes in linear growth, changes in weight, and body composition
2. Monitoring sexual maturity.

*Growth monitoring helps in:*
- Assessing whether the adolescents follow normal growth pattern, helping to pick up malnutrition and diseases as evidenced by failure to gain growth parameters lose weight specifically.
- Planning to educate the parents/adolescents regarding healthy food habits, immunization and other aspects of growth as well as development. This session serves to clear queries and alleviate anxiety about issues related to growth.

### Indices for Growth Monitoring

Basic anthropometric indices for regular monitoring in adolescents are height (Ht.), weight (Wt.), and body mass index (BMI). Other indices are midparental height (MPH) predicting target height, upper segment lower segment ratio, waist circumference (WC), skinfold thickness (SFT), bone age, etc., which are required in specific situations where it is a "planned assessment of growth" and it is not considered as regular growth monitoring.

The growth evaluation can be:
- A structured one as "growth monitoring" to identify whether they are following normal pattern of growth and to identify whether there is any growth faltering leading to evaluation for the cause for the same.
- Assessment of growth in conditions such as under nutrition, chronic illnesses, endocrine disorders, etc. where growth faltering is expected.

## Specific Indications for Assessment
- Arrest at same stage of puberty for >2 years
- Micropenis
- Unilateral or bilateral gynecomastia in boys
- Hirsutism and menstrual irregularities in girls
- Delayed puberty—in girls with no breast budding by 14 years and no menarche by 15 years and in boys with no signs of puberty by 16 years.

Regular growth monitoring is advocated every year for children/adolescents in the age group of 6-18 years with the anthropometric assessment of height, weight, and BMI basically. Additional frequency and indices are based on the identification of any deviation from normal growth. Sexual maturity rating (SMR) is to be done yearly between 9 and 18 years.

## Process of Growth Monitoring
### Monitoring of Linear Growth, Weight, and Body Composition
This can be carried out in three steps (1) measuring anthropometric indices, (2) plotting in appropriate charts, and (3) interpretation to identify the pattern of the growth.

*Measurement of anthropometric indices:*
*Weight:* Adolescent is made to stand still over the weighing scale in the center after removing foot wear and outer clothing with feet slightly apart. Adolescent is requested to remain still until the weight is displayed. Take care to set the reading at the number 0.0, whether it is digital or mechanical weighing scale. Record the child's weight to the nearest 0.1 kg.

*Height:* Footwear, socks, and hair ornaments to be removed. Adolescent stands on the stadiometer baseboard with feet slightly apart. Back of the head, scapula, buttocks, calves, and heels should touch the vertical measuring board. Do not allow to lean back or forward. A helper can hold the adolescent's knees and ankles to keep the legs straight and feet flat, helps heels, and calves to touch the vertical board. The head should be kept such that an imaginary horizontal line from the external ear canal to the lower border of the eye socket (Frankfurt plane) is parallel to the base board. To ascertain this, hold the bridge between accessor's thumb and forefinger over the adolescent's chin. It can push abdomen gently in to help the adolescent stand erect. Bring the headboard to top of the head to fit in snugly. Record the height accurately in centimeters to the last completed 0.1 cm.

*Body mass index:* Body mass index is a simple index of weight-for-height arrived out of the formula—weight (kg)/height (m)$^2$.

The following are the other indices needed when we suspect faltering of growth to aid in further evaluation of the cause, as applicable.

*Midparental height/target height:*
Target height calculation:
Target height in boys = Father's height + mother's height +13/2
Target height in girls = Father's height + mother's height – 13/2

*Steps to plot target height:* Measure the parents height. Calculate the child's target height and plot it at 18 years and mark it with an arrow on the growth chart. The target range is produced by plotting two points 6 cm above and below the target height and this represents the 3rd and the 97th centile for that child. Taking those two points above and below the target height 97th and 3rd centiles are constructed by tracing lines backward to match the current age.

*Upper segment and lower segment length and ratio:* Upper segment is the length between vertex and upper border of pubic symphysis and lower segment is between upper border of pubic symphysis and heel. Measure the height, then lower segment and arrive at upper segment as height (cm)—lower segment.

*Waist circumference:* Waist (midway point between lowest rib cage and iliac crest) circumference to be measured with a special tension tape. Make the adolescent to wear only underclothes, and make him stand with feet together and arms relaxed. Tape is kept horizontally just above the upper lateral border of the right ileum. While the adolescent breathing normally, measure the WC at the end of normal expiration and measure to the nearest mm. Take an average of three measurements. If wearing a shirt or undergarment, subtract 1 cm before recording.

*Triceps skinfold thickness:* Skin fold (double fold of skin along with subcutaneous fat, excluding muscle) is an important index for assessment of body fat composition in adolescents and is an independent predictor for hypertension. It can be measured using Harpenden calipers **(Fig. 1)**. Commonly used are triceps and subscapular skinfold thickness measurements. Make the one adolescent more relaxed. Mark the center of triceps on the nondominant arm (usually left arm). Using your left thumb and index finger, grasp a fold of skin and underlying subcutaneous fat 2 cm above the marking. With examiner's right hand, the caliper is held and its jaws applied perpendicular to the fold at the marked site. Release the caliper and allow the jaws to close on the fold. Measure to the nearest millimeter roughly after 3 seconds.

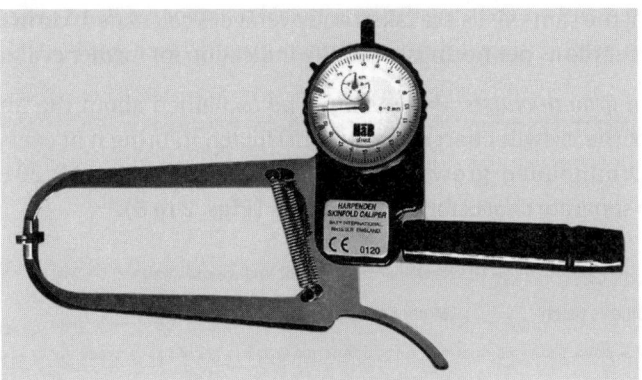

**Fig. 1:** Harpenden calipers.

*Bone age:* Bone age is an expression of biological age of the adolescent when it comes to investigating an adolescent for disorders of growth and puberty. It is a size-independent indicator of biological maturity. Many parameters correlate to bone age rather than chronological age namely height velocity, menarche, muscle mass, and bone mineral mass.

The tools usually used are Greulich and Pyle (GP) atlas which is available online on amazon.in and Gilsanz and Ratib (GR) atlas, which can be downloaded free on internet. Bone age assessment is carried out in cases of short stature, disorders of puberty, medicolegal issues, etc.

*Growth velocity:* A single height/weight measurements only identifies children whose height/weight is outside the normal range for their age. In contrast, repeated height measurements over time allow calculation of a growth velocity and can find abnormal growth in terms of a crossing of the height centiles, thereby identifying abnormalities in the pattern of growth within the individual.

Growth velocity charts exist for height and weight, specific for males and females.

*Uses:* Help to differentiate those with normal variant of growth and pubertal development such as constitutional delay of growth and puberty who are expected to grow at a normal height velocity, from those with pathological short stature. It helps in identification of population requiring follow up and investigation. Useful to assess early effectiveness of a medical intervention and predicting final stature (using height velocity and peak height velocity)

*Measurement:* Height velocity is calculated as the difference between two height measurements divided by the time interval between the two measurements and is generally expressed as centimeter per year. Height velocities are measured at an interval of 6 months. Accurate measurement of height using proper device is essential, as even change of 1–2 cm can lead to error and problem in arriving at diagnosis. To avoid errors in measurement, two or three readings at the same visits are taken and average is calculated. Growth velocity <25th percentile as per norm is a definite indication for further evaluation.

*Plotting in growth charts:* Parents must be explained about the importance and use of the growth chart as well as instructed to bring it at every hospital visit. Recommended growth charts for adolescents is IAP 2015 charts. There are separate charts for boys and girls **(Figs. 2 to 5)**.

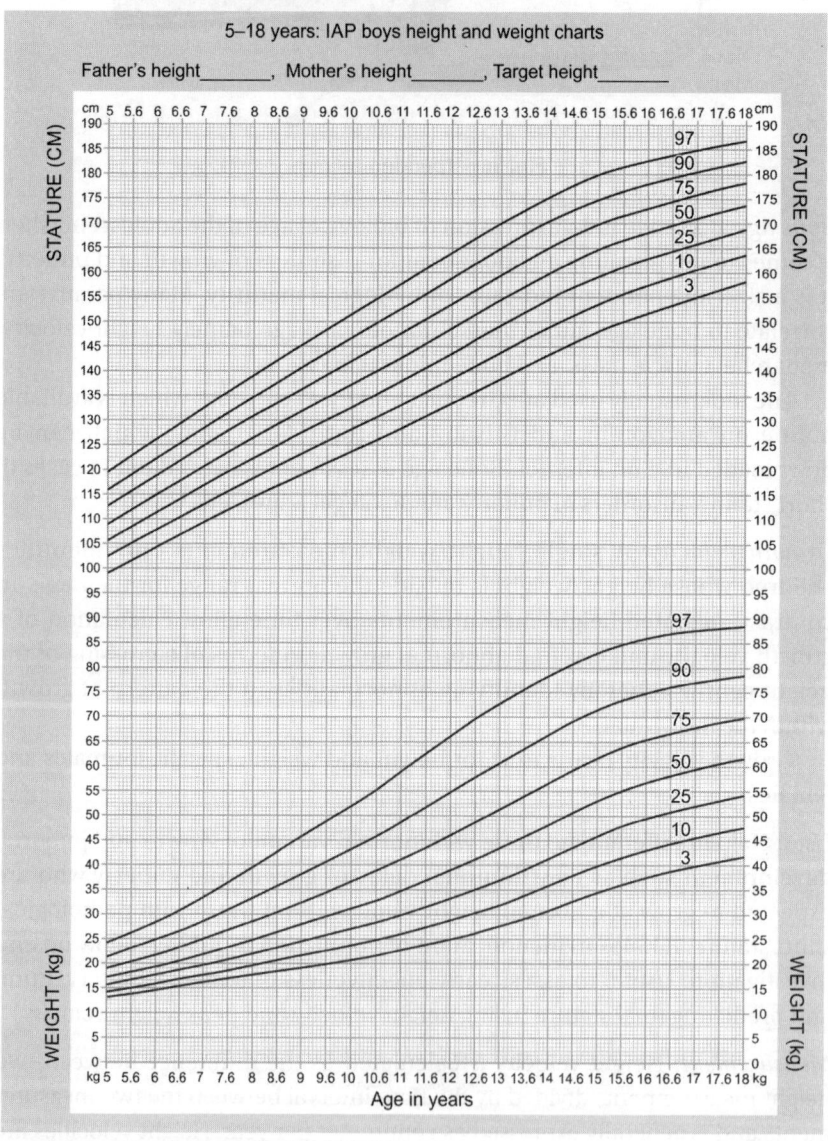

**Fig. 2:** Weight and height for age chart (boys).

*Source:* Revised IAP growth charts for height, weight and body mass index for 5 to 18 years old Indian children. V. Khadikar et. al. from Indian academy of pediatrics growth chart committee Indian pediatrics. Jan 2015, volume 52.

# CHAPTER 8: Monitoring Physical Growth of Adolescents

Name and date of birth should be written in the chart for arriving at exact age. At every visit growth parameter marked in a growth chart appropriate for age and gender with a dot and these is dots connected with a line to study the pattern of growth of the child. From the marked weight or height, a horizontal line is drawn to the 50th centile and from there vertically downward to X-axis. The point of intersection on X-axis corresponds to the weight age/height

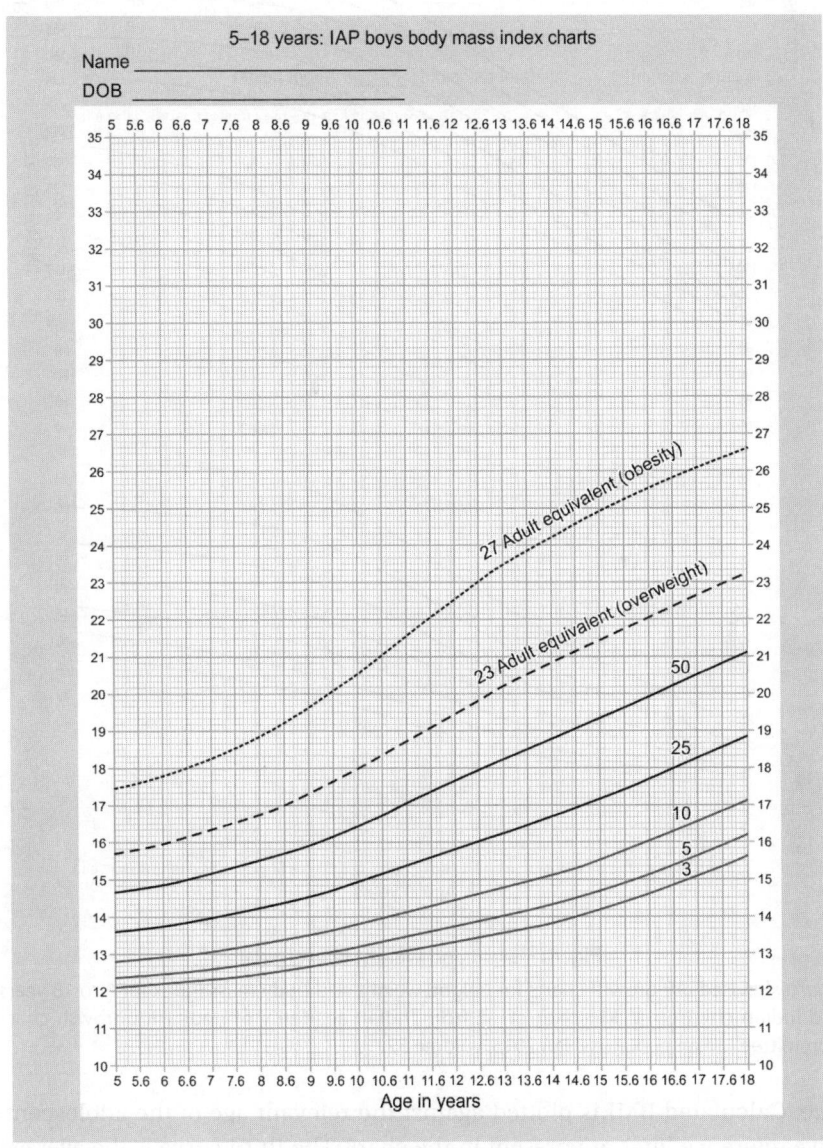

**Fig. 3:** Body mass index chart (boys).

*Source:* Revised IAP growth charts for height, weight and body mass index for 5 to 18 years old Indian children. V. Khadikar et. al. from Indian academy of pediatrics growth chart committee Indian pediatrics. Jan 2015, volume 52.

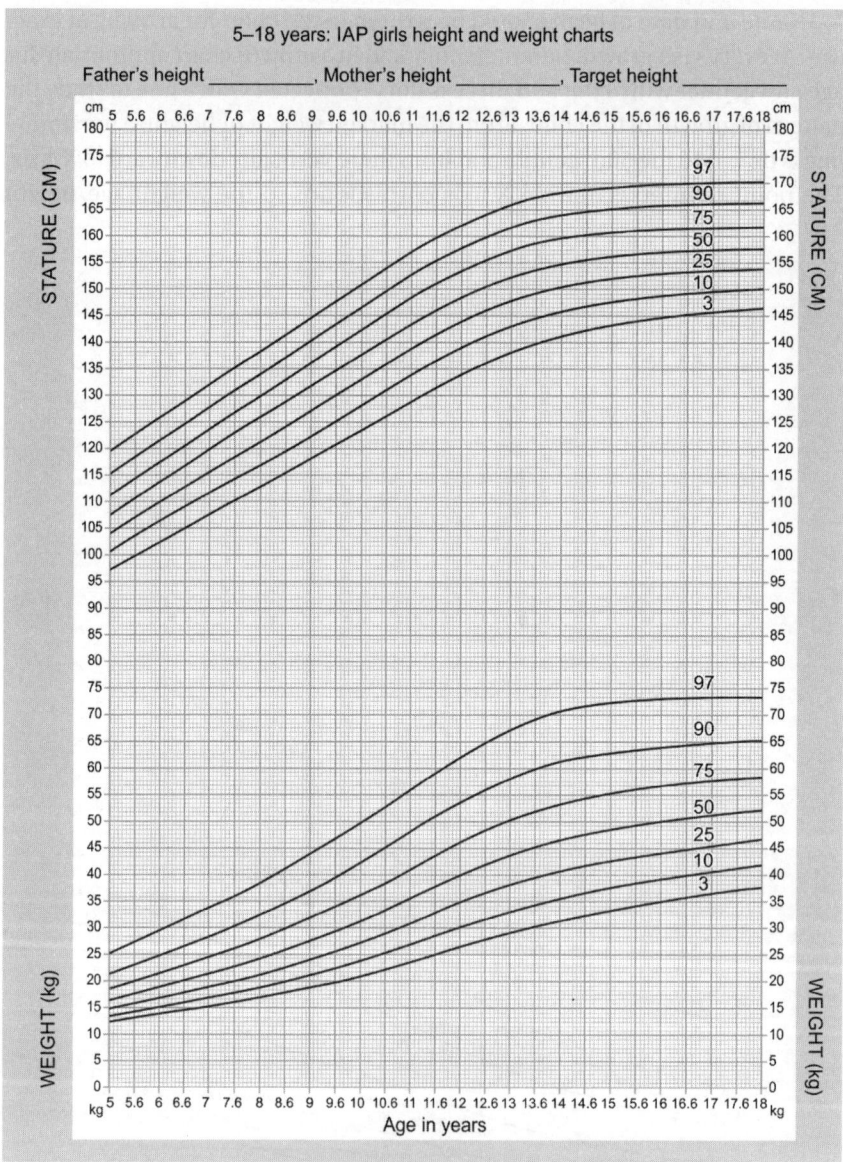

**Fig. 4:** Height and weight chart (girls).

*Source:* Revised IAP growth charts for height, weight and body mass index for 5 to 18 years old Indian children. V. Khadikar et. al. from Indian academy of pediatrics growth chart committee Indian pediatrics. Jan 2015, volume 52.

age. Calculated BMI is plotted against the relevant age of the adolescent. Five reference lines are present in the chart. The third curve is the average or the median. The plotted point should be between the second and fourth curves of the graph. If it falls above second curve it is over nutrition and if below fourth curve it is under nutrition. Both need to be evaluated further.

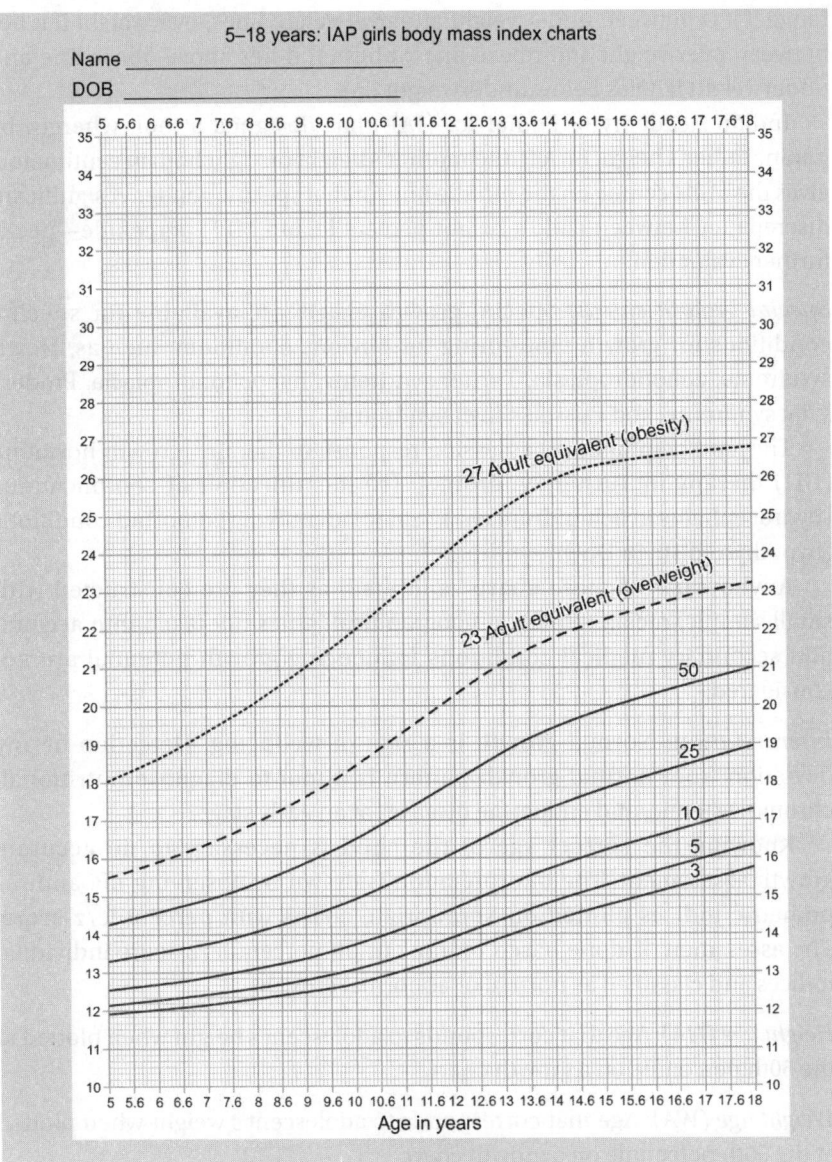

**Fig. 5:** Body mass index chart (girls).

*Source:* Revised IAP growth charts for height, weight and body mass index for 5 to 18 years old Indian children. V. Khadikar et. al. from Indian academy of pediatrics growth chart committee Indian pediatrics. Jan 2015, volume 52.

*Pediatrician friendly growth charts:* A quick BMI screening tool is also available on the chart based on weight for height. It has three lines which show overweight, obese, and underweight, the overweight line is orange, and obese line is red. Based on where child's weight lies on Y-axis for the height on X-axis, the adolescents should be classified to have BMI within normal range if it is between underweight and overweight lines; overweight if it lies between overweight and obese lines; obese if it lies above obese line and underweight if it lies below underweight line.

Indian Academy of Pediatrics (IAP) has designed a tool, wherein by joining father's height on left and mother's height on right both in centimeters gives the MPH centile on the middle line for that specific gender. A significant discrepancy between child's height percentile and MPH percentile—needs further evaluation.

*Special growth charts:* Special growth charts are available for specific conditions for growth monitoring for obvious conditions such as, Down syndrome, achondroplasia, Turner syndrome, hypochondroplasia, Prader-Willi syndrome, and Russell-Silver syndrome.

They are helpful in (a) assessing response to therapy [growth hormone (GH) therapy in Turner syndrome], (b) identification of complications (hydrocephalus in achondroplasia), and (c) identifying comorbid conditions (hypothyroidism in Down syndrome).

Anyhow use of these charts is limited, as they are constructed with small sample; racial, ethnic, or geographical issues not taken into account and secondary medical conditions influencing growth potential are not considered.

*Interpretation:* Normal growth is a sign of wellbeing. Detection of any deviation from normal growth pattern is a tool to diagnose nutritional, chronic systemic, and endocrine diseases at an early stage.

Knowing the correct age of the child is necessary to do accurate growth assessment. The interpretation is drawn by observing the anthropometric indices plotted on appropriate charts with percentile/z-score. The assessment is done based on the cut-off percentile/z-score individual indices and classified as normal or abnormal growth.

*Height age (HA):* Age that corresponds to adolescent's height when plotted at the 50th percentile on a growth chart.

*Weight age (WA):* Age that corresponds to adolescent's weight when plotted at the 50th percentile on a growth chart.

The interpretation of the observations based on comparison of chronological height and weight ages are shown in **Table 1**.

## Monitoring of Sexual Maturity

The monitoring of sexual maturity during puberty in adolescence is with SMR labeled usually as "Tanner staging". Sexual maturation is correlated well with linear growth, weight, body composition, and hormonal changes. Tanner staging comprises assessing development of breast/pubic hairs in girls and testicular size/pubic hair in boys. Physical changes observed in girls

**TABLE 1:** Interpretations based on comparison of chronological, weight, and height ages.

| Observation | Interpretation |
|---|---|
| CA = HA = WA | Normal |
| CA > HA > WA | Malnutrition or systemic disease |
| CA > WA > HA | Endocrine disease |
| HA > WA > CA | Precocious puberty |
| WA > CA > HA | Endocrine obesity |
| WA > HA > CA | Nutritional obesity |

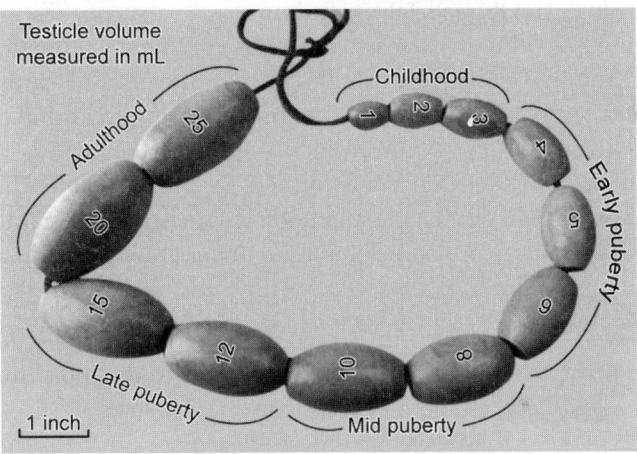

**Fig. 6:** Prader orchidometer.

are beginning of growth spurts, pubertal changes in breasts/genitalia/pubic hair, weight changes-body shape/size.

The pubertal changes observed in boys include development of the testes and scrotum (as the first sign of puberty), pubic hair, voice changes, and sometimes gynecomastia. The testicular volume is measured with the help of Prader orchidometer **(Fig. 6)**. Stretched penile length and penile circumference have to be measured by using a plastic tape measure and interpreted. Stretched penile length is measured from the pubopenile junction (pubic ramus) of the penis to the tip of the glans on the dorsal surface with the prepubic fat pad pushed to the bone, fully stretched but in a still flaccid state with maximal extension of the penis. Penile circumference is measured at the middle of the shaft.

The average time line of events in girls and boys during adolescence is summarized in **Table 2 and Figure 7**.

In a nut shell, the puberty is assessed by (a) detailed medical history, (b) detailed physical examination including anthropometry and SMR,

**TABLE 2:** Average timings of pubertal events in adolescent girls and boys.

| Events | Timing |
|---|---|
| **Girls** | |
| • Onset of breast development | 10 years |
| • Age at menarche | 12 years |
| • Tanner stage 2 to menarche | 2 years duration |
| • Start to finish (end of growth) | 3 years |
| **Boys** | |
| • Onset of testicular enlargement | 11.5 years |
| • Time from onset of puberty to Tanner stage 4 (beginning of growth spurt) | 2 years |
| • Start to finish (end of growth) | 4 years |

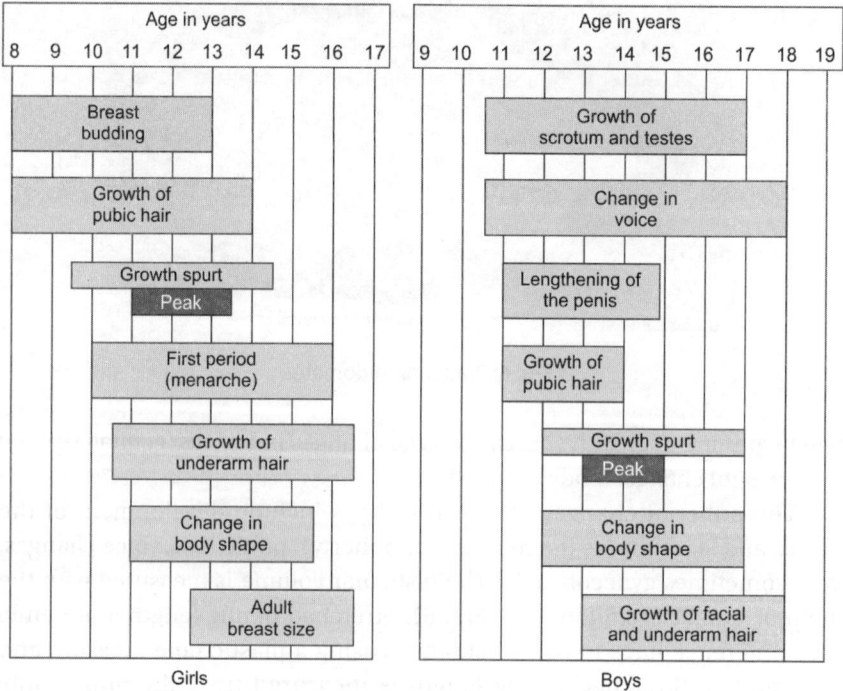

**Fig. 7:** Average timing of pubertal changes in girls and boys.

as well as (c) bone age and (d) focused laboratory evaluation, in case of any deviation from normal growth pattern.

## ■ COUNSELING ON GROWTH AND RELATED ISSUES

Appropriate counseling to be given to the parents as regards to:
- The importance of regular growth monitoring.

- The interpretation of the growth pattern noticed, and about the timing of anticipated body changes (even if normal growth pattern, still insist on further regular monitoring).
- The need for further evaluation, in case of deviation of growth pattern from normal.
- Adhering to interventions recommended (depending upon the cause for growth faltering).

## SUGGESTED READING

1. Abbassi V. Growth and normal puberty. Pediatrics. 1998;102(2 Pt 3):507-11.
2. Agarwal DK, Agarwal KN, Upadhyay SK, Mittal R, Prakash R, Rai S. Physical and sexual growth pattern of affluent Indian children from 5-18 years of age. Indian Pediatr. 1992;29:1203-82.
3. Agarwal KN, Saxena A, Bansal AK, Agarwal DK. Physical growth assessment in adolescence. Indian Pediatr. 2001;38:1217-35.
4. Bhave SY, Yadav S. Normal adolescent development. Indian J Pract Pediatr. 2015;17(2):85-9.
5. Horton WA, Rotter JI, Rimoin DL, Scott CI, Hall JG. Standard growth curves for achondroplasia. J Pediatr. 1978;93:435-8.
6. Indian Academy of Pediatrics Growth Charts Committee; Khadilkar V, Yadav S, Agrawal KK, Tamboli S, Banerjee M, et al. Revised IAP growth charts for height, weight and body mass index for 5-18 year old Indian children. Indian Pediatr. 2015;52:47-55.
7. Khadilkar A, Ekbote V, Chiplonkar S, Khadilkar V, Kajale N, Kulkarni S, et al. Waist Circumference Percentiles in 2-18 Year Old Indian Children. J Pediatr. 2014;164(6):1358-1362.e2.
8. Khadilkar V, Khadilkar A, Arya A, Ekbote V, Kajale N, Parthasarathy L, et al. Height Velocity Percentiles in Indian Children Aged 5-17 Years. Indian Pediatr. 2019;56(1):23-8.
9. Khadilkar VV, Karguppikar MB, Ekbote VH, Khadilkar AV. Turner Syndrome Growth Charts: A Western India Experience. Indian J Endocrinol Metab. 2020;24(4):333-7.
10. Myrelid A, Gustafsson J, Ollars B, Annerén G. Growth charts for Down's syndrome from birth to 18 years of age. Arch Dis Child. 2002;87(2):97-103.
11. National Institute of Public Cooperation and Child Development. Growth Monitoring Manual. New Delhi: National Institute of Public Cooperation and Child Development.
12. Parekh BJ, Khadilkar V. Pediatrician-Friendly IAP Growth Charts for Children Aged 0-18 Years. Indian Pediatr. 2020;57(11):997-8.
13. Park SK, Ergashev K, Chung JM, Lee SD. Penile circumference and stretched penile length in prepubertal children: a retrospective, single-center pilot study. Investig Clin Urol. 2021;62(3):324-30.
14. Rogol AD, Clark PA, Roemmich JN. Growth and pubertal development in children and adolescents: effects of diet and physical activity. Am J Clin Nutr. 2000;72(2 Suppl):521S-528S.
15. World Health Organization. Training Course on Child Growth Assessment. WHO Child Growth Standards. Geneva: World Health Organization; 2008.

# 9

# Adolescent Counseling

*Atul M Kanikar, CP Bansal*

## ■ INTRODUCTION AND DEFINITIONS

Counseling psychology is one of the largest subfields in psychology. It is centered on offering therapy and aiding clients who suffer from mental illness and psychological distress. According to the Society of Counseling Psychology, the goal of counseling psychology is to improve personal functioning by focusing on social, emotional, educational, health, developmental, family, and work-related issues. Some amount of depression, thought distractions, anxiety, phobias, tendency to experiment, and even blues (sadness) are normal for teenagers. Intervention is needed only when these troubles augment to cause emotional disturbance and hinder the mental growth and potential of the individual. The purpose of intervention counseling is prevention, remediation, learning new skills (behavior modification), growth, and personality development.

Various thinkers, theories, languages, and cultures have given different meanings to the word "counseling". Like the terms "personality" or "intelligence", many scholars have defined counseling in various ways. However, all the psychologists agree on the ultimate purpose or aim of counseling, i.e., helping the individuals to overcome future problems. The Oxford dictionary definition mentions counseling as "the provision of professional assistance and guidance in resolving personal or psychological problems".

Perez (1965) gave a popular definition of counseling as an interactive process conjoining the counselee who needs assistance and the counselor who is trained and educated to offer this assistance. This interactive process needs to be initiated, facilitated, and maintained by the counselor through feelings of spontaneity, warmth, tolerance, respect, and sincerity. Carl Rogers in his book "Counseling and Psychotherapy", has defined counseling as a process consisting of a definitely structured permissive relationship which allows the client to gain an understanding of self to a degree which enables the client to take positive steps in the light of his/her new orientation. Rogers also adds that in the process of counseling, the

# CHAPTER 9: Adolescent Counseling

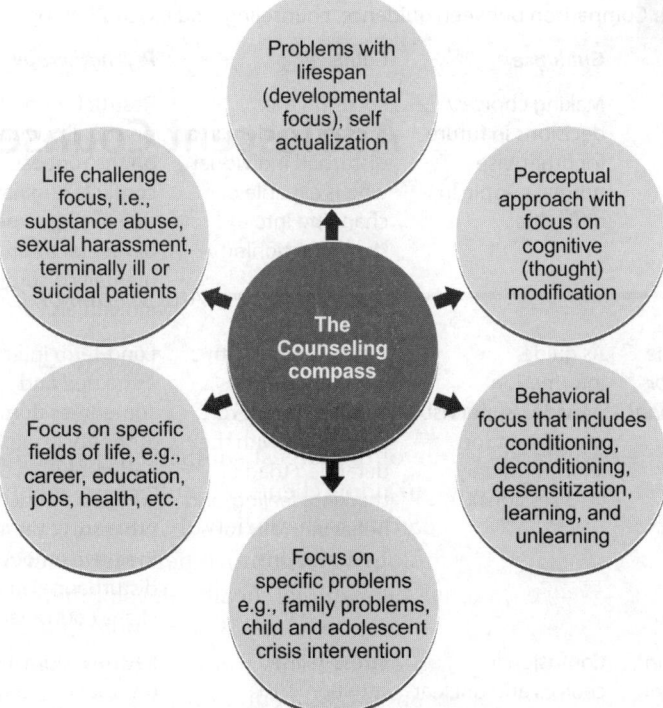

**Fig. 1:** The scope of counseling.

structure of the self is relaxed in the safety of the client's relationship with the therapist and previously denied experiences are perceived and then integrated into an altered self.

Most of the definitions proposed by renowned scholars maintain that counseling is a process which involves bringing about sequential changes over a period of time, leading to a set goal. Over the years, due to exponential growth of various old and new stressors, the scope of counseling has evolved into multiple fields of human life and at all ages. This can be illustrated as shown in **Figure 1**.

Counseling, guidance, and psychotherapy are terminologies which are used synonymously by many, although their meanings differ practically **(Table 1)**.

For the benefit of practitioners, researchers, and theoreticians, the Western Interstate Commission for Higher Education (WICHE) led by Parker (1974) has proposed a three-dimensional model for the functions or roles of a counselor **(Fig. 2)**. This further elaborates and specifies the scope of counseling in the modern world.

Mental health professionals employ various theories of counseling in dealing with their clients with an approach that keeps the "best benefit of

**TABLE 1:** Comparison between guidance, counseling, and psychotherapy.

|  | Guidance | Counseling | Psychotherapy |
|---|---|---|---|
| Aim | Making choices/decisions in future for otherwise normal people in difficulties | Focus on the present problem in a disturbed individual who is capable of changing into a "fully functioning individual" | Restructuring of personality with focus on the root causes/conflicts originating due to past experiences or mental trauma in mentally disordered individuals |
| Role of the director or professional | As guide, information provider, supervisor or assistant for short term only (1–3 sessions). | Purely mental with communicator's and facilitator's role for dealing with the deranged triad of thinking, feeling, and behaving. May take 1–15 sessions | Long-term intervention as trained and sometimes dominant authority in exploration and resolution of conflicts or unconscious processes that resulted in severe emotional disturbances in the client/counselee |
| Problem in the patient or client | Confusion in choices and unclear vocational ideas or concepts. | Stress-related situation/crisis which could be due to intrapersonal or interpersonal disturbances. | Severe mental health disorder (psychosis, severe anxiety, phobias, severe depression, etc.) usually needing pharmacotherapy and/or electroconvulsive therapy (ECT) in addition |
| Process | Quantitative analysis, problem solving techniques, and listing of possibilities using information pool | Qualitative as well as quantitative tools and specialty skills which may be cognitive, emotive, or behavioral | Mostly qualitative, directive, and interpretative due to severity of disorders. Psychoanalysis including dream therapy or cognitive behavior therapy in conjunction with ECT and drugs |
| Objectives | Educational or vocational or career improvement | Positive self-esteem, capacity building, and autonomy for becoming a fully functional and responsible human | Empowerment for adjustment, functionality, and improved mental health |

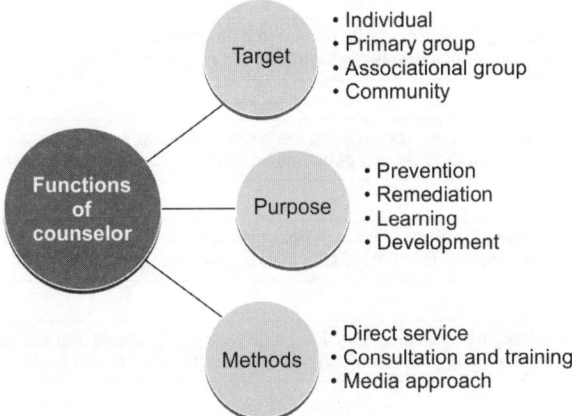

**Fig. 2:** Three-dimensional model for counselor's role proposed by Western Interstate Commission for Higher Education (WICHE).

client's growth in focus" (eclectic approach). The choice and combination of the theories lies with the professional only and depends on the case at hand. Although different concepts are used either singly or in combination, many professionals follow selective theories only.

## ■ SPECIAL ISSUES IN COUNSELING ADOLESCENTS

Many adolescents are at times difficult to counsel. The obvious reasons are unwillingness for therapy, unfriendly attitudes of the therapist, nonacceptance of problem leading to resistance, tendency to blame the caretakers, social stigma, poor compliance leading to drop-outs, peer influence and a feeling of being victimized by parents or teachers. However, the positive points about adolescent counseling cannot be ignored. Adolescents are quite receptive to the process provided the counselor exhibits skillful and adolescent friendly interview. Further, because adolescence is a period of storm and stress with multiple happenings, adolescents are looking for someone who will understand them and be with them unconditionally and with respect. Frontalization of brain and pruning (unused neuronal connections are chopped off) occur during adolescence which contributes to the development of adult personality. For a counselor and caretaker, adolescence should be looked upon as a period when basic life philosophies take shape and interventions done during this period will have a long-term benefit, provided the counselor is adolescent friendly. Principles and basic skills of counseling are depicted in **Figure 3**. The different stages of the counseling process are listed in **Box 1**.

The counselor should be interested in helping adolescents, have perceptual sensitivity, normally adjusted in his/her personal life, genuine, and well trained with congruence and good emotional control. A lot of

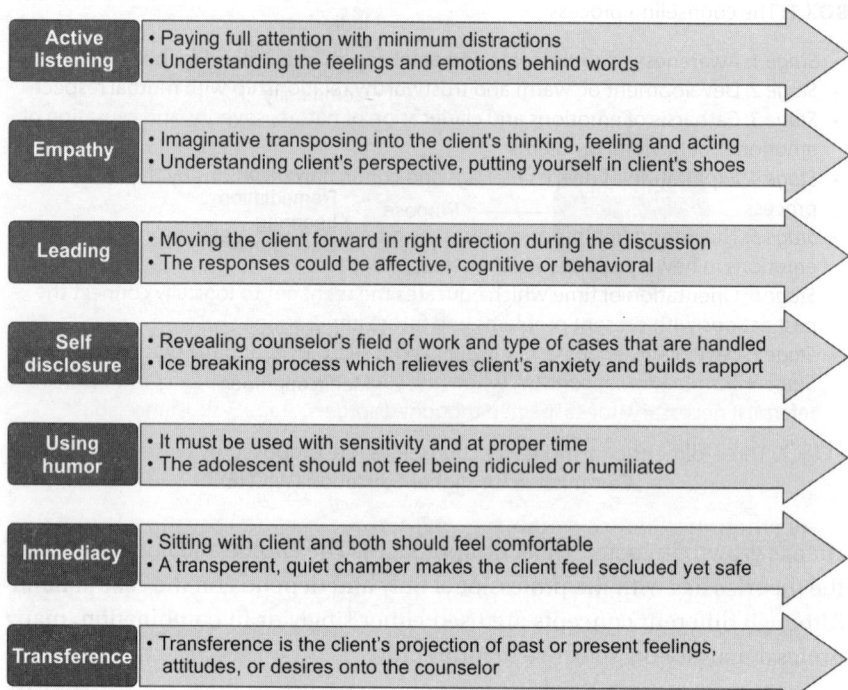

**Fig. 3:** Principles and basic skills of counseling.

importance is given by Carl Rogers to the term "acceptance". He defined acceptance as "a warm regard for the client as a person of unconditional self-worth and of value under any condition, behavior, or feelings". Acceptance implies helping an individual and not controlling him/her.

A counselor should follow work ethics such as anonymity, confidentiality, and record keepings. Advice giving, lecturing, excessive questioning, storytelling, etc., should be avoided.

The effective communication skills that work wonders with an adolescent client are:

- *Nonverbal tools:* These account for nearly 80% of total interaction and include eye contact, smile, unfolded arms with flexed knees, minimum body movements, and safe physical proximity.
- *Active listening:* This process which aims at understanding the feelings and emotions along with spoken words and includes means to minimize ambient distractions, facilitating responses, paraphrasing or reflecting the feelings and words for the adolescent, and summarizing the key points. Silence at certain moments is a very effective tool that aids in ventilation of clouded emotions, gives breathing space for restructuring words, putting thoughts sequentially, and understanding the exact flow

**BOX 1:** The counseling process.

- *Stage 1:* Awareness of adolescents and gatekeepers about need for help
- *Stage 2:* Development of warm and trustworthy relationship with mutual respect
- *Stage 3:* Catharsis of emotions and clarification of nature, severity, and causation of emotional/behavioral problems
- *Stage 4:* Exploration of deeper feelings and conflicting situations by the "analysis" process
- *Stage 5:* The integration process where the adolescent can objectively assess his emotions in new perspective without fear or withdrawal
- *Stage 6:* Orientation of time which educates the teenager to logically connect the past actions with present problems and future implications
- *Stage 7:* Developing awareness or insight about self, others, and the present problems
- *Stage 8:* Termination of contract when the session goals are met and prompt referral if necessary (for suspected thought disorders, stage 3 substance abuse, suicidal ideation, severe anxiety, etc.)

of emotions. Silence can thus be paradoxically called the most useful tool in interpersonal communication.
- *Verbal tools:* A right choice of words and questions in a soft tone which facilitate communication must be learnt for proper counseling. Open-ended questions (can you describe your feelings?, what do you think about your relationship with parents?, what is it that you do not like about your school?, and what are the ways a teenager can enjoy life?), yield descriptive answers unlike parallel closed-ended questions (did you feel sad?, is your relationship with your parents fine?, do you like your school?, and do you enjoy life?), which yield yes or no responses and are not helpful.

Role of pediatrician has extended from school health check-up to imparting family life education (or premarital counseling for college graduates) and helping teacher counselors to improve scholastic performance in children. Life skills education (LSE) is also an important tool for improving mental health.

Life skills education is a didactic, psychoeducational, active-directive, and eclectic approach of counseling adolescents. The World Health Organization (WHO) defines life skills as the abilities for adaptive and positive behavior that enable individuals to deal effectively with the demands and challenges of everyday life **(Box 2)** while the United Nations Children's Fund (UNICEF) defines life skills based education as being a behavior change approach, designed to a balance of knowledge, attitude, and skills. Life skills are usually used in combination to deal with real life situations.

The goals of LSE are: (1) Curative (pertaining to present problems) and (2) Preventive (to avoid future problems). LSE is one of the useful tools for imparting sexuality education, teaching responsible behaviors, and adolescent counseling individually or in groups.

**BOX 2:** Ten basic life skills (World Health Organization).

1. *Self awareness:* Recognition of our character, strength, weakness, likes, and dislikes. A prerequisite for effective communication
2. *Empathy:* Imagining what is life for another person. It helps us understand and accept others and develops a nurturing attitude
3. *Interpersonal relations:* It helps us develop and nurture supportive networks and also enables to end sore relationships constructively
4. *Effective communication:* Capacity to express ourselves both verbally and nonverbally in culturally appropriate ways and situations
5. *Critical thinking:* Ability to analyze information and experiences in an objective manner. Helps to develop right attitudes and behaviors
6. *Creative thinking:* It enables us to explore available options, view consequences of actions, and respond adaptively and flexibly
7. *Decision making:* It involves defining the problem, considering consequences, family values, and preferences to make right decisions
8. *Problem solving:* Involves identifying needs and attitudes, detailed definition of problem, brainstorming, and evaluation of various solutions
9. *Coping with emotions:* Identifying effects of emotions on self and others. Understanding the triad of thinking, feeling, and behaving
10. *Coping with stress:* Identifying the stressors, time management, positive thinking, behavior modification, and relaxation techniques

The latest coronavirus disease (COVID) pandemic has drastically changed the needs of counselee as well as counselors. Teleconsultations and online counseling sessions are being widely used but with limitations. It has been documented that counseling of COVID cases (hospitalized and at home) improved the patient outcome in many cases. Empathetic active listening and "giving hope" seem to empower COVID cases to deal more effectively with situations at hand.

Psychoeducation (suggested by Albert Ellis) for school children and adolescents along with anticipatory guidance for parents are two vital tools for pediatricians in their office practice. Adolescent counseling by a well-trained professional is the need of the hour and pediatricians, as primary mental health caretakers of children and adolescents, need to take this responsibility.

## ■ POINTS TO REMEMBER

- Adolescent counseling is the need of the hour.
- Special skills must be learnt beforehand.
- Pediatricians are the key persons in early detection, management, and timely referrals for mental health problems in adolescents.

## ■ ACKNOWLEDGMENT

The authors wish to acknowledge the unconditional love and guidance of our teachers Dr MKC Nair, Dr Swati Bhave, and the family named Adolescent

Health Academy (AHA), who have inspired us to perform our duties toward the betterment of at least few adolescents in India.

## ■ SUGGESTED READING
1. Corey G. Theory and Practice of Counseling and Psychotherapy, 9th edition. Boston, United States: Cengage Learning; 2012.
2. Hurlock EB. Developmental Psychology: A Life Span Approach. The McGrawHill Publishing Company Ltd, New Delhi, 1980.
3. Indian Academy of Pediatrics. "Mission Kishore-Uday", Trainer's Manual on Comprehensive Adolescent Care. Mumbai, India: Indian Academy of Pediatrics; 2013.
4. Kanikar A. From Terrible to Terrific Teens. Chandigarh: White Falcon Publishing; 2019.
5. Kanikar A, Bhave S. Positive Discipline. Bhave's Textbook of Adolescent Medicine. Jaypee Brothers Medical Publishers. 2006:854-59.
6. Nagpal J, Prasad DS. Life skills training programs, Chapter in Bhaves Text Book of Adolescent Medicine, 1st ed. Jaypee Brothers Medical Publishers. 2006;8(4):299-303.
7. Nair MKC, Paul MK. Scholastic Backwardness Guidance, PGD-AP Course Manual. Thiruvananthapuram: University of Kerala and Child Development Center.
8. Piedmont. Managing stress during the ongoing COVID-19 pandemic. [online] Available from https://www.piedmot.org/living-better/managing-stress-during-the-covid-19-pandemic. [Last accessed January, 2023].
9. Preeti M. Galagali, Swati Y. Bhave, Motivation, Bhave's textbook of adolescent medicine. Jaypee Brothers Medical Publishers. 897-906.
10. Rao SN, Sahajpal P. Counseling and Guidance, 3rd edition. New Delhi: Tata McGraw Hill education private limited; 2017.
11. Scott E. (2020). The main causes of stress—what impacts you most may not be the same for the same as for someone else. [online] Available from https://www.verywellmind.com/what-are-the-main-causes-fo-stress-3145063. [Last accessed January, 2023].
12. Swati Bhave, Helen Pratt, Atul Kanikar. Adolescent Parenting: How and Why is it different?, Bhave's textbook of adolescent medicine, .Jaypee Brothers Medical Publishers. 875-85.
13. WHO. Life skills education program in schools, Program on mental health. Geneva: WHO; 1993.

# 10

# Motivational Interviewing

*Swati Ghate, Sreyoshi Ghosh*

## ■ INTRODUCTION

Motivational interviewing (MI) is a collaborative conversation style used by counsellors for strengthening a person's motivation and commitment to change. It was proposed by Bill Miller and Stephen Rollnick, in the 1980s.

It is a person-centered counseling style based on humanistic theories of psychology. These theories, most notably the one proposed by Carl Rogers, believe that individuals have immense potential and that the client should be kept at the center stage in the process of counseling. MI tries to address the common problem of ambivalence about change in behavior, by motivating the clients taking into consideration their personal attributes.

## ■ DEFINITION

Motivational interviewing is a collaborative and goal oriented style of communication, with particular attention to the language of change, designed to strengthen personal motivation for and commitment to a specific goal, by eliciting and exploring the person's own reasons for change, within an atmosphere of acceptance and compassion.

## ■ THEORETICAL BACKGROUND

Many people, especially adolescents, who indulge in harmful behaviors, are not aware of or are not willing to accept that these are detrimental to their health. These clients are often on different stages of "the continuum of change" and need to be approached differently according to their stage. The transtheoretical model by Prochaska and DiClemente describes the various "stages of change", which is a continuum of readiness to change one's behavior.

There are five stages in the process of change **(Fig. 1)**:
1. *Precontemplation:* Not realizing the cons of behavior, not considering change in near future
2. *Contemplation:* Intending to make a healthier change in behavior, could be in two minds

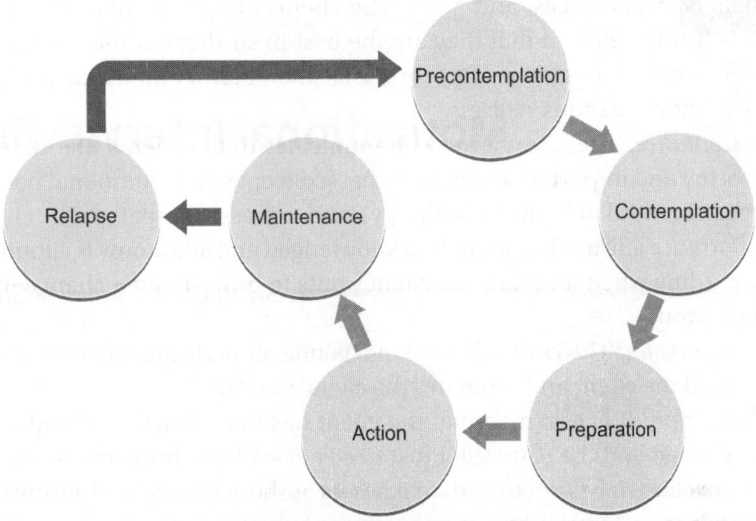

**Fig. 1:** Stages of change in behavior.

3. *Preparation:* Determination and planning to take small steps
4. *Action:* Executing the plan to bring about the change
5. *Maintenance:* Stabilizing and continuing the change in behavior and avoiding relapse.

While generally, it is assumed that the client who has walked in for counseling, is willing and ready for change, it may not be always so. Most adolescents come to the counsellor only because their caretakers want them to do so. They could be positioned anywhere on the continuum of change. Further, clients may not feel confident enough to embark on their journey of change. Identifying their stage and moving them gently toward the attainment of desirable changes is what MI attempts to do. It refrains from being judgmental about the client, does not label him (for example, "a smoker"), and does not take a prescriptive or directing stance. MI is ready to offer help to people who are more passive and therefore unsuitable for more structured therapies like cognitive behavioral therapy (CBT). It does not rely on skill building or didactic information sharing, but believes in exploring and reinforcing the client's intrinsic motivation for adopting healthy behaviors while respecting their autonomy. It offers a good option for helping clients who are ambivalent and lack self-efficacy.

## ■ SPIRIT OF MOTIVATIONAL INTERVIEWING

The spirit of MI encompasses the following:
- *Collaboration:* The counsellor establishes a partnership with the clients where they are positioned as experts with regard to their own values,

beliefs, experiences, and goals. The clients are given equal status and it is firmly believed that they are the best in sorting out their problems. The counsellor assumes the role of a facilitator rather than that of a guide or a tutor of various skillsets.

- *Acceptance:* The interviewer communicates to the clients that they are worthy and important no matter what (concept of unconditional positive regard central to humanistic theory), and expresses empathy. The client's efforts are affirmed, genuinely acknowledged and autonomy is supported regarding when and how the client wants to bring about a change in his behaviour.
- *Compassion:* The counsellor is kind, gentle, noncritical, and considerate toward the client and promotes the client's welfare.
- *Evocation:* It is assumed that the client has the strength and capacities to change and the counsellor just needs to evoke or bring them out. The counsellor's job is not to find weaknesses or shortcomings and ensure their rectification. Instead, by using open-ended questions, the counsellor makes the clients articulate their values and goals and brings out the discrepancies between them and the current lifestyle, thus motivating for change.

## PRINCIPLES OF MOTIVATIONAL INTERVIEWING

Motivational interviewing uses the following five principles while working toward the goal of bringing out behavioral change **(Fig. 2)**.

1. *Expressing empathy:* This principle emphasizes accepting the values and behaviors of the client nonjudgmentally. Persuading for change typically results in rebelliousness and resistance from the adolescents and is avoided.
2. *Developing discrepancy:* This principle is about bringing out inconsistencies between the current status or behavior of the clients and

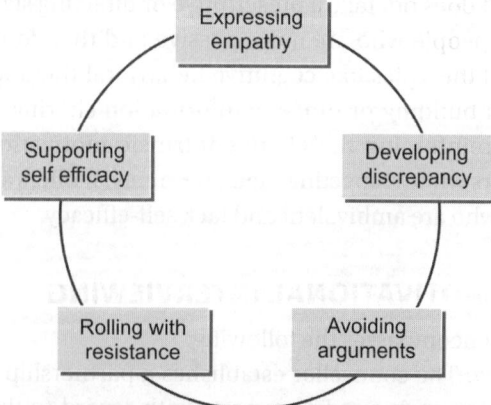

**Fig. 2:** Principles of motivational interviewing.

their important goals and values. While the session goes on, the counsellor tactfully identifies such discrepancies and communicates them to the client in a nonthreatening manner. The clients are also offered objective information regarding consequences of their behavior, if they are willing for the same.
3. *Avoid argumentation:* Arguing with the client is considered counter-productive and may increase resistance. The clients must be listened to and allowed to voice their views in a safe space without fear of judgement or reproof.
4. *Rolling with resistance:* Clients with problematic behaviors are often in two minds (ambivalence) regarding whether they want to change or not. MI believes that recognizing and accepting where the client stands and starting from there, is a better strategy than being pushy and demanding. Thus arguing or persuading is avoided and the clients are given time to make their decision.
5. *Supporting self-efficacy:* Self-efficacy is the person's own belief that he can accomplish a given task (Bandura). When the clients contemplate a change, the best way to help them is to boost their confidence in achieving their target. Hence, in MI, the counsellor makes all efforts to reinforce optimism by describing the client's strengths and past successes. Most importantly, counsellor accepts and expresses that change is not an all or none phenomenon but a slow process.

## ■ STRATEGIES USED IN MOTIVATIONAL INTERVIEWING

The strategies used in MI that can be remembered by the mnemonic OARS.
- **O**pen-ended question for elaboration or examples
- **A**ffirming the client's strengths and ability
- **R**eflecting the client's self-confidence statements
- **S**ummarizing the client's reasons for optimism about change.

Open-ended questions are the ones where elaborate or descriptive answers are elicited rather than a monosyllabic yes or no. They help the counsellor to develop an understanding of the young person's patterns of the problematic behavior including antecedents or triggers for the behavior and consequences of the same. An example of an open-ended question could be "Can you tell me about the impact of smoking on your life?" as opposed to "You do agree that smoking has a detrimental impact on health, right?" which is a closed-ended question. Another example of open-ended questioning would be to discuss parents' and friends' attitudes toward the problem behavior and how those attitudes might affect their behavior toward the client. The counsellor is respectful of the young persons' experiences, and does not make disapproving statements about their behavior.

Affirmations express appreciation. For example, "I really appreciate your being so honest with me!" Affirmations should be genuine and should be used sparingly. Their overuse may sound inauthentic.

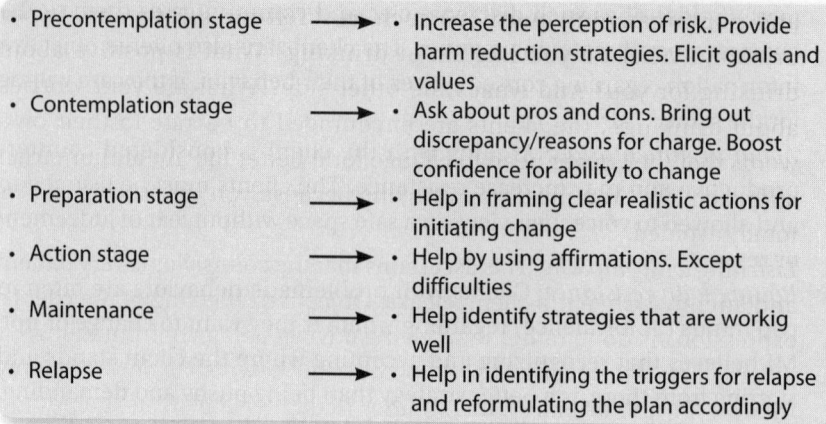

**BOX 1:** Tasks for counsellors during motivational interviewing sessions.

- Precontemplation stage ⟶ • Increase the perception of risk. Provide harm reduction strategies. Elicit goals and values
- Contemplation stage ⟶ • Ask about pros and cons. Bring out discrepancy/reasons for charge. Boost confidence for ability to change
- Preparation stage ⟶ • Help in framing clear realistic actions for initiating change
- Action stage ⟶ • Help by using affirmations. Except difficulties
- Maintenance ⟶ • Help identify strategies that are workig well
- Relapse ⟶ • Help in identifying the triggers for relapse and reformulating the plan accordingly

Reflective listening calls for a warm, nonjudgmental restatement, enhancement, or expansion of what the client has said. Such paraphrasing of the client's talk ascertains that the counsellor has understood precisely what the client wants to convey. Many adolescents find it difficult to put into words their thoughts, emotions, or experiences. Younger adolescents are respond better to reflections of emotion which essentially means to point out the emotions that the client may be expressing implicitly. For example, in the case of an adolescent boy seeking to cut down on drinking and expressing concerns about missing classes due to his problematic drinking, a reflection of emotion might be: "You are disappointed and upset when you miss out on things like participating in sports or academic classes because of your drinking". Picking out the strengths that the client has expressed during his flow of narration are used to build up his confidence. "So, last year you could manage to get selected in the sports team by practicing hard. You showed a great determination".

Summaries can be used during the process of exploration to gather together the patient's statements regarding his thoughts and feelings. "This behavior has become a cause of your underperformance in school as well as sports, which you wish to improve" **(Box 1)**.

During MI sessions, the counsellor gently and respectfully communicates with the clients regarding the difficulties that they face in initiating and maintaining a change in his behavior.

## ■ PHASES OF MOTIVATIONAL INTERVIEWING

### Phase 1: Building Motivation for Change

This phase consists of shifting the balance from "status quo" to "the change in behavior" using the following strategies.

- *Eliciting self-motivational statements:* By using nonaccusing and nonthreatening questions such as, "Tell me a little about your drinking. What do you like about drinking? What is positive about drinking for you? And what's the other side? What are your worries about drinking?", the clients are encouraged to narrate in their own words that they might need to change for a better life. An authoritarian approach like "You must stop drinking because you are scoring low" is totally avoided.
- *Listening with empathy:* This ascertains that the counsellor is very patient and attentive while the client speaks. Objective reflecting of the client's expressions is done rather than giving advice, being confrontational or judgmental. If the client says, "I do not know how I shall do without my friends, if I quit drinking", then, rather than advising, "You should find new friends", the counsellor here says, "It is hard for you to see yourself living without alcohol".
- *Questioning:* Rather than telling the clients how they should feel and think, the client is asked to elaborate on various aspects of themselves and their problems which are then reflected and affirmed.

    "Decision balance" is brought about, by asking relevant open-ended questions to elicit information from the client for and against quitting the problem behavior, with an attempt to illustrate to the client that the reasons for change may outweigh the reasons for maintaining the status quo. Presenting a personal feedback, on the basis of information gathered from various sources such as the client and his caretakers, an objective picture is presented to the client about the nature and magnitude of his problem.
- *Affirming the client:* Judicious appreciation of the good thoughts and actions that the clients share are used in building a healthy relationship with the client.
- *Handling resistance:* Resistance is shown by the clients in the form of denial, belittling the problem, arguing, interrupting, side-tracking the conversation, etc. They might miss appointments or arrive late. This resistance is believed to stem from the counsellor's faulty, confrontational directive style, rather than the personal attributes of the client. Hence, the motivational-reflective style of conversation is desirable. Rolling with resistance implies that the counsellor reframes the problem positively in such a way that the client feels the need to change. "So, you do not want to disturb your parents with your personal problems and so you drink. But then they are disturbed by your drinking".
- *Summarizing:* This is done at intervals during the sessions or at the end of it to bring out clarity regarding the narratives and exchanges between the client and the counsellor.

**SECTION 2:** Dealing with Adolescent Client

**BOX 2:** The change plan.

> The changes I want to make are:
> - The most important reasons to make these changes are
> - The specific steps I plan to take in making the change are
> - Some people who can support me are
> - They can help me by
> - I will know my plan is working when
> - Things that could interfere with my plan (barriers) and possible solutions include

## Phase 2: Strengthening Commitment to Change

- *Recognizing readiness for change:* This is the determination stage and is identified by the clients' behavior. They appear settled and calm, asks fewer questions, do not resist, and makes self-motivational statements indicating a desire to change.
- *Discussing a plan:* The counsellor now shifts from "reasons to change" to "action plans" that are convenient to the client.
- *Communicating free choice:* The clients are given a choice to implement the change the way they desire. They are given a sense of responsibility to bring about the change. "It is totally up to you as to how and when to go about this plan".
- *Consequences of action and inaction:* A written list of fears and expectations of the client as well as the pros and cons of change in behavior is made.
- Sharing a worksheet on planning the change **(Box 2)**.
- *Providing relevant information:* If the counsellors wish to share, they first ask permission from the clients and then share information. Clients' ignorance is not taken for granted. Their thoughts on the recently acquired information are also asked. Thus an "Ask Share Ask" strategy is applied.
- *Supporting to continue the change:* The clients are encouraged and helped in continuing the change by various strategies that involve affirmation, focusing on his goals, respecting values, etc.

## STRENGTHS AND WEAKNESSES OF MOTIVATIONAL INTERVIEWING

### Advantages

Motivational interviewing is a client centric, gentle approach and hence acceptable to most people who are struggling with problem behaviors. It is useful for patients who are low on motivation, have a hesitancy to engage in treatment plans, or for those who face difficulties in changing their unhealthy behavior. It comes in handy when clients are not willing for structured therapies like CBT, where a lot of active participation by the client is expected. It appears to be less time consuming as research has shown that four MI sessions had equivalent effects to 12 sessions of CBT and alcoholics anonymous facilitation on treating disordered drinking.

## Areas of Application

Motivational interviewing is useful across a wide variety of issues and conditions related to health care, rehabilitation, public health, social work, dentistry, social rehabilitation, coaching, and academics.

Motivational interviewing has been extensively studied and found useful in substance abuse including alcohol, tobacco, and illicit drug dependence. It has also been shown to be effective in the treatment of addictive behaviors such as gambling. It is also very useful in making healthy lifestyle changes in physical disorders like diabetes where adherence to a healthy diet and exercise plan is an integral part of the treatment.

It is useful in improving treatment compliance for other chronic disorders like asthma, which require regularity and strict adherence to treatment plans for long periods. It has a definite role in dieting, eating disorders, dental hygiene, reducing sexual risk behaviors, and domestic violence. Some studies reveal that improving academic performance is highly likely by using MI techniques for middle and high school students, though these findings need further research.

Incorporating MI strategies into parenting approaches for toddlers, middle school students, and parents of children with disruptive behaviors like attention-deficit hyperactivity disorder (ADHD) have also been investigated.

## Disadvantages

Motivational interviewing counsellor needs to get himself in depth acquainted with and trained in all the nuances of MI.

In many countries, a specific tool, the scale of Motivational Interviewing Treatment Integrity (MITI) is applied to assess the MI skills of persons conducting MI sessions. It is difficult sometimes to follow the principle of equity as the practitioners have already embodied an expert role. MI is hardly of any use in mental disorders such as severe depression and suicidality. Since most of the neurodevelopmental and executive functioning required for MI develop only by 12 years of age, it is less likely to be useful for adolescents younger than 12.

## ■ RELEVANCE IN ADOLESCENT OFFICE PRACTICE

Motivational interviewing is an adolescent friendly style of intervention that respects their autonomy and is far from being directive and preachy. It does not expect them to learn any skill sets and there are no assignments. Learning MI is helpful for clinicians as they get to learn good communication skills and relationship building. This would in all likelihood increase patients' compliance to therapeutic interventions. The patients are more likely to continue to remain in touch with the healthcare system and thus learning and using MI techniques is rewarding and highly satisfying to practicing doctors.

## ■ CONCLUSION

Motivational interviewing is a useful tool for counseling adolescents in the clinic. The collaborative nature of MI can engender interactions that are mutually rewarding and fun. It is amazing to see how resourceful adolescents can be when their opinions are elicited and lecturing is eliminated from the office encounter. Thus, MI enables the pediatrician to support the adolescent's autonomy, facilitate development of important life skills such as problem solving and decision making, and promote healthy choices. Most importantly, problem behaviors like substance use can be effectively addressed as MI promotes a strong alliance between clinician and client which will enhance retention within the health care system and thus nip the problem in the bud before downstream complications ensue.

## ■ POINTS TO REMEMBER

- MI is a client centric communication that respects their values and autonomy.
- It involves the use of MI spirit, principles, and strategies which help bring in desirable behavioral changes in ambivalent clients.
- It has wide applications in physical and mental health sectors.
- It is an adolescent friendly counseling style.
- The patients are likely to be more compliant and adhere better to treatment plans when MI is used in office practice.

## ■ SUGGESTED READING

1. Barnett E, Sussman S, Smith C, Rohrbach LA, Spruijt-Metz D. Motivational Interviewing for adolescent substance use: a review of the literature. Addict Behav. 2012;37(12):1325-34.
2. Cushing CC, Jensen CD, Miller MB, Leffingwell TR. Meta-Analysis of Motivational Interviewing for Adolescent Health Behavior: Efficacy Beyond Substance Use. J Consult Clin Psychol. 2014;82:1212-8.
3. Gold M, Kokotailo P. (2007). Motivational Interviewing Strategies to Facilitate Adolescent Behavior Change. [online] Available from https://pubs.niaaa.nih.gov/publications/practitioner/youthguide/aapadolescenthealthupdatebmi.pdf. [Last accessed January, 2023].
4. Hall K, Gibbie T, Lubman D. Motivational Interviewing Techniques: Facilitating Behaviour Change In The General Practice Setting. Aust Fam Physician. 2021;41(9):660-7.
5. Miller WR, Rollnick S. Motivational Interviewing: Preparing People for Change, 2nd edition. New York, NY: Guilford Press; 2002.

6. Miller WR, Zweben A, DiClemente CC, Rychtarik RG. Motivational Enhancement Therapy Manual: A Clinical Research Guide for Therapists Treating Individuals With Alcohol Abuse and Dependence. [online] Available from https://pubs.niaaa.nih.gov/publications/projectmatch/match02.pdf. [Last accessed January, 2023].
7. Naar-King S, Suarez M. Motivational Interviewing with Adolescents and Young Adults. New York: Guilford Press; 2011.
8. Naar-King S. Motivational interviewing in adolescent treatment. Can J Psychiatry. 2011;56(11):651-7.
9. N'zi AM, Lucash RE, Clionsky LN, Eyber SM. Enhancing Parent–Child Interaction Therapy With Motivational Interviewing Techniques. Cogn Behav Pract. 2017;24(2):131-41.
10. Prochaska J, Norcross J, Saul S. (2020). American Psychologist Generating Psychotherapy Breakthroughs: Transtheoretical Strategies From Population Health Psychology. [online] Available from https://www.researchgate.net/publication/344862542_American_Psychologist_Generating_Psychotherapy_Breakthroughs_Transtheoretical_Strategies_From_Population_H. [Last accessed January, 2023].
11. Rüsch N, Corrigan PW. Motivational interviewing to improve insight and treatment adherence in schizophrenia. Psychiatr Rehabil J. 2002;26(1):23-32.
12. Strait G, Smith B, McQuillin S, Terry J, Swan S, Malone P. A Randomized Trial of Motivational Interviewing to Improve Middle School Students' Academic Performance. J Community Psychol. 2012;40(8):1032-9.
13. Szczekala K, Wiktor K, Kanadys K, Wiktor H. Benefits of Motivational Interviewing Application for Patients and Healthcare Professionals. Polish J Public Health. 2018;128(4):170-3.
14. Wikipedia. Self-efficacy. [online] Available from https://en.wikipedia.org/wiki/Self-efficacy. [Last accessed January, 2023].
15. Winters KC, Leitten W, Wagner E, Tevyaw T. Use of Brief Interventions for Drug Abusing Teenagers Within a Middle and High School Setting. J Sch Health. 2007;77:196-206.

# CHAPTER 11

# Making Pediatric Practice Adolescent Friendly

*Kritika Agarwal, Rajiv Mohta*

## ■ INTRODUCTION

At 253 million, India has the largest adolescent population in world. Every fifth person in India is an adolescent between the age of 10 and 19 years. Mental, behavioral, and sexual disorders can begin in adolescence. Health services which cater to the needs of adolescents are scanty and concentrated in urban areas. Focusing on adolescent health is an investment for a healthy adulthood and for future generations.

Behaviors established in adolescence have long-term effects. Tobacco use, alcohol consumption, reduced physical activity, unsafe sex, unhealthy eating habits, and violence during adolescence contribute to 33% of total adult disease burden and 66% of premature deaths. Therefore, adolescent period can be considered as key to future health. We need to reach out to adolescents and enable them to adopt healthy choices in terms of eating, exercising, sexual behaviors, and to avoid addictive substances and excessive risk taking.

The outreach of adolescent health services in India is very low. Studies show that only 2-10% of adolescents consulted the outpatient services of the Primary Health Center for the treatment of their health problems. It was observed that the overall utilization of Adolescent Friendly Health Clinic (AFHC) services was low (15% among girls and zero among boys).

The Indian Academy of Pediatrics (IAP) in association with the Adolescent Health Academy (AHA) has been conducting many skills building programs for professionals and community-oriented activities to promote adolescent health. Mission Kishore Uday 2013, 2018-19 and awesome adolescent and young adults' module (Awesome AYA 2020) are examples of such programs. Consensus guidelines for establishing adolescent friendly health services (AFHS) were released by the IAP in 2022. Active involvement of pediatricians in adolescent healthcare is the need of hour to bridge this gap of health services available and required for adolescents.

**BOX 1:** Problems faced by adolescents in India.

- Socioeconomic disparities
- Undernutrition
- Infectious diseases
- Noncommunicable diseases
- Poor access to health services
- Gender discrimination
- Psychosocial conflict
- Adjustment problems
- Identity crisis
- Scholastic problems
- Early marriage
- Poor sexual and reproductive health

## ■ PROBLEMS FACED BY ADOLESCENTS IN INDIA

According to the National Family Health Survey-5 (NFHS-5), 59% of girls and 31% of boys aged between 15 and 19 years are anemic, 23% were married before 18 years, and 6.8% were already mothers or pregnant before 19 years leading to increase in low-birth-weight babies and in maternal, neonatal, and infant mortality. The adolescent girl therefore needs additional nutritional support and reproductive healthcare services. Adolescent boys in India have inhibitions and hesitate in expressing their problems and needs. Among boys of 10–14 years, injuries and communicable diseases cause disabilities and death while disabilities due to high-risk sexual behavior and mental illnesses are seen in boys of 15–19 years. Problems faced by adolescents in India are listed in **Box 1**.

## ■ ADOLESCENT FRIENDLY HEALTH SERVICES IN INDIA

Promotion of AFHS has been a key focus area for India and several middle- and low-income countries for nearly 20 years. There have been many studies highlighting the need for AFHS in the community attached to health facilities. Some evaluations have demonstrated an increase in adolescent knowledge and health behaviors with AFHS.

The Rashtriya Kishor Swasthya Karyakram (RKSK) was launched by the government of India in 2014 to strengthen and scale up adolescent friendly clinics. It is a comprehensive plan which aims to provide preventive, diagnostic, and curative services in six key areas: substance misuse, sexual and reproductive health and mental health, noncommunicable diseases, nutrition, violence, and injury prevention.

## ■ BARRIERS TO UTILIZATION OF ADOLESCENT FRIENDLY HEALTH SERVICES

Studies done in India have highlighted many barriers to adolescent health.

Most of the adolescents and youth in the study settings were not aware of AFHCs. Awareness about AFHCs was found only in 8% of young women and 5% of young men in the villages where study was carried out. Though all these villages were in the vicinity (within 5–10 km) of the AFHCs the access and awareness was poor.

Lack of seriousness about health issues, social stigma in seeking treatment, poverty, absence of family support, and lack of quality care were some of the major reasons why young adults did not seek advice/treatment from AFHCs.

The youth highlighted lack of privacy (presence of other people), different staff asking for the reasons for visit, and short consultation time as some of the deterrents for visiting the AFHCs. Explanations provided to them were not comprehensive and seemed preachy and judgmental.

Only 62% of doctors and 49% of paramedical staff had knowledge regarding services under the Adolescents Reproductive and Sexual Health (ARSH).

Several facility-level barriers such as lack of privacy, inconvenient operating hours, and long waiting times also contributed to insufficient service utilization by adolescents.

## ATTITUDES AND PREFERENCES OF ADOLESCENTS FOR AFHS

### Healthcare Environment

Based on study on adolescent preferences about offices and waiting:
- Making the interior design less childish, more teen-oriented
- Teens preferred artwork portraying realistic images
- Modifying interior decor with neutral colors, constructing smaller sub-waiting areas
- Medical paraphernalia to be hidden
- Decreasing waiting time and enhancing waiting experience by providing teen diversions (e.g., magazines, television, and games)
- Incorporating diversions that are teen oriented.

## DOMAINS OF ADOLESCENT FRIENDLY CARE

Indicators were drawn from a systematic review on young people's perspective on assessment of youth-friendly healthcare. Eight domains stood out as central to young people's positive experience of care:
1. *Accessibility of healthcare:* Services should be affordable and location should be easy to reach.
2. *Attitude of staff:* Should be friendly, respectful, trustworthy, and supportive.

3. *Communication:* Clinician should have good listening skills; technical information should be clear without lecturing and "straight talk" was preferred for bad news.
4. *Medical competency:* Technical skills of the doctor (physical examination, pain management, and procedures) should be of high quality.
5. *Guideline-driven care:* Maintaining confidentiality, especially while taking sexual history and psychosocial assessment. In chronic illness, transition to adult health and comprehensive care should be provided. Adolescents wanted to gain autonomy in emotional management and good communication skills.
6. *Age-appropriate environment:* Appointment times should be flexible. Health information which is teen oriented should be available. Clinic should be clean and should have separate physical space for teens. Long waiting time means that they are not respected by the clinician. For development of trust and privacy following up with the same clinician was considered important.
7. *Involvement in healthcare:* Adolescents wanted to have good understanding of their illness and treatment plan.
8. *Health outcomes:* Rating for the health service was dependent on emotional wellbeing. Teens who perceived a positive outcome of their care were more satisfied and wanted to adhere to treatment plan, whereas those who suffered from severe mental illness, had long treatment course or had low quality of life were less satisfied with the services provided.

Different group of adolescents have different preferences and expectations from healthcare, but across the world, different group of adolescents identified two key common characteristics. They want to be treated with respect and wanted to be sure that their confidentiality is protected.

## ROLE OF A PEDIATRICIAN

With IAP's inclusion of "care of a child up to 18 years", pediatricians need to change their perspective toward adolescents and keep in mind the developmental stages of the adolescent while providing healthcare and counseling.

## ROLE OF AN ADOLESCENT FRIENDLY CLINIC

An adolescent friendly clinic should have health professionals who:
- Understand the physical, emotional, and behavioral problems of an adolescent
- Understand mental and reproductive health issues and deviation, if any
- Do psychosocial evaluation by HEEADSS
- Provide anticipatory guidance
- Provide parental guidance
- Give age-appropriate immunization.

## HOW TO MAKE A PEDIATRIC CLINIC INTO AN ADOLESCENT FRIENDLY CENTER?

Any existing pediatric clinic can be converted into an adolescent clinic through some minor changes in the structure and by adopting an adolescent friendly approach as follows:
- Pediatricians should familiarize themselves with common adolescent health issues.
- With parental consent pediatrician should spend few minutes alone with all children above age 10 and elicit a brief HEEADSSS history **(Table 1)**.

**TABLE 1:** HEEADSSS: Psychosocial interview of adolescents.

| | *Potential first line questions* |
|---|---|
| H: Home | Who all live with you? How are the relationships at home? Has any person joined/left the family? Who do you share your stress with? |
| E: Education/ employment | How is your school? How is your relationship with students, teachers? How are you doing in school? Who can you talk to in school? How are your grades? Any failing in grades? What are your future plans? Are you working? Where/how much? |
| E: Eating | Does your weight concern you? How do you feel when you see yourself in the mirror? Have you anytime tried to manage your weight? Outline your exercise routine? What do you think a healthy diet is as compared to your diet? Are there any recent changes in your appetite? |
| A: Activities | How do you spend your time (with family/friends)? How many hours do you spend on screen? What do you use internet for? What are your hobbies (music/art/books)/For how long do you sleep? Do you have any difficulty in sleeping? |
| D: Drugs | Do any of your family members or friends use tobacco/drugs/alcohol? Do you drink or use drugs? (to assess severity of drug use CRAFFT screening tool) |
| S: Sexuality | Are you involved romantically? Are you physically intimate with anyone? If yes, with whom? How do you express affection? Do you use any precautions? Have you had any discomfort in passing urine? Do you have any genital discharge or itching? Have you ever been touched in a manner that made you uncomfortable? Elicit menstrual history |
| S: Suicide | Have you ever felt hopelessness, sadness, and a failure in life? Any recent changes in mood, behavior, sleep, appetite, or academic performance? Is there anyone in whom you confide your problems? Have you thought about hurting someone or yourself? |
| S: Safety | Do you feel safe when you are at home/school? Have you been bullied? Do you drive any vehicle? While riding a vehicle do you use seat belt/helmet? Have you sat in a car with someone who has taken alcohol/drug? Have you ever been in serious accidents? |

- Assign a day and time in a week exclusive for adolescent care that should be displayed on the clinic's notice board.
- Train the staff to be friendly and respectful in their approach.
- The clinic should display services offered in the waiting area.
- Provide health education material, posters, leaflets, and magazines that are age-appropriate.
- Care provided should be respectful and appropriate in terms of culture, values, religion, gender, moral values, and educational level of each adolescent.
- Confidentiality, assent, and consent should be explained to the parents and adolescent. Maintain privacy and confidentiality of the medical records of the patients.
- Be an empathetic listener and encourage open communication to build rapport with the adolescent. To break the ice, initial conversation should be informal about friends, family, and their likes/dislikes. Once rapport is established, discuss difficult and sensitive issues such as drugs and relationship. Conversations between teens and providers are two-way, where teens should feel respected and not judged.
- Equipment and materials at the clinic should include adult examination table, IAP growth charts, body mass index (BMI) charts, blood pressure (BP) charts, weighing machine, orchidometer, adult-sized stethoscope, and BP cuff. Questionnaires such as HEEADSSS for psychosocial issues, Patient Health Questionnaire-2 (PHQ-2) to screen depression, Screening for Childhood Anxiety Related Emotional Disorders (SCARED) to screen for anxiety, Screening to Behavior Intervention (S2BI) for drug use, and Ask Suicide-Screening Questionnaire (ASQ) for suicidal behavior should be available.
- Examination of a female/male client by the doctor to be done in the presence of the same sex chaperone. A separate examination area (separate room/area cordoned off by a screen) should be used for allowing privacy.
- Give accurate scientific information and counsel. Counseling should take into account the psychosocial, financial, and spiritual needs of the adolescent while guiding them through the steps of decision making.
- Interview adolescent and parents separately; understand their problems, requirements, and plan further intervention. Plan should be first discussed with adolescents and later with parents.
- Develop a multidisciplinary team of adolescent friendly health professionals, including gynecologist, dermatologist, psychiatrist, psychologist, endocrinologist, remedial educator, dietician, and other health professionals.

## ANTICIPATORY GUIDANCE

By providing preventive health education and counseling to adolescents many anticipated problems can be prevented. Components of anticipatory guidance include:
- Insights on normal development during adolescence. Importance of nutrition and physical activity should be emphasized.
- Information on menstrual calendar and hygiene should be given.
- Discussions on using appropriate safety measures to avoid injuries with helmets, safety belts, speed limits while driving, and avoiding drunken driving should be done.
- Coping methods with skills to handle bullying and peer pressure.
- Information on safe media usage.
- Discuss responsible sexual behavior and give knowledge on safe sex and prevention against sexually transmitted diseases STDs.
- Information should be provided on drug use and adverse effects. Assistance for deaddiction, if required, is given.
- Parents should be educated on the normal developmental stages of adolescence and how to communicate with their children supporting independence and nurturing their holistic development.

## HEALTH CHECKUPS

It is recommended that all adolescents should come for an annual health visit. Adolescents should have thrice complete physical examination during these annual visits. Once during early adolescence (11–14 years), once during middle adolescence (15–17 years), and once during late adolescence (18–21 years) unless more frequent examinations are warranted. During annual visits, age-appropriate anticipatory guidance should be done and health promotion messages should be reinforced. Adolescents who have initiated with health risk behaviors or having any physical or emotional disorders should be identified and counseled. **Table 2** presents health services for adolescents during annual visit.

## CONCLUSION

This chapter discusses the key points about including adolescent friendly care in routine pediatric practice. India has a large population of young people; adolescents constitute 18% of our population. If pediatricians and other medical experts concentrate on the health and well-being of these 253 million strong and vulnerable groups, this demographic bulge will be transformed into a bountiful reward. Although adolescence is normally a healthy stage of life, adolescent diet and health have an impact on future generations also. Thus, in order to enhance results for both health and development, it is crucial that we work with teenagers to mentor them and

**TABLE 2:** Health services for adolescents during annual visit.

| Physical examination | Development/behavior screening | Anticipatory guidance | Laboratory tests (as indicated) |
|---|---|---|---|
| • Weight, height, BMI, SMR<br>• Systemic examination, BP, eye checkup<br>• Hearing assessment<br>• Dental checkup<br>• Breast/testicular examination | HEEADSSS | • Nutrition<br>• Normal development<br>• Injury prevention<br>• Physical activity<br>• Safe sexual behavior<br>• Substance use (including tobacco and alcohol) | • Annual hemoglobin, lipid profile (if obese or has positive family history of early cardiac events)<br>• STI/HIV (if sexually active) |

(BMI: body mass index; BP: blood pressure; HIV: human immunodeficiency virus; SMR: sleeping metabolic rate; STI: sexually transmitted infection)

meet their health and developmental needs. Here lies the role of a pediatrician and IAP in general for advocating for adolescent health at all levels.

## POINTS TO REMEMBER

- Investing in adolescent health has a triple dividend—ensuring health in adolescence, in adulthood, and over generations.
- Pediatricians should actively participate and help in promoting adolescent health.
- All adolescents should be advised an annual health maintenance visit.
- Privacy, confidentiality, and rapport building are pillars of AFHS.
- Anticipatory guidance and counseling are keys to adolescent healthcare.

## ACKNOWLEDGMENT

The authors wish to express sincere thanks to Dr Preeti Galagali for sharing her expertise and guidance during the process of developing this article.

## SUGGESTED READING

1. Ambresin A-E, Bennett K, Patton GC, Sanci LA, Sawyer SM. Assessment of Youth-Friendly Health Care: A Systematic Review of Indicators Drawn From Young People's Perspective. J Adolesc Health. 2013;52(6):670-81.
2. Ambresin AE, Christopher G, Kristina P, Lena B, Sanci A. Global Consultation on adolescent-friendly health services. A consensus statement. Geneva: World Health Organization; 2002.
3. Azzopardi PS, Hearps SJC, Francis KL, Kennedy EC, Mokdad AH, Kassebaum NJ, et al. Progress in adolescent health and wellbeing: tracking 12 headline indicators for 195 countries and territories, 1990-2016. Lancet. 2019;393:1101-18.

4. Bansal CP. Mission Kishore Uday: Getting IAP ready to meet the challenge of adolescent health. Indian Pediatr. 2013;50:831-2.
5. Bhave SY, Galagali PM. Setting up adolescent health clinics in private and public environment. In: Bhave SY (Ed). Bhave's Textbook of Adolescent Medicine, 1st edition. New Delhi: Jaypee Brothers Medical publishers (P) Ltd.; 2006. pp. 9-16.
6. Galgali PM, Rao C, Dinakar C, Gupta P, Shah D, Chandrashekaraiah S, et al. Indian Academy of Pediatrics Consensus Guidelines for Adolescent Friendly Health Services. Indian Pediatr. 2022;59:477-84.
7. Hayrumyan V, Grigoryan Z, Sargsyan Z, Sahakyan S, Aslanyan L, Harutyunyan A. Barriers to utilization of adolescent friendly health services in primary healthcare facilities in Armenia: a qualitative study. Int J Public Health. 2020;65(8):1247-55.
8. Hoopes AJ, Agarwal P, Bull S, Chandra-Mouli V. Measuring adolescent friendly health services in India: A scoping review of evaluations. Reprod Health. 2017;14(1):43.
9. Kumar T, Pal P, Kaur P. Health seeking behaviour and health awareness among rural and urban adolescents in Dehradun District, Uttarakhand, India. Int J Adolesc Med Health. 2017;29(2):/j/ijamh.
10. Mehta R. Preconception care for adolescent in clinical practice. In: Bhave SY (Ed). Bhave's Textbook of Adolescent Medicine, 1st edition. New Delhi: Jaypee Brothers Medical publishers (P) Ltd.; 2006. pp. 43-8.
11. Ministry of Health and Family Welfare. Strategy Handbook. Rashtriya Kishor Swasthya Karyakram. Government of India: Ministry of Health and Family Welfare; 2014.
12. Nair MKC, George B, Thankachi Y, Swamidhas P, Russel S. ARSH 6: Reproductive health needs assessment of adolescents and young people (15-24 y): a qualitative study on perceptions of program managers and health providers. Indian J Pediatr. 2013;80 Suppl 2:S222-8.
13. Nair MKC, George B, Thankachi Y, Swamidhas P, Russel S. Reproductive health needs assessment of adolescents and young people (15-24 y): a qualitative study on 'perceptions of community stakeholders'. Indian J Pediatr. 2013;80 (Suppl 2): S214-21.
14. Santhya KG, Prakash R, Jejeebhoy SJ, Singh SK. Accessing Adolescent Friendly Health Clinics in India: The Perspectives of Adolescents and Youth. New Delhi: Population Council; 2014.
15. Thulasingam M, Premarajan KC, Soundappan K, Rajarethinam K, Krishnamoorthy Y, Rajalatchumi A, Mathavaswami V, et al. A Mixed Methods Evaluation of Adolescent Friendly Health Clinic Under National Adolescent Health Program, Puducherry, India. Indian J Pediatr. 2019;86(2):132-9.
16. Tivorsak T, Britto MT, Klostermann BK, Nebrig DM, Slap GB. Are pediatric practice settings adolescent friendly? An exploration of attitudes and preferences. Clin Pediatr (Phila). 2004;43(1):55-61.

# CHAPTER 12

# Psychopharmacological Interventions in Children and Adolescents

*Tejas Golhar, Shashi Kiran, Shoba Srinath*

## ■ INTRODUCTION

In 1937, Charles Bradley, a psychiatrist, administered dl-amphetamine to "problem" children in Rhode Island (USA), to alleviate headaches. Bradley noticed an unexpected effect: improved school performance, social interactions, and emotional responses (Lorberg, 2020). From that serendipitous discovery by Bradley to the multisite well-designed placebo-controlled clinical trials of the 21st century, psychopharmacology in children and adolescents has evolved from an area of research to a standard of clinical care. Evidence-based pharmacotherapy in child and adolescent mental health conditions can be found summarized in evolving practice guidelines and treatment algorithms.

The psychiatric assessment of children/adolescents is a complex one. It explores in detail:
- The presenting problems, what patterns of emotional/behavioral/cognitive difficulties are recurring
- The predisposing, precipitating, and perpetuating factors for the current presentation—they could be biological, developmental, temperamental, cultural factors, or systemic influences (such as adverse childhood experiences and psychosocial and relational difficulties)
- Risk of harm to self or others, risk of developmental arrest or future derailment from developmental trajectory; as well as
- Strengths of the child and of the system around the child (protective factors).

A recent clinical practice guideline for clinical assessment of child/adolescent mental health conditions (Srinath, 2019) is suggested to the readers to assist with drawing up a comprehensive and considered plan of intervention for young people and their families. Evidence-based pharmacotherapy in children/adolescents, always adjuvant to psychosocial management strategies, forms an important part in such an intervention plan. Pharmacotherapy is either directed toward management of a psychiatric disorder or directed at specific target symptoms to support reduction of risks, improvement of functioning, and hastening recovery.

Except for medication for attention deficit hyperactivity disorder (ADHD), most psychopharmacological interventions in children/adolescents are extrapolated from their use in adult psychiatric conditions. There is notable research on the short-term efficacy of many of these psychotropics in children/adolescents. As yet though, there is not adequate research on the long-term impact of pharmacotherapy in children/adolescents. Children/adolescents continue to be considered "therapeutic orphans" due to paucity of interest in research into medication in this politically voiceless group. This adds to the natural reluctance of caregivers to use psychotropic medication in children/adolescents.

A general concern is that agents acting on neurotransmitter systems during rapid development may interfere with normal processes and result in unwanted long-lasting changes. A high level of concern is warranted when treating children with medication, especially when the treatment is at an early age (under age 6 years) or long-term. Studying the long-term effects of treatments poses many challenges from practical and methodological perspectives. From clinical experience, it appears to be clear that what is safe for adults may not necessarily be safe for children. It is important to be mindful about reaching out "too quickly" for medication for children/adolescents with mental health difficulties, especially when adequate psychosocial intervention strategies may not be in place.

That said, the following *general approach* (**Flowchart 1**) and key steps are suggested to assist a clinician to prescribe psychotropic drugs in children/adolescents.

## KEY STEPS TO GUIDE THE PSYCHOPHARMACOLOGICAL INTERVENTION IN CHILDREN/ADOLESCENTS

- Complete a comprehensive diagnostic evaluation documenting the presence of a condition for which medication is indicated.
- The **Flowchart 1** should assist with judicious use of medication. In case the child/adolescent's mental health symptoms are too severe, or risk is too high to wait for a comprehensive diagnostic evaluation or for effects from psychosocial interventions, PRN/"SOS" medication targeting specific symptoms can be effectively used (see ahead in "special consideration").
- Resources like Maudsley Prescribing Guidelines can be referred to for regularly updated guidance on prescribing for various child and adolescent mental health disorders and conditions.
- When in doubt before (or even after) starting the medication, do not hesitate to refer to a higher center with more expertise or communicate

# CHAPTER 12: Psychopharmacological Interventions in Children and Adolescents

**Flowchart 1:** A general approach to starting medication in young people for mental health conditions (Lorberg, 2020).

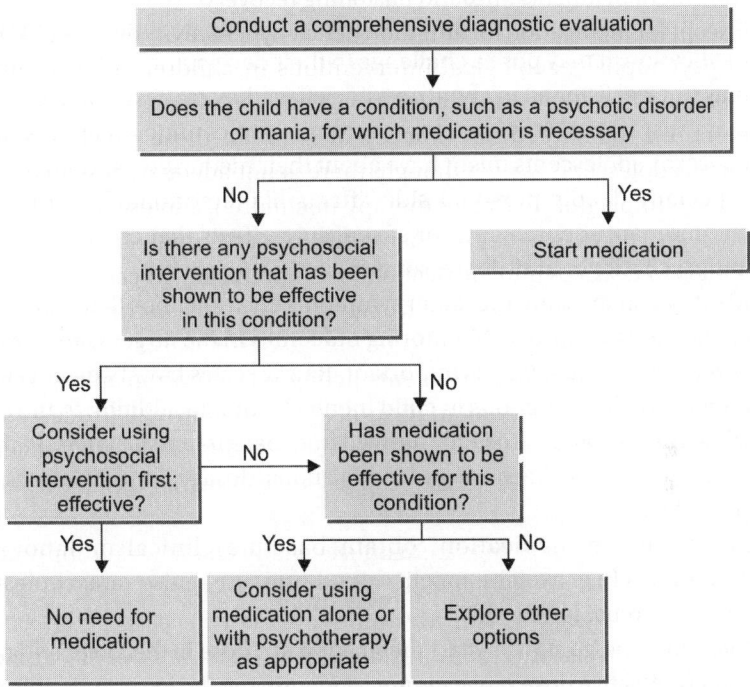

with a child and adolescent psychiatrist or another pediatrician with significant experience in child and adolescent mental health.
- Inform parents and child (especially a teenager) of the potential benefits and risks of medication as compared with alternative options. Consent from a parent and assent of the child/adolescent should be documented.
- It is important to emphasize to parents that all medication interventions in children are "a trial"—based on guidelines, a medication can be chosen, but we need to establish its effectiveness and tolerability in *their* child/adolescent.
- If the medication does not have a regulatory-approved indication for use in children with the condition, inform parents that the medication is being used "off-label".
- Medicolegal documentation of the discussion with parents and children is important.
- Any parent can be worried about their children being given tablets to alter their minds or behavior. One needs to discuss their worries and, if they still have strong negative feelings, a healthcare professional may not be able to prescribe the medication. It may be helpful to say things like *"I think you are quite right to worry about 'x' going on to tablets. I would worry too giving a child some medication. I put in a lot of thought before deciding to*

*prescribe medication for children. I would think your child deserves a fair trial to reduce his suffering. I can help monitor the risks".*

- It is not uncommon to find adolescents struggle with adherence to medication; it may pose a challenge to their developing autonomy or they may not feel listened to about any side effect they may experience, or they may "just forget". It is wise to *invest* time into confidentially discussing concerns adolescents might have about their medication and side effects, especially deeply personal side-effects like emotional blunting with common anti-depressants, or sexual side-effects that could occur with antipsychotics or anti-depressants.
- Identify and measure the target symptoms and functions that medication is expected to improve. Monitoring outcomes in the *target symptoms* and in *more than one setting* is important. Rating scales have been developed for most of the conditions in child mental health. In addition to the child, clinical information is usually derived from parents and teachers. Parents/adolescents could keep a log of medications, dosage, improvements, and side effects.
- Based on the medication, obtain baseline clinical or laboratory parameters (e.g., weight, height, blood pressure, pulse rate, cholesterol level, and renal function).
- "Start low and go slow"—start medication at a dose in the lower end of the usually effective dose range aiming at identifying the lowest possible dose that produces the desired outcome. Increase the doses very gradually with frequent monitoring.
- Monitor effects, side effects and, if appropriate, plasma levels (e.g., lithium levels) in the first few weeks of treatment, and adjust the dose appropriately.
- Allow time for an "adequate trial" before deciding to change the medicines, especially in chronic disorders (e.g., it may take 6–8 weeks for a child with depression/anxiety or schizophrenia to respond to the medication).
- Monotherapy is ideal. But in young people, due to multiple comorbid conditions, multiple medications can be required so extra caution is needed regarding interactions and side effects.
- Where needed, try and limit changing of medication to one medication at a time.
- If there is improvement, optimize the dose aiming at maximum resolution of symptoms and improvement in functioning.
- Determine the maintenance dose; and based on the condition and medication, establish a tentative duration of treatment.
- As appropriate, periodically consider the need for continuing treatment versus discontinuation.
- When discontinuing treatment, examine the need for a gradual taper, which is recommended for most medications after chronic treatment

(e.g., antidepressants, lithium, and antipsychotics) versus abrupt discontinuation, which can be appropriate for some medications (e.g., methylphenidate).

## SPECIFIC CLASSES OF PSYCHOTROPICS COMMONLY USED FOR CHILDREN/ADOLESCENTS

Following is a brief description of various classes of psychotropic drugs commonly used for children/adolescents. Additional reading is suggested (Taylor, 2021) to guide the prescribing of these drugs in various child/adolescent mental health conditions.

### Psychostimulants

Stimulants such as methylphenidate, dexamphetamine, and lisdexamfetamine are the most studied psychotropic medication used for children/adolescents. The approved indications for these are ADHD, narcolepsy, and binge eating disorder.

Methylphenidate is available in a short-acting preparation (2–4 hours duration of action) and long-acting preparations (up to 12 hours duration of action). Dexamphetamine has a short duration of action. Lisdexamfetamine is a prodrug of dexamphetamine, broken down in red blood cells so that dexamphetamine is gradually made available over 12 hours. But this may vary in individual children/adolescents as they might either be "fast metabolizers" or "slow metabolizers" of stimulant medication. Common side effects of stimulant medications are appetite suppression, insomnia (avoid night doses), hypertension, tachycardia, and growth deceleration. Mood changes, perceptual disturbances, obsessive symptoms, and tics could occur as well. They could also reduce seizure threshold. The younger the child, the higher is the risk of side effects. Baseline medical fitness to start these drugs is essential. Overall, children/adolescents with a clinical diagnosis of moderate-to-severe ADHD respond very well to stimulants; stimulants are considered first-line medication for ADHD along with the other interventions needed for the comorbid conditions such as specific learning disability and oppositional and defiant disorder.

### Nonstimulant Medication for Attention Deficit Hyperactivity Disorder

These drugs are second-line medication for ADHD. They are useful when stimulants are not tolerated, or are not safe to use (e.g., with comorbid inadequately controlled anxiety/psychosis/seizures or risk of diversion of stimulants to peers), or there is nonresponse to stimulants, or to augment the effect of stimulants when dose of stimulants cannot be increased. Unlike the immediate effects noted for stimulants, these drugs may take 2–4 weeks to show a difference.

Atomoxetine is a nonepinephrine reuptake inhibitor (NRI). One needs to specifically monitor for emergent suicidal thinking and liver disease when using atomoxetine. It should be avoided in children under 8 years of age. It can help when anxiety is comorbid with ADHD.

Clonidine and guanfacine are alpha-2 adrenergic agonists. While using these drugs, it is important to monitor for sedation, hypotension, and rebound hypertension with abrupt cessation. These drugs can also help with tics and Tourette's syndrome.

## Selective Serotonin Reuptake Inhibitors

The most widely studied and used selective serotonin reuptake inhibitor (SSRI) is fluoxetine. It is the first-line medication for depression and anxiety disorders in children/adolescents including obsessive-compulsive disorder (OCD). Other indications are disruptive mood dysregulation disorder, stereotyped movement disorder, bulimia nervosa, binge eating disorder, impulsivity, and repetitive behaviors (including "compulsive" self-injurious behaviors) in children/adolescents with intellectual disability (ID) or autism spectrum disorder (ASD). Its half-life is long so in case of missed doses (which can commonly occur in adolescent population) there are no major withdrawal side effects. It can raise the serum levels of drugs such as sodium valproate, phenytoin, and carbamazepine by virtue of its hepatic metabolic pathway. Overall its safety is well established.

Other SSRIs studied and used in children/adolescents are fluvoxamine, sertraline, and escitalopram. They can be used if fluoxetine is not tolerated or effective after an adequate trial of 8–12 weeks. Fluvoxamine is usually administered at night while other SSRIs are usually administered in the mornings. Emotional blunting (cannot feel any emotions) is not an uncommon side effect heard from teenagers, some of whom may prefer to bear with their anxiety and stop using SSRIs in order to "at least feel something".

Selective serotonin reuptake inhibitors can cause paradoxical activation and agitation or worsening in anxiety disorder if doses are rapidly increased. Fortnightly instead of weekly dose increments can help prevent this.

A major reported concern with SSRIs can be the increase in suicidal thoughts reported in young people, though the actual risk of suicide behavior may not increase. It is prudent to at least fortnightly monitor mental state and risks during the first couple of months of SSRI trial.

## Serotonin and Norepinephrine Reuptake Inhibitors

Drugs such as venlafaxine, desvenlafaxine, and duloxetine are similar to SSRIs in their effects and side effects except that they can also have cardiovascular side effects due to noradrenergic actions (especially venlafaxine) and that they are not found to be effective in depression in children/adolescents but can be used as second-line agents in anxiety disorders in older adolescents.

## Antipsychotic Drugs

These drugs heralded the advent of adult psychopharmacological interventions. Their use in children/adolescents is far less common and the main reason for controversy is the potentially severe neurological and developmental adverse effects as well as metabolic syndrome with long term use. There is also a risk of unpleasant short-term side effects like extrapyramidal syndrome (which can occur in children with antipsychotics that usually will not be suspected to cause this side effect). There is a need to monitor for severe and life-threatening side effects like neuroleptic malignant syndrome (NMS). The commonly used antipsychotics in children/adolescent are risperidone, olanzapine, quetiapine, aripiprazole, and clozapine. Their current long-term use in children is restricted to severe psychotic disorders such as schizophrenia and severe mood disorder like bipolar disorder. These severe mental illnesses should ideally be treated with the involvement of a psychiatrist. Risperidone, quetiapine and olanzapine are used for short-term tranquilization for severe mood dysregulation and severe anxiety. Olanzapine and quetiapine assist with comorbid insomnia. Risperidone and aripiprazole are used for severe self-injurious stereotypic behaviors and aggression in children with ID and ASD. Risperidone and haloperidol low doses are used in severe tics and Tourette's syndrome.

## Mood Stabilizers

Lithium is a drug with proven efficacy even in children for the treatment of bipolar disorder and of depressive disorder with high suicidality. Antiepileptics such as sodium valproate, carbamazepine, topiramate, and lamotrigine have found a place in the treatment of bipolar disorder as mood stabilizers. Bipolar disorder should ideally be treated with the active involvement of a psychiatrist.

## Anxiolytics and Sedatives

Benzodiazepines such as diazepam, lorazepam, and clonazepam assist with acute reduction in severe unmanageable anxiety and panic attacks. They are also used in management of withdrawal symptoms in substance use disorders as well as for severe insomnia resistant to sleep hygiene and melatonin. Lorazepam has a special use in a severe condition like catatonia. Due to the addiction potential, benzodiazepines are sparingly used in children/adolescents and not recommended to use beyond 2–4 weeks. Paradoxical agitation is not uncommon in children/adolescents with benzodiazepines, monitoring is required for the same if first time users.

### Melatonin

Most of the mental health conditions in children/adolescents present with insomnia as a co-occurring symptom. Insomnia makes coping with the psychosocial and relational stressors more challenging thereby worsening the stress and mental health disorder. Many a times, initiating pharmacotherapy just with melatonin helps to improve sleep and to improve the uptake of the psychosocial intervention. It is relatively safe, nonaddictive, and has been found to be quite acceptable to families, especially when sleep hygiene has not worked or when it is hard for the child/adolescent to "shut off" from the worries and racing mind at night. Melatonin also has been found helpful in insomnia related to ADHD and ASD.

## SPECIAL CONSIDERATIONS WHILE USING PSYCHOPHARMACOLOGICAL INTERVENTION IN CHILDREN/ADOLESCENTS

### Rapid Tranquilization and PRN/"SOS" Use of Medication

Pro re nata (PRN) use of medication (when the medication is not a regular prescription; sometimes called as "SOS" use of medication) can be helpful in children and adolescents, especially when particular symptoms such as severe mood dysregulation episodes, unmanageable aggressive outbursts, or severe anxiety/panic attacks cannot be managed with psychosocial interventions but occur too infrequently to warrant a regular medication. Lorazepam, diazepam, risperidone, quetiapine, and olanzapine can help with such PRN use. It is unwise to use PRN medication beyond rapid tranquilization. For example, it is not advisable to use stimulants as PRN for improving concentration only during examinations or only on certain days of the week. Any felt-need for PRN use of medication beyond rapid tranquilization, or frequent need for PRN medication should prompt a referral to a higher center or to a child psychiatrist or seeking an opinion from experienced colleagues.

### Children/Adolescents with Neurodevelopmental Disorders

Children/adolescents with ID or ASD are noted to be more susceptible to experiencing side effects with commonly prescribed psychotropics mentioned earlier. They need an enhanced level of monitoring, recognition of clear target symptoms, and evidence-based practice for diagnostic clarification.

### Preschoolers and Toddlers

The use of psychotropics in preschoolers and toddlers is unproven at best and is controversial. Evidence suggests that these children are receiving psychotropic drugs despite limited support for their safety and efficacy. This is quite alarming as the potential hazards appear to outnumber benefits. These youngsters need a specialist or a second opinion.

## Role of Psychotherapy

Decisions about prescribing medication must also consider the availability of effective nonpharmacological interventions. Though generally found less effective at decreasing acute and severe symptoms in most conditions, psychotherapy should always be considered in lieu of, or in combination with medication. Psychotherapy, used either sequentially (i.e., start first with psychotherapy, then add medication if insufficient) or in combination (i.e., start both psychotherapy and medication concurrently), may be able to shorten time to recovery and reduce the total dose of medication needed to control symptoms.

## Training in Mental Health for Nonmental Health Clinicians

The Henrikje Klasen iCAMH Training is a free 24-30 hours competency-based training aimed at practitioners around the world who have no specific training in child psychiatry, but nevertheless see children with mental health problems (e.g., pediatricians, general psychiatrists and their final year trainees; mental health officers, etc.). This program can assist with improving confidence to identify and manage mental health conditions in children/adolescents. More details can be found on the following link: https://iacapap.org/resources/henrikje-klasen-icamh-training.html.

## ■ CONCLUSION

It is very important to understand that medication is neither a panacea nor a bane in treatment of children/adolescents with psychiatric conditions. A thoughtful use of psychotropics may be warranted, despite a paucity of long-term studies. It is understandable to feel pressured (or being made to feel so by various stakeholders involved in the care of our young patients) about wanting "quick recovery" or needing to "do something" for a child/adolescent in distress. The child/adolescent *deserves* a confident diagnosis and a confident review of existing guidelines before starting medication whose long-term safety has not been confidently established yet. While it may appear feasible to initiate psychopharmacological treatment after just a brief evaluation, it is often unrealistic and undermines quality of care in the long run for the child/adolescent/family.

Child psychiatrists are scarce in numbers; so, while not all psychotropics for children/adolescents can be realistically started or supervised by these specialists, it would be prudent to appropriately and timely escalate cases to a child psychiatrist where treatment as per existing guidelines is not working as expected.

It is also important to remember that in psychiatric disorders of childhood/adolescence, the use of drugs is always a supplement to psychosocial intervention such as individual therapy, family therapy, counseling, socioenvironmental modification/accommodations, and behavior modification. When there is ongoing impairment/risk of substantial nature, judicious use of psychotropics is to be seriously considered in view of serious prognosis for many of these disorders affecting children/adolescents. In the meantime, these drugs would need to be tested for empirical evidence on long-term outcomes in children/adolescents. They would have to stand the test of time and demonstrate their utility as the use of these drugs is likely to increase even further in the future.

## POINTS TO REMEMBER

- Psychopharmacological intervention in children and adolescents has a growing evidence base though long-term outcomes on the developing brain are yet not adequately established.
- Psychotropic drugs, when judiciously used, adhering to existing guidelines and in active collaboration with families, can be very helpful in children and adolescents struggling with mental health conditions.
- Psychosocial interventions targeting individuals, families, and/or systems are essential for all children and adolescents for their mental health recovery; medication can complement psychosocial interventions to hasten recovery and prevent severe decline in functioning.
- All psychotropic drug use in children and adolescents is a "trial" to begin with and requires close monitoring. Younger children and those with neurodevelopmental disorders need closer monitoring due to their sensitivity to experience side effects.
- Resources and practice guidelines are available to support evidence-based psychopharmacotherapy practice for children and adolescents.

## SUGGESTED READING

1. Avasthi A, Sharma A, Grover S. Clinical practice guidelines for the management of obsessive-compulsive disorder in children and adolescents. Indian J Psychiatry. 2019;61(Suppl 2):306-16.
2. Coté CJ, Kauffman RE, Troendle GJ, Lambert GH. Is the "therapeutic orphan" about to be adopted? Pediatrics. 1996;98(1):118-23.
3. Garfield LD, Brown DS, Allaire BT, Ross RE, Nicol GE, Raghavan R. Psychotropic drug use among preschool children in the Medicaid program from 36 states. Am J Public Health. 2015;105(3):524-9.
4. Gautam S, Jain A, Gautam M, Gautam A, Jagawat T. Clinical practice guidelines for bipolar affective disorder (BPAD) in children and adolescents. Indian J Psychiatry. 2019;61(Suppl 2):294-305.
5. Grover S, Avasthi A. Clinical practice guidelines for the management of depression in children and adolescents. Indian J Psychiatry. 2019;61(Suppl 2):226-40.

## CHAPTER 12: Psychopharmacological Interventions in Children and Adolescents

6. Grover S, Avasthi A. Clinical practice guidelines for the management of schizophrenia in children and adolescents. Indian J Psychiatry. 2019;61(Suppl 2): 277-93.
7. Lagerberg T, Fazel S, Sjölander A, Hellner C, Lichtenstein P, Chang Z. Selective serotonin reuptake inhibitors and suicidal behaviour: a population-based cohort study. Neuropsychopharmacol. 2022;47(4):817-23.
8. Lorberg B, Davico C, Martsenkovskyi D, Vitiello B. Principles in using psychotropic medication in children/adolescents. In: Rey JM, Martin A (Eds). JM Rey's IACAPAP e-Textbook of Child and Adolescent Mental Health. Geneva: International Association for Child and Adolescent Psychiatry and Allied Professions; 2020.
9. McClellan J, Kowatch R, Findling RL. Practice parameter for the assessment and treatment of children and adolescents with bipolar disorder. J Am Acad Child Adolesc Psychiatry. 2007;46(1):107-25.
10. National Institute for Health and Clinical Excellence. (2018). Attention Deficit Hyperactivity Disorder: diagnosis and management. [online] Available from https://www.nice.org.uk/guidance/ng87. [Last accessed January, 2023].
11. National Institute for Health and Clinical Excellence. (2019). Depression in Children and Young People: Identification and Management. [online] Available from https://www.nice.org.uk/guidance/ng134. [Last accessed January, 2023].
12. Nischal A, Tripathi A, Nischal A, Trivedi JK. Suicide and antidepressants: what current evidence indicates. Mens Sana Monogr. 2012;10(1):33-44.
13. Pliszka S; AACAP Work Group on Quality Issues. Practice parameter for the assessment and treatment of children/adolescents with attention-deficit/hyperactivity disorder. J Am Acad Child Adolesc Psychiatry. 2007;46(7):894-921.
14. Shah R, Grover S, Avasthi A. Clinical practice guidelines for the assessment and management of attention-deficit/hyperactivity disorder. Indian J Psychiatry. 2019;61(Suppl 2):176-93.
15. Srinath S, Jacob P, Sharma E, Gautam A. Clinical practice guidelines for assessment of children and adolescents. Indian J Psychiatry. 2019;61(Suppl 2): 158-75.
16. Taylor DM, Barnes TRE, Young AH. The Maudsley Prescribing Guidelines in Psychiatry. New Jersey: Wiley-Blackwell; 2021.
17. Walter HJ, Bukstein OG, Abright AR, Keable H, Ramtekkar U, Ripperger-Suhler J, et al. Clinical practice guideline for the assessment and treatment of children and adolescents with anxiety disorders. J Am Acad Child Adolesc Psychiatry. 2020;59(10):1107-24.

# SECTION 3

# Common Medical Problems

13. **Adolescent Headache**
    Amitha Rao Aroor, Preeti M Galagali
14. **Adolescent Sleep Problems**
    Jayashree K, Preeti M Galagali
15. **Dermatological Issues in Adolescence**
    Shivangi Bora, Mary Augustine
16. **Irritable Bowel Syndrome in Children and Adolescents**
    Ramaswamy Ganesh, Suresh Natarajan, Malathi Sathiyasekaran
17. **Adolescent Obesity**
    Viji Thirugnanam, Hemchand K Prasad
18. **Adolescent Polycystic Ovary Syndrome**
    MKC Nair, Sheila Balakrishnan, Varsha Bharti
19. **Coping Strategies in Adolescents: Developmental Issues**
    Shashi Kiran, Shekhar Seshadri
20. **School Performance in Adolescence**
    Preeti M Galagali, Newton Luiz
21. **Adolescent Anxiety and Depression**
    MKC Nair, Shyamal Kumar
22. **Disruptive Behavior Disorders in Adolescents: Management**
    Harish K Pemde, Prerna Kukreti
23. **Management of Adolescent Suicidal Behavior in Office Practice**
    Preeti M Galagali, Amitha Rao Aroor
24. **Anemia in Adolescents**
    Piyali Bhattacharya
25. **Menstrual Disorders in Adolescence**
    J Shyamala, Chitra Dinakar, Shilpa Chandrashekhar
26. **Relationship Counseling**
    MKC Nair, Shyamal Kumar, Riya Lukose
27. **Office Management of Substance Abuse**
    Jayashree K, Preeti M Galagali

# CHAPTER 13

# Adolescent Headache

*Amitha Rao Aroor, Preeti M Galagali*

## ■ INTRODUCTION

Headache disorders are ranked by the Global Burden of Diseases as the second leading cause of years lived with disability and are prevalent in 60–80% of children. Most are primary headache disorders which are less serious but can have impact on the quality of life. However, a small percentage of children may have secondary headache which could indicate a serious underlying condition.

## ■ CLASSIFICATION

Based on the etiology, headache may be classified as primary and secondary. Primary headache has no causative etiology and arises from an intrinsic process, while secondary headache is a part of symptomatology of another disorder such as trauma, vascular causes, infection, and tumors. Criteria for diagnosis of primary headache disorders are outlined in the International Classification of Headache Disorders, 3rd edition, beta version (ICHD-3 beta).

Based on their temporal pattern, headache may be classified as **(Fig. 1)**:
- Acute
- Acute recurrent (episodic) ⎤
- Chronic nonprogressive      ⎦ Commonly due to primary headache disorder
- Chronic progressive.

### Primary Headache

Migraine and tension-type headaches (TTHs) are the most common primary headache disorders observed in children and adolescents. Headache type may evolve during adolescence and is influenced by hormonal changes and stressors. Prevalence of migraine is approximately 10% among children aged 5–15 years and reaches to adult levels by late teens. Conversion to chronic headache is seen in about 2% of children. Primary headache disorders are diagnosed clinically based on the ICHD-3 criteria **(Table 1 and Box 1)**.

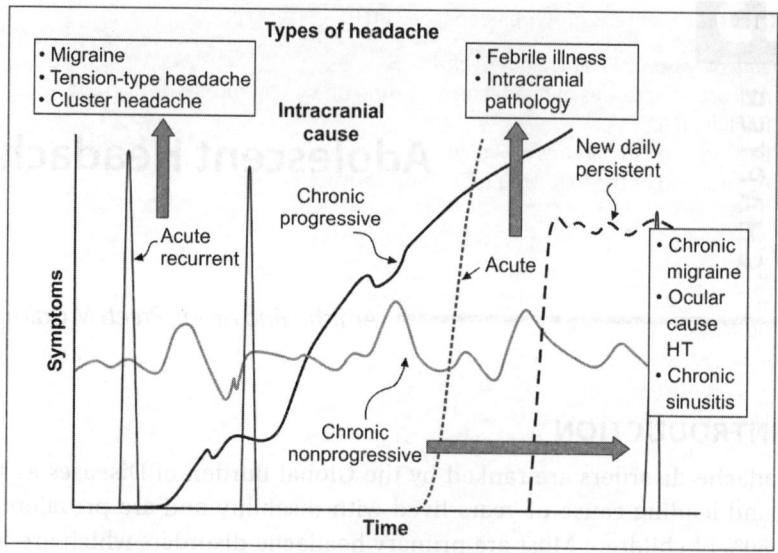

**Fig. 1:** Headache types based on the temporal pattern. (HT: hypertension)

**TABLE 1:** Criteria for migraine with and without aura.

| Migraine without aura | Migraine with aura |
|---|---|
| A. At least five attacks fulfilling criteria B–D<br>B. Headache attacks lasting 2–72 hours<br>C. Headache has at least two of the following four characteristics:<br>  1. Unilateral location<br>  2. Pulsating quality<br>  3. Moderate to severe pain intensity<br>  4. Aggravation by routine physical activity<br>D. During headache at least one of the following:<br>  – Nausea and/or vomiting<br>  – Photophobia and phonophobia<br>E. Not better accounted for by another International Classification of Headache Disorders, 3rd edition (ICHD-3) diagnosis | A. At least two attacks fulfilling criteria B and C<br>B. One or more of the following fully reversible aura symptoms:<br>  – Visual<br>  – Sensory<br>  – Speech and/or language<br>  – Motor<br>  – Brainstem<br>  – Retinal<br>C. At least two of the following four characteristics:<br>  1. At least one aura symptom spreads gradually over ≥5 minutes and/or two or more aura symptoms occur in succession<br>  2. Each individual aura symptom last 5–60 minutes<br>  3. At least one aura symptom is unilateral<br>  4. The aura is accompanied or followed within 60 minutes by headache<br>D. Not better accounted for by another ICHD-3 diagnosis<br>*Typical aura symptoms:* Fully reversible visual, sensory, and/or speech/language symptoms; no motor, brainstem, or retinal symptoms<br>*Brainstem aura symptoms:* No motor or retinal symptoms and at least two of the following: dysarthria, vertigo, tinnitus, hyperacusis, diplopia, ataxia not attributable to sensory deficit, decreased level of consciousness |

**BOX 1:** Criteria for tension-type headache (TTH).

*Infrequent episodic TTH (<12 days/year)*
A. At least 10 episodes of headache occurring on <1 day/month on average, fulfilling B–D
B. Lasting from 30 minutes to 7 days
C. At least two or the following four characteristics:
   1. Bilateral location
   2. Pressing or tightening (non-pulsating) quality
   3. Mild or moderate intensity
   4. Not aggravated by routine physical activity
D. Both of the following:
   – No nausea or vomiting
   – No more than one of the following: photophobia or phonophobia
E. Not better accounted for by another International Classification of Headache Disorders, 3rd edition (ICHD-3) diagnosis

*Frequent episodic TTH:* Above criteria 1–14 days/month for >3 months

*Chronic episodic TTH:* Above criteria 15 days/month or more for >3 months

Pediatric migraine may differ clinically from those reported in adults. It may be of shorter duration, frontal instead of temporal and bilateral rather than unilateral **(Table 2)**. Exact reason for this difference is not known; however, has been attributed to differences in degree of brain maturation including myelination and synaptic reorganization.

## Chronic Migraine

Headache occurring on ≥15 days/month for >3 months, with characteristics of migraine on at least 8 days/month delineates chronic migraine. It may be complicated by medication overuse headache (MOH).

## Medication Overuse Headache

Identification and effective treatment of MOH leads to reduction in number of episodes and better response to preventive therapy. The diagnostic criteria are:
- Headache occurring on at least 15 days per month in a patient with a preexisting headache disorder
- Regular overuse for >3 months of one or more drugs taken for acute/symptomatic treatment
- Not better accounted for by another ICHD-3 diagnosis.

## Cluster Headache

Cluster headache is the most common type of trigeminal autonomic cephalalgias and the most painful of the primary headache disorders. Age of onset is usually 20–40 years of age. It is uncommon in children with a frequency of approximately 0.03–0.1%. It is always unilateral on or around an

**TABLE 2:** Adult versus pediatric migraine.

| Feature | Adult migraine | Pediatric migraine |
|---|---|---|
| Side | Unilateral | Can be bilateral |
| Site | Frontotemporal | Often bifrontal |
| Duration | 4–72 hours | 2–72 hours |
| Associated symptom | As mentioned in **Table 1** | Nausea/vomiting more prominent |
| Visual aura | Fortification spectra, shimmering scotoma. Involve only half the visual field | Photopsia is more common. Randomly dispersed in the field |

eye, lasting 15–180 minutes and is associated with autonomic features on the same side of the pain (tearing, congestion, pallor, sweating, and rhinorrhea) and a sense of restlessness or agitation. However, pediatric cluster headache tends to be associated with less restlessness, less prominent autonomic features, a lower frequency of the clusters, and a shorter duration of the cluster attack.

## ■ APPROACH TO AN ADOLESCENT WITH HEADACHE

Approach to an adolescent with headache involves detailed history and systemic examination.

### Characteristics of Headache

The location, type, and character of the headache point to the clinical diagnosis. The following details about the headache need to be asked in detail:
- *Location:* Migraine is typically bifrontal or temporal while TTH is often diffuse. Occipital headache may be indicative of intracranial pathology. However, occipital headache alone, with normal neurological examination, is not an indication for imaging.
- *Pattern and duration:* Primary headaches are usually acute-recurrent or chronic-nonprogressive. Chronic progressive headache may point toward a secondary cause. Sudden-onset severe headache (thunder clap headache) may indicate vascular etiology.
- *Character:* Migraine is usually characterized by throbbing type whereas tension headache is usually pressing or tightening in character.
- *Severity:* Severe headache impedes all activities during attacks, moderate headache impedes some but not all activities, and mild headache dose not interfere with normal daily activities. Frequency of use of medications for treatment should be asked.
- *Aura:* Aura in migraine may precede or occur during migraine attack, evolves over minutes and is of short duration. Rapid progression of the aura over seconds and longer duration may indicate a secondary cause.

**BOX 2:** The Pediatric Migraine Disability Assessment (PedMIDAS) questionnaire.

- How many full days of school were missed in the last 3 months due to headache?
- How many partial days of school were missed in the last 3 months due to headaches?
- How many days, in the last 3 months, did you function at less than half your ability in school because of a headache (do not include days counted in the first two questions)?
- How many days were you not able to do things at home due to a headache?
- How many days did you not participate in other activities due to headaches?
- How many days did you participate in these activities, but functioned at less than half your ability (do not include days counted in the fifth question)

- Headache worsening with sneezing/coughing/Valsalva/exercise may indicate intracranial hypertension
- *Precipitating factor:* Various triggers include stress, anxiety, lack of sleep, fasting, dehydration, caffeine, certain food, media use, etc.
- History of periodic syndrome during childhood may hint toward a diagnosis of migraine during adolescence. These are referred to as "episodic syndromes that may be associated with migraine" in ICHD-3, including benign paroxysmal torticollis, benign paroxysmal vertigo, abdominal migraine, and cyclical vomiting syndrome.
- History of poorly controlled medical disorder such as asthma, Juvenile idiopathic arthritis (JIA), or diabetes mellitus.
- Family history of migraine.
- *Level of disability:* The Pediatric Migraine Disability Assessment (PedMIDAS) score can be used to assess the level of disability and is validated for children aged 4–18 years. It has total of six questions for the same **(Box 2)**. Disability is graded as little or none (score of 1–10), mild (score of 11–30), moderate (score of 31–50), and severe (score of >50). It can also be used to monitor response to therapy.

## Medical History
Suggestive of acute and chronic conditions that can present with headache.

## HEEADSSS Screening
It identifies comorbid conditions such as depression, anxiety, substance use, sexual abuse, and other contributory psychosocial stressors.

## Detailed Physical Examination
Fever, pallor, hypertension, obesity, sinus tenderness, eye examination, dental caries, and neurocutaneous markers should be looked for. Endocrine changes such as growth retardation, pubertal abnormalities, and obesity may be clinical pointers toward intracranial space occupying lesion involving hypothalamus or pituitary.

**TABLE 3:** General characteristics of primary versus secondary headache.

| Characteristics | Primary headache | Secondary headache |
|---|---|---|
| Location | Frontal/temporal | Occipital |
| Temporal pattern | Acute recurrent/chronic nonprogressive | Acute/subacute/chronic progressive |
| Quality | Pulsating/throbbing/squeezing | Pressure |
| Intensity | Mild to severe | Usually severe |
| Time of the day | Any time | Usually in the morning |
| Duration | Hours to days | Continuous |
| Emesis | Nausea > vomiting | Vomiting > nausea |
| Neurological examination | Normal | Normal/abnormal |
| Visual symptom | Visual aura | Diplopia |
| Phonophobia/photophobia | Can be present | Absent |

## Neurological Examination

Abnormalities in neurological examination such as altered mental state, vision disturbances (decreased visual acuity/field of vision, nystagmus, and diplopia), lateralizing signs, cranial nerve deficits (especially II, III, IV, and VI cranial nerves), papilledema, meningeal signs, and alteration in balance and coordination indicate intracranial pathology. However, focal neurological deficit with or without vision disturbances lasting for a short duration can also be a part of migraine aura.

Differentiating points between primary and secondary headache are shown in **Table 3**.

## Investigations

Investigations are routinely not indicated in primary headache, but neuroimaging should be considered in those with an abnormal neurological examination, in migraine with unusual neurological features, and when there are red flags indicating secondary headache. MRI is the imaging modality of choice whenever feasible. Further investigations depend on the suspected etiology.

## Red Flag Signs of Secondary Headache

A detailed headache history involves asking about red flag signs (**Box 3**). Presence of these features indicates underlying brain abnormalities and need for detailed evaluation.

Mnemonic SNOOPPPY (**S**ystemic symptoms, Abnormal **N**eurologic signs, Acute **O**nset, **O**ccipital headache, **P**recipitated by Valsalva, **P**ositional, **P**rogressive, Age <6 **y**ears) can be used for the red flag signs.

**BOX 3:** Red flag signs of secondary headache.

- Early morning headache or vomiting awaken patient from sleep
- Recent onset of severe headache
- Thunderclap headache
- Change in quality or frequency of headache
- Occipital headache
- Progressive headache
- Coexistence of seizures
- Changes in personality, behavior, and worsening school performance
- Worsening with cough/Valsalva
- Symptoms of systemic disease
- Abnormal neurological examination/fundus
- Abnormality in growth/puberty
- Hypertension
- Neurocutaneous markers
- Not responding to conventional therapy

## ■ TREATMENT OF PRIMARY HEADACHE

Usual reasons for clinic visits are impact of headache on education and fear of serious illness. Though primary headaches like migraine are usually intermittent, the risk of conversion to daily headache becomes more likely as the frequency increases or when the acute episodes are not effectively treated. Treatment is multitiered and includes pharmacologic as well as nonpharmacologic methods **(Table 4)**. Treatment should be individualized depending on type, severity, and frequency of headache and associated conditions.

### General Measures

These include educating the child and family about the benign nature of headache and counseling them to follow a healthy lifestyle. Adequate sleep with regular bedtime and wakeup time, drinking adequate fluids, consuming

**TABLE 4:** Treatment modalities for migraine.

| Tier level | Treatment | Measures |
|---|---|---|
| 1st | Lifestyle modification (SMART) | • **S**leep—good sleep hygiene<br>• **M**eals—regular healthy meals, hydration, limit caffeine intake<br>• **A**ctivity—regular exercise<br>• **R**elaxation—stress reduction<br>• **T**rigger avoidance |
| 2nd | Integrative therapies | • Behavioral therapies<br>• Nutraceuticals |
| 3rd | Pharmacotherapy | Abortive and preventive therapies |

a balanced diet, and reducing the screen time should be reinforced. Keeping headache diary helps in identifying the pattern of headache, triggers, and response to therapy.

## Integrative Therapies

### Behavioral Therapies

These include mindfulness, cognitive behavioral therapy (CBT), progressive muscle relaxation, and biofeedback training.

### Nutraceuticals/Supplements

Alone or in combination, magnesium, riboflavin, and coenzyme Q10 have all been suggested as preventives for migraine. Currently, there are no clinical guidelines to support the use of nutraceuticals and/or supplements in children and adolescents with migraine.

## Pharmacotherapy

There is lack of clinical studies on treatment and prevention of adolescent migraine and the available studies show conflicting results. This may be partly attributed to the power of placebo effect in reducing both frequency and duration of migraine attacks in children.

### Abortive Therapy

The aim of abortive therapy should be to obtain adequate response with minimal side effects and return to normal functioning as fast as possible. Recommendations by American Academy of Neurology (AAN) for acute treatment focus on the importance of early treatment, choosing the route of administration based on characteristics of the migraine attack, and providing counseling on lifestyle factors that can exacerbate migraine. Drugs commonly used are nonsteroidal anti-inflammatory drugs (NSAIDs) and triptans. Systematic review has shown both NSAIDs and triptans to have good efficacy in relieving migraine pain. To prevent the development of MOH, "3 to 10 rule" should be followed, i.e., not to use headache medications for >3 successive days and not >10 days per month.

- *NSAIDs:* These are used in mild-to-moderate headaches. Drugs commonly used are ibuprofen (10 mg/kg/dose), acetaminophen (15 mg/kg/dose), and naproxen (5–7 mg/kg/dose).
- *Triptans:* These are indicated in moderate-to-severe migraine attacks and in mild headaches unresponsive to NSAIDs. There are four triptans approved by the Food and Drug Administration (FDA) for children >12 years of age and rizatriptan is approved for children >6 years. These include sumatriptan, almotriptan, zolmitriptan, and rizatriptan. They are available for oral (almotriptan, rizatriptan, and sumatriptan) and

**TABLE 5:** Triptans in adolescent migraine.

| Drug | Dose and route |
|---|---|
| Sumatriptan (10–17 years) | PO: 50–100 mg<br>IN: 10 mg |
| Rizatriptan (>6 years) | PO: 5 mg (<40 kg), 10 mg (>40 kg) |
| Zolmitriptan (>12 years) | PO: 2.5–5 mg<br>IN: 5 mg, maximum 10 mg/day |
| Almotriptan (>12 years) | PO: 6.25–12.5 mg |
| Sumatriptan/naproxen | 10 mg/60 mg, maximum 85 mg/500 mg |

(IN: intranasal; PO: per oral)

intranasal (zolmitriptan and sumatriptan) use **(Table 5)**. Pregnancy, cardiovascular/cerebrovascular disease, and uncontrolled hypertension are contraindications for their use.

As per the Cochrane review, triptans are safe, well tolerated in the adolescent population without significant increase in serious adverse events. In case of unsatisfactory response to monotherapy with triptans, a combination of NSAID with triptan can be used. The combination of sumatriptan 85 mg and naproxen sodium 500 mg has shown good efficacy in adolescent migraine.

- *Antiemetics:* These are used as adjuncts to therapy, especially in those with significant nausea and vomiting. Commonly used drugs are prochlorperazine and metoclopramide.
- *Calcitonin gene-related peptide (CGRP) receptor antagonists:* Though approved in adults, their use is not yet approved in children and adolescents.

## Preventive Therapy

Preventive therapy for migraine includes following a healthy lifestyle, pharmacotherapy, and behavioral therapy. Preventive medications can be considered in those patients with increased disability or frequency despite lifestyle modification and behavioral therapy. Indications for the use of preventive medications include high frequency of migraine attacks (1-2/week or >3-4/month), impairment of both the quality of life and the daily activities or PedMIDAS score >20, severe and prolonged attacks (>4 hours), and ineffective/not tolerated/contraindicated/overused acute treatment. Goal of therapy should be to reduce both frequency of attacks (1-2 headaches or fewer/month) and disability level (PedMIDAS score <10). Treatment should be evaluated for 6-12 weeks before considering ineffective. Prophylaxis treatment can be interrupted when frequency of severe migraine attacks is reduced to 1-2/month for 3-6 months.

There are four main classes of medications used for preventive therapy: antihistamines, antiepileptics, antidepressants, and antihypertensives **(Table 6)**. There is no standard guideline for choosing a preventive drug and

**TABLE 6:** Commonly used drugs for migraine prophylaxis.

| Medication | Titration | Dose | Side effects |
|---|---|---|---|
| Amitriptyline | Starting dose | 0.25–0.5 mg/kg (5–10 mg qhs) | Dry mouth, constipation, dizziness, and prolonged QT interval |
| | Increase by | 0.25 mg/kg (5–10 mg) q 2 weeks | |
| | Maintenance dose | 1 mg/kg qhs* | |
| | Maximum dose | 1 mg/kg/dose up to 150 mg/day | |
| Topiramate | Starting dose | 0.5–1 mg/kg (12.5–25 mg qhs) | Paresthesia, drowsiness, cognitive dysfunction, weight loss, and metabolic acidosis |
| | Increase by | 0.5–1 mg/kg (12.5–25 mg) q 2 weeks | |
| | Maintenance dose | 2–3 mg/kg (50–150 mg qhs) | |
| | Maximum dose | 4 mg/kg/day up to 200 mg/day | |
| Valproate | Starting dose | 250 mg/day | Alopecia, weight gain, thrombocytopenia, elevated pancreatic enzymes, and teratogenicity |
| | Increase by | 250 mg q weekly | |
| | Maintenance dose | 15–20 mg/kg | |
| | Maximum dose | 45 mg/kg/day | |
| Cyproheptadine | Starting dose | 0.2 mg/kg (2–4 mg qhs) | Sedation and weight gain |
| | Increase by | 2–4 mg q week | |
| | Maintenance dose | 0.2–0.4 mg/kg (4–8 mg qhs) | |
| | Maximum dose | 8 mg 12 hourly | |
| Propranolol | Starting dose | 10 mg tid | Hypotension and bradycardia |
| | Increase by | 10 mg q 3 weeks | |
| | Maintenance dose | 1–4 mg/kg (20–40 mg tid) | |
| | Maximum dose | 4 mg/kg/day up to 40 mg tid | |
| Flunarizine | | 5–10 mg/day | Constipation and weight gain extrapyramidal symptoms |

*At bed time

benefits of preventive medications have to be weighed against the potential harm.

Amitriptyline, a tricyclic antidepressant, is one of the most common drugs used. The most recent guidelines from the AAN suggest that there is not enough evidence to use amitriptyline alone; however, in combination with cognitive behavioral therapy, the drug was found to be effective in reducing frequency of attacks. Sodium valproate and topiramate were evaluated for prophylactic therapy of pediatric migraine in some controlled studies. Topiramate is the first drug approved by FDA in 2014 for prevention of migraine in children >12 years. Cyproheptadine is an antihistamine used for migraine prophylaxis, especially in young children. Propranolol is a nonselective beta antagonist and only a few studies have supported its efficacy in migraine prevention. Flunarizine is a calcium channel blocker with effects on cerebrovascular circulation and has shown good efficacy with evidence level A.

The Childhood and Adolescent Migraine Prevention (CHAMP) trial published in 2017 in children and adolescents aged 8–17 years showed that reduction in migraine frequency was similar in amitriptyline, topiramate, and placebo groups. More side effects were noted in the drugs group when compared to placebo. Counseling about lifestyle factors at each visit and timely abortive therapy could have contributed to the high placebo response seen in this group. As per the systematic review of randomized controlled trials (RCTs) by AAN preventive medications failed to demonstrate superiority to placebo. They recommended counseling on lifestyle and behavioral factors that influence headache frequency along with treatment of comorbid disorders associated with headache persistence. Locher et al. conducted a review and meta-analysis of various prophylactic drugs compared to placebo and concluded that prophylactic pharmacotherapy has little evidence supporting efficacy in pediatric migraine. Monoclonal antibodies to CGRP have been approved in adults for the preventive treatment of migraine headaches. Trials are being done in adolescent population and consensus statement on its recommendation was published, stating that it can be considered in postpubertal adolescents with ≥8 headaches/month, PedMIDAS score ≥30, and failure of two preventive therapies.

## ■ CONCLUSION

A systematic approach to an adolescent with headache helps in providing effective care and relief **(Flowchart 1)**.

## ■ POINTS TO REMEMBER

- Primary headache is more common than secondary headache during adolescence, migraine being the most common.

**Flowchart 1:** Approach to an adolescent with headache.

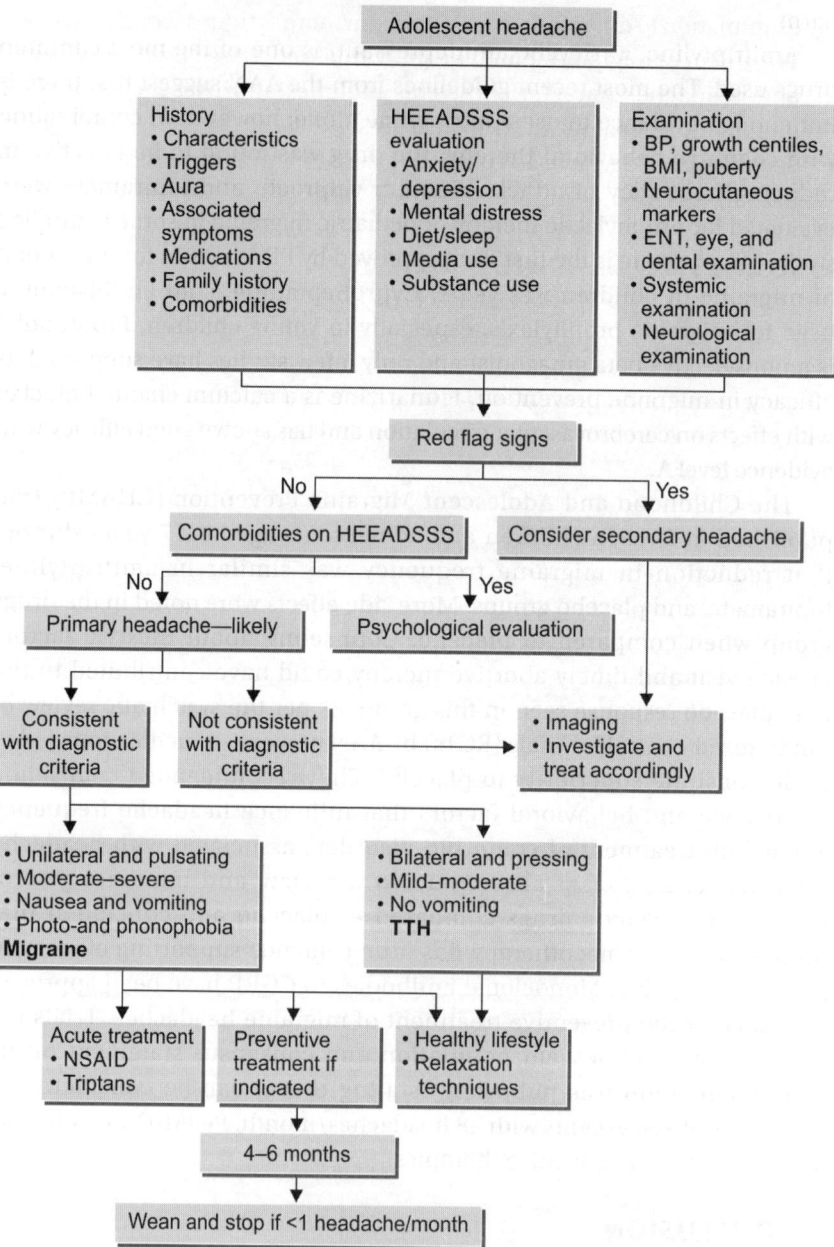

(BMI: body mass index; BP: blood pressure; ENT: ear, nose, and throat; NSAID: nonsteroidal anti-inflammatory drug; TTH: tension-type headache)

- Evaluation requires detailed history, HEEADSSS screening and physical examination to differentiate primary from more serious secondary causes.
- Treatment of migraine should be individualized, based on the individual and headache characteristics. This includes abortive and preventive therapy along healthy lifestyle measures.
- Secondary headache needs detailed evaluation with imaging and specific investigations.

## SUGGESTED READING

1. Arafeh IA, Valariani M, Prabhakar P. Headache in children and adolescents: A focus on uncommon headache disorders. Indian Pediatr. 2021;58:757-63.
2. Blume HK. Pediatric headache: a review. Pediatr Rev. 2012;33:562-76.
3. Dao JM, Qubty W. Headache diagnosis in children and adolescents. Curr Pain Headache Rep. 2018;22:17.
4. Derosier FJ, Lewis D, Hershey AD, Winner PK, Pearlman E, Rothner AD, et al. Randomized trial of sumatriptan and naproxen sodium combination in adolescent migraine. Pediatrics. 2012;129(6):e1411-20.
5. Headache Classification Committee of the International Headache Society (IHS). The International Classification of Headache Disorders, 3rd edition (beta version). Cephalalgia. 2013;33:629-808.
6. Kacperski J, Kabbouche MA, O'Brien HL, Weberding JL. The optimal management of headaches in children and adolescents. Ther Adv Neurol Disord. 2016;9(1):53-68.
7. Klein J, Koch T. Headache in Children. Pediatr Rev. 2020;41(4):159-71.
8. Kliegman R, St. Geme J. Nelson Textbook of Paediatrics, 21st edition. Philadelphia: Elsevier/Saunders; 2019.
9. Locher C, Kossowsky J, Koechlin H, Lam TL, Barthel J, Berde CB, et al. Efficacy, Safety, and Acceptability of Pharmacologic Treatments for Pediatric Migraine Prophylaxis A Systematic Review and Network Meta-analysis. JAMA Pediatrics. 2020;174:341-9.
10. Nieswand V, Richter M, Gossrau G. Epidemiology of headache in children and adolescents—another type of Pandemia. Curr Pain Headache Rep. 2020;24:62.
11. O'Donnell DM, Agin A. Management of headaches in children and adolescents. Curr Probl Pediatr Adolesc Health Care. 2021;51(7):101034.
12. Oskoui M, Pringsheim T, Holler-Managan Y, et al. Practice guideline update summary: Pharmacologic treatment for paediatric migraine prevention: report of the Guideline Development, Dissemination, and Implementation Subcommittee of the American Academy of Neurology and the American Headache Society. Neurology. 2019;93;500-9.
13. Oskoui M, Pringsheim T, Holler-Managan Y, Potrebic S, Billinghurst L, Gloss D, et al. Practice guideline update summary: acute treatment of migraine in children and adolescents: report of the Guideline Development, Dissemination, and Implementation Subcommittee of the American Academy of Neurology and the American Headache Society. Neurology. 2019;93:487-99.
14. Papetti L, Ursitti F, Moavero R, Ferilli MAN, Sforza G, Tarantino S, et al. Prophylactic Treatment of Pediatric Migraine: Is There Anything New in the Last Decade? Front Neurol. 2019;10:771.

15. Pasculli M, Striano P, Ledda MG. Pediatric migraine treatment: an updated review. Neonat Pediatr Med. 2019;5:178.
16. Popova V, Berk T. Pediatric Migraine—An Updated Review. US Neurology. 2019;15(2):68-73.
17. Powers SW, Coffey CS, Chamberlin LA. Ecklund DJ, Klingner EA, Yankey JW, et al. Trial of Amitriptyline, Topiramate, and Placebo for Pediatric Migraine. N Engl J Med. 2017;376:115-24.
18. Prezioso G, Suppiej A, Alberghini V, Bergonzini P, Capra ME, Corsini I, et al. Pediatric headache in primary care and emergency departments: consensus with RAND/UCLA Method. Life (Basel). 2022;12:142.
19. Richer L, Billinghurst L, Linsdell MA, Russell K, Vandermeer B, Crumley ET, et al. Drugs for the acute treatment of migraine in children and adolescents. Cochrane Database Syst Rev. 2016 4:CD005220.
20. Saylor D, Steiner TJ. The global burden of headache. Semin Neurol. 2018; 38(2):182-90.
21. Szperka CL, Vander Pluym J, Orr SL, Oakley CB, Qubty W, Patniyot I, et al. Recommendations on the use of anti CGRP monoclonal antibodies in children and adolescents. Headache. 2018;58(10):1658-69.

# CHAPTER 14

# Adolescent Sleep Problems

*Jayashree K, Preeti M Galagali*

## ■ INTRODUCTION

Sleep is integral to the health and survival of human beings. Adequate quantity and quality of sleep rejuvenates, restores, and maintains the optimal functioning of the body. About 8–10 hours of daily sleep is needed for adolescents to be in good health. Using pooled mean estimates, it has been calculated that globally, adolescents between 12–17 years of age sleep for 7 hours in the night on school days. When adolescents are allowed to sleep, they slept for almost 9.25 hours in a study conducted on adolescents yearly from 10 to 12 years till 15–18 years of age with no relation to age and stage of pubertal maturation. Ohayon et al. showed that on school days there is a reduced duration of sleep with no change on leave days, and reduced sleep duration on school days is dependent on environmental demands. Study from urban region of Kerala suggests 60% of the adolescents were sleeping for a period of <8 hours with a mean duration of 7.2 ± 1.26 hours. Another study from Delhi found that the preteens had better sleep compared to teens. A community study from Tamil Nadu revealed that over 64% of adolescents sleep <8 hours at night and 5.6% sleep <6 hours.

Due to the pandemic-related lockdown and online schooling many adolescents reported better quality and quantity of sleep with less daytime sleepiness. Also, there is a delay in the onset of sleep and wake time. Mostly the preparation needed to attend online classes were less and allowed them to get few extra hours of sleep. However, there is increase in the incidence of anxiety/depression and media/gadgets use.

## ■ FACTORS AFFECTING SLEEP IN ADOLESCENCE

Sleep regulation has two basic processes acting concurrently that control sleep and wakefulness. As the child grows into adolescence, duration of sleep hours gets reduced. During puberty there is a slow change in bedtime and wake time due to circadian sleep rhythm shift. There are various factors that affect sleep. Internal factors are a puberty-related shift in the biological clock resulting in delayed bedtime/wake times and decreased internal drive to sleep. Various studies reveal positive effects of delaying school start time initially on sleep patterns and secondly on daytime functioning. A systematic review by Prono F et al. suggests that vitamin D is involved in sleep regulation and vitamin D deficiency <20 ng/mL is associated with a higher risk of sleep disorders in children. External factors known to interfere with adolescent sleep are early school hours, afterschool activities, high ambient temperature, poor exposure to sunlight, vigorous exercise and emotional confrontations before bedtime, academic pressure, caffeine intake, alcohol and drug use, anxiety, depression, allergic rhinitis, chronic adenoid hypertrophy, anomalies of the airway, chronic diseases like asthma, obesity, psychological trauma, and too much screen time. In adolescents, higher level of physical fitness is associated with longer night sleep; better sleep quality was observed in a few studies. The results by Mayne et al. suggest that the neighborhood-built environment, particularly noise and green space, should be considered when intervening to support healthier sleep among adolescents. In adolescence, lack of sleep is attributed to the various changes occurring during this period at the physical and mental level, also a shift of circadian sleep rhythm. Adolescents tend to sleep for longer duration during holidays to compensate for inadequate sleep during school days which further disturbs the circadian rhythm and results in poor sleep. A study by Sarah et al. shows that parental rule-setting for bedtimes, healthy parental sleep, and parental warmth can play an important role in adolescent sleep with longer sleep duration, quality, and better adolescent daytime functioning.

The protective factors, such as parent-set bedtimes and good sleep practices, decline as adolescents grow older. Moreover, sleep competes with increasing school demands and the pervasive use of information and communication technology (ICT). In the Tamil Nadu study, 43% of adolescents had disturbed sleep, 64% watched television and 23% used mobile phones in bed before sleeping. Using screens at bedtime impairs sleep because of physiological arousal, increasing alertness and engagement, and results in the delay of secretion of melatonin due to the blue light emitted from the devices. During the transition from late childhood to early adolescence period, they are vulnerable to internalizing disorders which are exacerbated by sleep related problems (SRPs), which may interrupt intrinsic brain networks dynamics and increase internalizing symptoms. This is well explained by a novel developmental model, Sleep to Internalizing Pathway in Young Adolescents (SIPYA) model. Internalizing disorders can be severe and are associated with significant personal distress, poor academic performance, social withdrawal, as well as suicidal thoughts and behaviors.

## ■ IMPORTANCE OF SLEEP

In adolescents, sleep is needed to maintain various physical, mental/emotional health, and vital brain functions such as attention, memory,

**BOX 1:** Effects of insufficient sleep.

- *Morning tiredness:* Negative effects on cognitive function, mood, and motivation
- *Day sleepiness:* Delay in sleep onset in adolescents has been associated with fatigue, mood disorders, and anxiety
- Classroom inattentiveness and difficulty in learning an instrument or any new skill
- Obesity and diabetes mellitus
- Road traffic accidents
- Impulsive behavior, anger, aggression, and violence
- Immune dysregulation
- Suicidal behavior

thinking, learning new skills, and self-regulation. During sleep, growth hormone, testosterone, cortisol, ghrelin, leptin, and insulin are secreted, and immune regulation takes place. The process of pruning or synaptic reorganization, which is maximum in adolescent period, is responsible for maturation of sleep architecture.

Effects of insufficient sleep in adolescents are given in **Box 1**. Lack of sleep is linked with higher occurrence of overweight and obesity and an increased risk of prehypertension and hypertension independent of obesity putting these children at risk for long-term cardiovascular morbidity. In a recent study from Mumbai, it was reported that <7 hours of sleep and a poor quality of sleep in adolescents was a risk factor for obesity. It was also seen that there was a clustering of risk factors in 18.8% adolescents in terms of physical inactivity, increased screen time, and poor sleep leading to obesity.

## SLEEP DISORDERS

Many studies show various problems related to sleep duration, quality of sleep, patterns, and sleep lag. Bedtime autonomy increases and adolescents also have more autonomy in their evening activities.

The common sleep disorders seen are given in **Table 1**.

When an adolescent with delayed sleep-wake phase disorder (DSPD) is allowed to sleep at will, a normal quantity and quality of sleep are observed. DSPD occurs whenever the affected individual sleeps at odd hours as per social demands. In adolescents, the prevalence is as high as 14%. There is a well-established link between poor sleep and pain in healthy populations. However, it has also been demonstrated in conditions such as juvenile idiopathic arthritis, headaches, or as part of a pain syndrome (such as chronic widespread pain and fibromyalgia).

## ASSESSMENT OF SLEEP-RELATED ISSUES

This includes detailed history taking from parents and adolescents separately in privacy offering confidentiality. Sleep and media history forms a part of "activities" section of HEEADSSS psychosocial history taking. This is a clinical tool for screening for traumatic life events, scholastic and non-scholastic

**TABLE 1:** Common sleep disorders in adolescents.

| | |
|---|---|
| Psychophysiological insomnia (PI) | Difficulty in getting sleep or to stay in that state due to preoccupied with several thoughts leading to anxiety and stress during night |
| Delayed sleep-wake phase disorder (DSPD) | A delay in circadian physiology during adolescence can result in inability to sleep with delayed wake up time, called as night owl |
| Obstructive sleep apnea (OSA) | Usually associated with obesity. Ear, nose, and throat (ENT) causes of upper airway obstructions |
| Narcolepsy | Recurrent episodes of excessive daytime sleepiness with significant functional impairment |
| Restless leg syndrome | Uncontrollable desire to move legs urge to move along with uneasiness in lower limbs. Bedtime struggles and difficulty in falling asleep. Usually, manifestations start toward the end of the day, rest makes it worse, improves with limb movement |
| Sleep walking (somnambulism) | Seen 1–2 hours after sleeping. Getting out of bed, walking around with open eyes and difficult wake them during the episode, and short period of disorientation/confusion if awakened. No memory to the episode next morning |
| Excessive daytime sleepiness | • Feeling of sleepiness or easily falling asleep during daytime. Manifests as lethargy or moodiness, lack of interest and motivation, feelings of boredom, and depression. Poor academic or sports performance. Feels sleepy during class or while doing homework<br>• Puberty-related sleep phase delay, use of media—mobiles, television, video games, and internet compete with sleep time |

stressors, anxiety, depression, suicidality, aggression, and safety issues. On examination, evaluation of chronic medical disorders such as obesity, asthma, obstructive sleep apnea (OSA) and hypertension is essential. The following history should be elicited in detail:
- Sleep behavior (sleep time, falling asleep, and awake times)
- Bed type, sharing with others, surrounding light and sound, temperature, and routine around the sleep time
- Household structure, daily routines, and cultural practices may be important and influence the timing and ease of sleep (e.g., parental work patterns, evening activities, and number of household members)
- Dietary practices that influence sleep, including timing of meals and caffeine intake
- Assess symptoms of OSA (e.g., gasps, snorting noises and breathing pauses) in all children who snore regularly.

*Sleep diary* is important when the diagnosis cannot be made with history. Details of sleep diary are given in **Box 2**.

**BOX 2:** Details in typical sleep dairy.

- Bedtime and/or lights-out time
- Wake-up time
- How long it takes to fall asleep
- The number and duration of sleep interruptions
- The number and duration of daytime naps
- Perceived sleep quality
- Consumption of chocolate, caffeine, and/or tobacco
- Daily medications
- Daily exercise

The following sleep screening tools are available:
- BEARS sleep screening
- The Pittsburgh Sleep Quality Index (PSQI)
- Adolescent Sleep Hygiene Scale-revised (ASHSr).

The *BEARS sleep screening* tool is simple to use in office practice and provided in **Table 2**.

## BEARS Sleep Screening Tool

BEARS is divided into five major sleep domains (B = Bedtime Issues, E = Excessive Daytime Sleepiness, A = Night Awakenings, R = Regularity and Duration of Sleep, and S = Snoring) and helps clinicians evaluate potential sleep problems in children 2–18 years old. Each sleep domain has a set of age-appropriate "trigger questions" for use in the clinical interview.

Different ways to assess sleep are self-reports, actigraphy, and polysomnography (PSG). Assessment of perceived sleep difficulties and daytime functioning are easier with self-reports, also it is used in diagnosis of few psychiatric conditions. Actigraphy device is worn like a wristwatch which differentiates movements during sleep as well as while awake. It can measure duration of sleep with night awake period. It can provide sleep pattern over long periods of time like a few weeks to months. PSG needs concurrent tracings of electroencephalogram (EEG), electrooculogram (EOG), and electromyogram (EMG). It records the total duration of sleep, sleep lag, waking, and movement of limbs.

## ■ MANAGEMENT

Sleep hygiene and screen time guidelines should be advised by all pediatricians catering to adolescents. Evaluation of sleep-related issues must include the use of any of the scales mentioned earlier. If sleep disorders are detected, then appropriate therapy needs to be given. Iron deficiency may be responsible for restless leg syndrome. Iron supplementation is indicated if serum ferritin <50 mg/dL. Management of DPSD is given in **Box 3**. Appropriate treatment of ear, nose, and throat (ENT) causes responsible for OSA.

**TABLE 2:** BEARS sleep screening.

| | Toddler/preschool child (2–5 years) | School-aged child (6–12 years) | Adolescent (13–18 years) |
|---|---|---|---|
| **B**edtime problems | • Does your child have any problems going to bed?<br>• Falling asleep | • Does your child have any problems at bedtime? (P)<br>• Do you have any problems going to bed? (C) | Do you have any problems falling asleep at bedtime? (C) |
| **E**xcessive daytime sleepiness | • Does your child seem over tired or sleepy a lot during the day?<br>• Does she still take naps? | • Does your child have difficulty waking in the morning, seem sleepy during the day or take naps? (P)<br>• Do you feel tired a lot? (C) | Do you feel sleepy a lot during the day? In school? While driving? (C) |
| **A**wakenings during the night | Does your child wake up a lot at night? | • Does your child seem to wake up a lot at night? Any sleepwalking or nightmares? (P)<br>• Do you wake up a lot at night?<br>• Have trouble getting back to sleep? (C) | • Do you wake up a lot at night?<br>• Have trouble getting back to sleep? (C) |
| **R**egularity and duration of sleep | • Does your child have a regular bedtime and wake time?<br>• What are they? | • What time does your child go to bed and get up on school days?<br>• Weekends?<br>• Do you think he/she is getting enough sleep? (P) | • What time do you usually go to bed on school nights?<br>• Weekends? How much sleep do you usually get? (C) |
| **S**leep-disordered breathing | Does your child snore a lot or have difficulty breathing at night? | Does your child have loud or nightly snoring or any breathing difficulties at night? (P) | Does your teenager snore loudly or nightly? (P) |

([BEARS: Bedtime problems; Excessive daytime sleepiness; Awakenings during the night; Regularity and duration of sleep; Sleep-disordered breathing] C: child; P: parent)

Stress management and relaxation techniques along with life skills education should be imparted to adolescents with mental distress. Comorbidities such as obesity and hypertension should be managed according to standard clinical guidelines. Psychiatric issues should be managed appropriately by psychotherapy and psychopharmacology

**BOX 3:** Treatment of delayed sleep-wake phase disorder (DSPD).

- At least half hour prior to the planned bedtime bright lights should be avoided
- Sleep time needs to be shifted earlier; keep shifting 15–20 minutes early everyday
- Smaller doses of melatonin (0.5–1 mg can be considered). It must be taken 4–6 hours prior to the current bedtime
- Try to get an early morning sunlight; exposure to morning light helps in shifting circadian sleep rhythm to earlier time
- Schedule same work all through the week for sleep time as well as wake time

(*Source:* American Academy of Sleep Medicine. International Classification of Sleep Disorders: Diagnostic and Coding Manual, 2nd edition. Westchester, IL: American Academy of Sleep Medicine; 2005.)

**BOX 4:** Basic principles of sleep hygiene.

- Wake up and bedtime should be at the same time daily even on non-school days.
- To catch up lost sleep do not sleep on weekends
- Daytime naps should be short <1 hour (those with problems falling asleep at night should avoid napping) and early to mid-afternoon is ideal
- Spend time daily outside. Exposure to sunlight keeps circadian rhythm on check
- Regular exercise
- Bed must be used only for sleeping. The bedroom should have an ambient cool temperature
- Involve in relaxing, and enjoyable activities 0.5–1 hour before sleep time. Do not indulge in vigorous exercise or arguments
- One hour prior to bedtime do not engage in watching television or digital devices. Bedroom should be a media-free zone
- Eat regular meals and do not go to bed hungry
- Avoid eating or drinking caffeine-containing products such as cocoa beverages, coffee, or chocolates
- Do not consume alcohol and do not smoke
- Avoid using sleeping pills, melatonin, or other no-prescription sleep aids unless prescribed by doctor. These can be dangerous, and sleep problems often return when one stops taking the medicine

and referral to mental health professional, if required. As a step toward maintaining good quality and quantity of sleep it is advisable for later school start time for middle and high school.

## ■ SLEEP HYGIENE FOR ADOLESCENTS

Few basic principles for healthy sleep for adolescents are provided in **Box 4**.

## ■ CONCLUSION

Pediatricians need to stress on good sleep hygiene and provide anticipatory guidance to children, adolescents, and parents. It is important to screen for various sleep disorders and the comorbidities associated with unhealthy sleep patterns in office practice so that early interventions can be planned for better results.

## ■ POINTS TO REMEMBER

- Good quality and quantity of sleep forms the core for optimal functioning of an adolescent.
- Pediatricians should advice about sleep hygiene.
- BEARS sleep screening tool can be used in office practice.
- Adolescents with serious sleeping disorder need tailored therapy.
- Parents should be educated about instilling sleep hygiene from early childhood which needs to continue into adolescent life and thereafter.

## ■ SUGGESTED READING

1. Akbar SA, Mattfeld AT, Laird AR, McMakin DL. Sleep to Internalizing Pathway in Young Adolescents (SIPYA): a proposed neurodevelopmental model. Neurosci Biobehav Rev. 2022;140:104780.
2. Alfonsi V, Scarpelli S, D'Atri A, Stella G, De Gennaro L. Later school start time: the impact of sleep on academic performance and health in the adolescent population. Int J Environ Res Public Health. 2020;17(7):2574.
3. American Psychiatric Association. Diagnostic and Statistical Manual of Mental Disorders, 5th edition. Arlington: American Psychiatric Association Publishing; 2013.
4. Bartel K, Gradisar M, Williamson P. Protective and risk factors for adolescent sleep: A meta-analytic review. Sleep Med Rev. 2015;21:72-85.
5. Buchmann A, Ringli M, Kurth S, Schaerer M, Geiger A, Jenni OG, et al. EEG sleep slow-wave activity as a mirror of cortical maturation. Cereb Cortex. 2011;21(3):607-15.
6. Carskadon MA, Acebo C, Jenni OG. Regulation of adolescent sleep: implications for behavior. Ann N Y Acad Sci. 2004;1021:276-91.
7. Fatima Y, Doi SA, Mamun AA. Longitudinal impact of sleep on overweight and obesity in children and adolescents: a systematic review and bias-adjusted meta-analysis. Obes Rev. 2015;16(2):137-49.
8. Fonseca APLM, de Azevedo CVM, Santos RMR. Sleep and health-related physical fitness in children and adolescents: a systematic review. Sleep Sci. 2021;14(4):357-65.
9. Galland BC, Short MA, Terrill P, Rigney G, Haszard JJ, Coussens S, et al. Establishing normal values for pediatric night-time sleep measured by actigraphy: A systematic review and meta-analysis. Sleep. 2018;41(4).
10. Hale L, Guan S. Screen time and sleep among school-aged children and adolescents: A systematic literature review. Sleep Med Rev. 2015;21:50-8.
11. Khor SP, McClure A, Aldridge G, Bei B, Yap MB. Modifiable parental factors in adolescent sleep: A systematic review and meta-analysis. Sleep Med Rev. 2021;56:101408.
12. Kuciene R, Dulskiene V. Associations of short sleep duration with prehypertension and hypertension among Lithuanian children and adolescents: a cross-sectional study. BMC Public Health. 2014;14:255.
13. Lovato N, Gradisar M, Short M, Dohnt H, Micic G. Delayed sleep phase disorder in an Australian school-based sample of adolescents. J Clin Sleep Med. 2013;9(9):939-94.

14. Mathew G, Varghese AD, Benjamin AI. A Comparative Study Assessing Sleep Duration and Associated Factors among Adolescents Studying in Different Types of Schools in an Urban Area of Kerala, India. Indian J Community Med. 2019;44(Suppl 1):S10-3.
15. Mayne SL, Morales KH, Williamson AA, Grant SFA, Fiks AG, Basner M, et al. Associations of the residential built environment with adolescent sleep outcomes. Sleep. 2021;44(6):zsaa276.
16. Moitra P, Madan J, Verma P. Independent and combined influences of physical activity, screen time, and sleep quality on adiposity indicators in Indian adolescents. BMC Public Health. 2021;21:2093.
17. Murugesan G, Karthigeyan L, Selvagandhi PK, Gopichandran V. Sleep patterns, hygiene, and daytime sleepiness among adolescent school-goers in three districts of Tamil Nadu: a descriptive study. Natl Med J India. 2018;31:196-200.
18. Navarro-Solera M, Carrasco-Luna J, Pin-Arboledas G, González-Carrascosa R, Soriano JM, Codoñer-Franch P. Short sleep duration is related to emerging cardiovascular risk factors in obese children. J Pediatr Gastroenterol Nutr. 2015;61(5):571-6.
19. Ohayon MM, Carskadon MA, Guilleminault C, Vitiello MV. Meta-analysis of quantitative sleep parameters from childhood to old age in healthy individuals: developing normative sleep values across the human lifespan. Sleep. 2004;27:1255-73.
20. Owens J; Adolescent Sleep Working Group; Committee on Adolescence. Insufficient sleep-in adolescents and young adults: an update on causes and consequences. Pediatrics. 2014;134(3):e921-32.
21. Owens JA, Dalzell V. Use of the "BEARS" sleep screening tool in a pediatric residents' continuity clinic: a pilot study. Sleep Med. 2005;6(1):63-9.
22. Paruthi S, Brooks LJ, D'Ambrosio C, Hall WA, Kotagal S, Lloyd RM, et al. Consensus statement of the American Academy of sleep medicine on the recommended amount of sleep for healthy children: methodology and discussion. J Clin Sleep Med. 2016;12(11):1549-61.
23. Prono F, Bernardi K, Ferri R, Bruni O. The role of vitamin D in sleep disorders of children and adolescents: a systematic review. Int J Mol Sci. 2022;23(3):1430.
24. Ramos Socarras L, Potvin J, Forest G. COVID-19 and sleep patterns in adolescents and young adults. Sleep Med. 2021;83:26-33.
25. Schrimpf M, Liegl G, Boeckle M, Leitner A, Geisler P, Pieh C. The effect of sleep deprivation on pain perception in healthy subjects: a meta-analysis. Sleep Med. 2015;16:1313-20.
26. Singh R, Suri J, Sharma R, Suri T, Adhikari T. Sleep Pattern of Adolescents in a School in Delhi, India: Impact on their Mood and Academic Performance. Indian J Pediatr. 2018;85:1-8.
27. Tarokh L, Saletin JM, Carskadon MA. Sleep in adolescence: physiology, cognition, and mental health. Neurosci Biobehav Rev. 2016;70:182-8.
28. Tashjian SM, Mullins JL, Galvan A. Bedtime autonomy and cellphone use influence sleep duration in adolescents. J Adolesc Health. 2019;64:124-30.
29. Wheaton AG, Chapman DP, Croft JB. School start times, sleep, behavioural, health, and academic outcomes: a review of the literature. J Sch Health. 2016;86:363-81.
30. Willis TA, Gregory AM. Anxiety disorders and sleep in children and adolescents. Sleep Med Clin. 2015;10(2):125-31.

# CHAPTER 15

# Dermatological Issues in Adolescence

*Shivangi Bora, Mary Augustine*

## ■ DEFINING ADOLESCENCE

According to the World Health Organization (WHO), adolescence is the phase of life between childhood and adulthood, from ages 10 to 19 years. Adolescents experience rapid physical, cognitive, and psychosocial growth. Despite being thought of as a healthy stage of life, there is a fair share of health issues that adolescents face, some of which have long-term significant aftereffects. Ensuring appropriate health education, supportive environment and acceptable healthcare opportunities are vital in responding to adolescents' specific needs and rights.

An evolving concern regarding the external appearance, in terms of their skin, hair, or overall body image, is a hallmark of adolescence, and hence needs special attention.

## ■ SKIN CHANGES DURING ADOLESCENCE

Just as overall growth and maturation in adolescence are influenced by the hormonal variations, skin and its subunits also undergo significant alterations, primarily under the same hormonal influence. Increased circulating levels of androgens cause maturation of several skin appendages. Terminal hair growth is stimulated in the axillae and pubis in both sexes, and additionally on the face and chest in boys. Apocrine sweat glands, predominantly distributed in the axillae, pubic and perineal areas, begin functioning and produce an odorless liquid secretion that is altered by bacterial action to produce a body odor that is sometimes unpleasant. Sebaceous glands enlarge and increase the production of sebum, which is composed of triglycerides that yield free fatty acids when hydrolyzed by skin bacteria. The normal anatomy of skin is shown in **Figure 1**.

Most chronic skin conditions that may start in childhood or adolescence tend to cause severe psychological impairment in adolescents, as body image, self-esteem, and peer interaction suffers. Proper counseling and regular treatment with qualified dermatologists will help them cope with these issues. Some of the common skin diseases are typically associated with adolescence,

# CHAPTER 15: Dermatological Issues in Adolescence

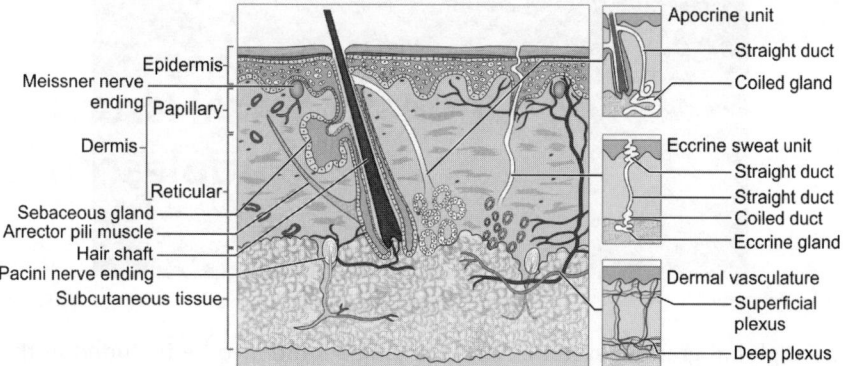

**Fig. 1:** Anatomy and physiology of the skin.
*Source:* Kolarsick PAJ, Kolarsick MA, Goodwin C. Anatomy and Physiology of the Skin. J Dermatol Nurses Assoc. 2011;3(4):203-13.

whereas certain diseases are common in them due to circumstances such as living in hostels and being active in sports.

## ◼ ACNE VULGARIS

Acne, one of the most common skin disease, is a chronic inflammatory disease of the pilosebaceous unit, with onset in adolescence and occurring in 80% of teenagers. It usually presents between the ages of 10 and 13 years in both sexes but at a younger age in girls aligning with earlier puberty. Prevalence of acne is more in females although that of severe acne is higher in males. Susceptibility to adolescent acne seems to be more strongly linked to the maternal than the paternal line. Acne results from the combination of increased sebaceous gland activity with seborrhea, abnormal follicular differentiation with increased keratinization, microbial hypercolonization of the follicular canal, and increased inflammation primarily through activation of the adaptive immune system.

### Clinical Features

Acne is characterized by open and closed comedones (blackheads and whiteheads) papules, pustules, and nodules of varying degree of inflammation and depth, most commonly affecting the face (99%) followed by back (60%) and chest (15%). The clinical picture varies from very mild comedonal acne, with or without sparse inflammatory lesions, to aggressive fulminant disease **(Fig. 2)**. Scarring is commonly seen as a consequence of acne and can present as atrophic scarring or hypertrophic or keloid scarring.

### Investigations

Severity is assessed visually according to the extent of disease and number of lesions. The Leeds photometric grading scale is the most commonly

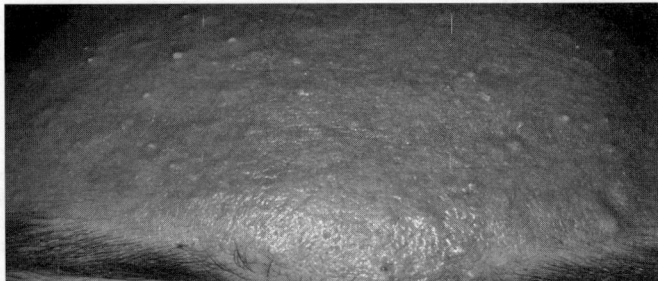

**Fig. 2:** Adolescent acne.

used global grading system. Acne scarring should also be included in the assessment of acne severity.

History should include use of occlusive topical applications, drug history including topical or systemic steroids, and features suggestive of underlying endocrinopathy.

## Psychosocial Complications

Acne and the resultant scarring lead to long-lasting psychosocial effects that affect the patient's quality of life. Depression, social isolation, and suicidal ideation are frequent comorbidities of acne, which should be addressed appropriately.

## Aims of Acne Management

- Alleviate symptoms
- Clear existing lesions
- Limit disease activity by preventing new lesions forming as well as scars developing
- Avoid negative impact on quality of life.

## Treatment Algorithm for Management of Acne

**Flowcharts 1 to 3** explain management of acne in general.

## Other Treatments

A variety of lasers and other light sources, chemical peels, and comedone extraction are also helpful, in combination with topical treatment.

Frequent cleansing, scrubbing, exfoliants, etc., will worsen acne. Skin and hair should be kept clean with the use of mild cleansers. Moisturizers can be used for dry skin, especially following topical retinoids. Liberal use of hair oil is to be discouraged. Cosmetics and sunscreens should be water based and noncomedogenic.

Although the role of diet in acne is still controversial, high glycemic index and carbohydrate intake have a modest yet significant proacnegenic effect.

**Flowchart 1:** Management of comedonal acne.

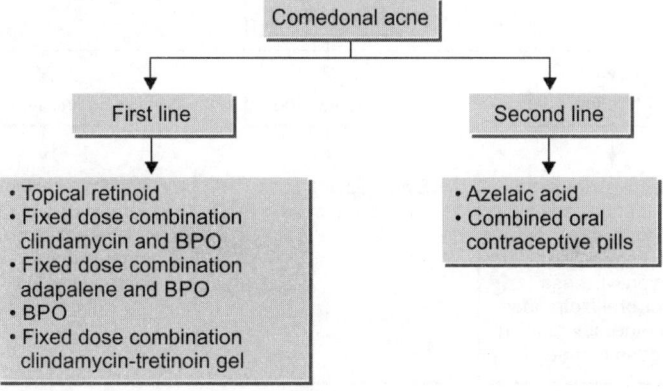

(BPO: benzoyl peroxide)

*Source:* Griffiths CEM, Bleiker TO, Creamer D, Ingram JR, Simpson RV. Rook's Dermatology Handbook, 1st edition. New York, United States: Wiley-Blackwell; 2021.

**Flowchart 2:** Management of mild-to-moderate papulopustular acne.

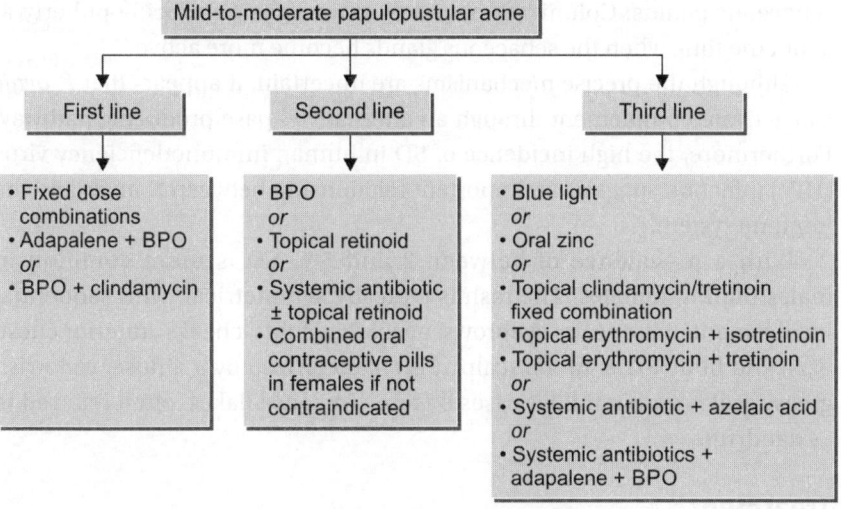

(BPO: benzoyl peroxide)

*Source:* Griffiths CEM, Bleiker TO, Creamer D, Ingram JR, Simpson RV. Rook's Dermatology Handbook, 1st edition. New York, United States: Wiley-Blackwell; 2021.

Dairy consumption is also implicated in populations with predominantly Western diet.

## ■ SEBORRHEIC DERMATITIS

Seborrheic dermatitis (SD) is a common inflammatory papulosquamous skin disease of the seborrheic areas, usually associated with the commensal

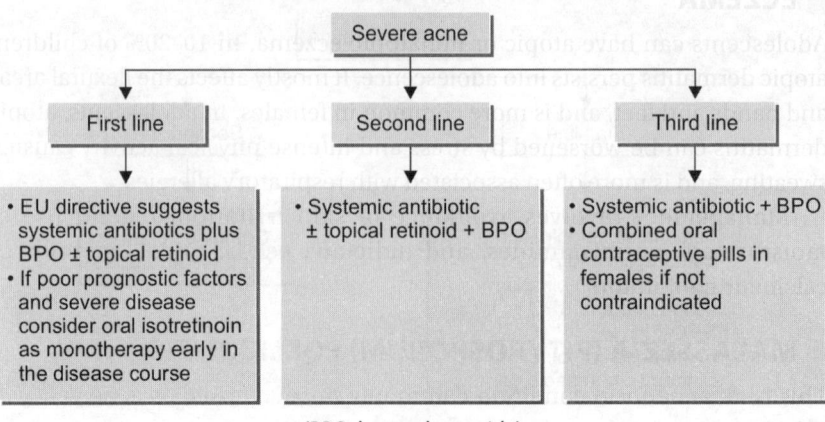

**Flowchart 3:** Management of severe acne.

(BPO: benzoyl peroxide)
*Source*: Griffiths CEM, Bleiker TO, Creamer D, Ingram JR, Simpson RV. Rook's Dermatology Handbook, 1st edition. New York, United States: Wiley-Blackwell; 2021.

lipophilic yeast *Pityrosporum ovale* found in the acroinfundibulum of sebaceous glands. Colonization with *P. ovale* increases during puberty at about the time when the sebaceous glands become more active.

Although the precise mechanisms are uncertain, it appears that *P. ovale* can activate complement through an alternative lipase producing pathway. Furthermore, the high incidence of SD in human immunodeficiency virus (HIV) infection suggests an important relationship between *P. ovale* and the immune system.

With a prevalence of between 2 and 5%, SD is more common in males than in females. The rash is typically symmetrical, with sequential involvement of the scalp, eyebrows, nasolabial folds, cheeks, anterior chest, ears, and body folds. In the scalp, it is characterized by a diffuse, yellowish greasy scales and in milder cases by fine, dry loose flakes, often referred to as dandruff.

## Treatment

Topical antifungals such as ketoconazole and ciclopiroxolamine in the form of shampoos, stay-on lotions, and cream are the mainstay of treatment for control of SD. These may have to be continued for long periods as SD is a chronic condition. Short exacerbations can be managed with mild topical steroids or calcineurin inhibitors such as tacrolimus and pimecrolimus.

Seborrheic dermatitis of the scalp should be differentiated from psoriasis which presents with well-defined plaques and dry white scales. The chronic and recurrent nature of SD should also be explained to the patient.

## ECZEMA

Adolescents can have atopic or nonatopic eczema. In 10-20% of children, atopic dermatitis persists into adolescence. It mostly affects the flexural areas and hands and feet, and is more common in females. In adolescents, atopic dermatitis can be worsened by stress and intense physical activity causing sweating, and is more often associated with respiratory allergies.

Management involves avoidance of skin irritation, regular use of moisturizers, antihistamines, and judicious use of topical steroids or calcineurin inhibitors.

## MALASSEZIA (PITYROSPORUM) FOLLICULITIS

This is an acneiform condition commonly misdiagnosed as acne vulgaris. It is caused by *Malassezia* species, commensal yeasts of seborrheic areas. These patients fail to respond to typical acne medications, and present with pruritic, 1-2 mm monomorphic papules, and pustules. The yeast can be demonstrated by direct microscopy. This disease occurs more commonly in hot and humid environments and is aggravated by occlusive clothing or topical applications and long-term antibiotics for acne. It responds well to antifungals, particularly to oral itraconazole.

## KERATOSIS PILARIS

This is a common autosomal dominant disorder of follicular hyperkeratosis, mostly beginning during adolescence. It is characterized by small, folliculocentric keratotic papules that may have surrounding erythema, giving the appearance of gooseflesh, most commonly affecting the extensor aspects of the upper arms, thighs, and buttocks. Treatment options include regular use of emollients and topical keratolytics such as salicylic acid, urea, retinoids, and chemical peels. The condition is chronic, although it may fade with time.

## STRIAE

Striae distensae, commonly referred to as stretch marks, is a sequelae of growth spurts, sudden weight gain or loss **(Fig. 3)**. Adolescent striae are most commonly found over the thighs, gluteal region, lumbosacral area, shoulders, and breasts. The incidence has been estimated to be up to 70% in females and 40% in males. During the earliest stages, patients may describe minor pruritus or irritation. As striae progress, they gradually fade in color and the end result is a white, atrophic, and depressed lesion, that is often subtle enough to be overlooked.

Striae distensae are often of primarily cosmetic concern to patients. As these stretch marks often tend to regress spontaneously with time, in most instances treatment is not recommended. Topical tretinoin cream (0.1%) has been shown to decrease the length and width of striae if applied during

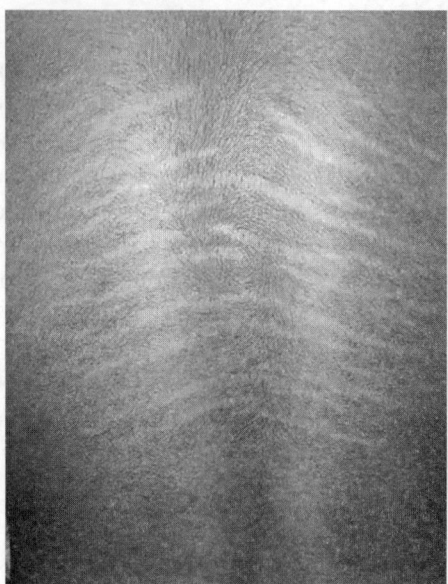

**Fig. 3:** Striae.

the early stages of evolution. Other topical therapeutic regimens, including 0.05% tretinoin, 20% glycolic acid, 10% L-ascorbic acid, and 20% glycolic acid, may also be effective.

## ■ FUNGAL INFECTIONS

Fungal infections are very common in the adolescent age group, especially those caused by dermatophytes. Dermatophytosis, also known as tinea, and commonly called ringworm, has specific predilection for different sites of the body. They spread by direct contact with soil, infected surfaces, or contact with infected body area. Sharing of clothes and common laundry in hostel settings make adolescents vulnerable to these infections. Rampant use of topical steroids makes the disease chronic, extensive, and recalcitrant. The common types of dermatophytosis in adolescence are the following:

- *Tinea cruris (commonly known as jock itch):* This is a superficial fungal infection of inguinal folds, perineal and perianal areas, common in adolescent males, and postpubertal females. Moist, nonaerated areas of skin such as in between skin folds can give rise to maceration which is a perfect breeding ground for dermatophytes. Summer, sweating, obesity, and tight fitting under garments increase the risk.
- *Tinea pedis (commonly known as athlete's foot):* Infection is usually in between toes where moist skin nurtures dermatophytes, producing itchy, macerated lesions with fissuring and often a foul odor. Common risk

factors are use of community shower stalls at schools, swimming pools, sports clubs, sharing slippers, socks and shoes, and wearing shoes for long time.

## Management

Most infections are diagnosed purely on clinical judgment, although a potassium hydroxide (KOH) preparation can provide a cheap, quick, and highly sensitive (88%) method of confirming the diagnosis.

Treatment is with topical (e.g., clotrimazole, miconazole, luliconazole, sertaconazole, terbinafine, and amorolfine) and systemic (e.g., terbinafine, itraconazole, and griseofulvin) antifungals. These should be used for adequate period of time, depending upon the area involved, irrespective of clinical clearance. Equally important is general measures such as daily bath, keeping skin dry, proper washing and drying of clothes, especially undergarments, treatment of infected contacts, and avoiding sharing of clothes and personal items.

## ■ SCABIES

Scabies, caused by an arthropod *Sarcoptes scabiei var hominis*, affects people of all social classes and ages, but it is more commonly seen in children and adolescents, because of close physical contact. Typical lesions are small linear brownish lesions called burrows, most commonly seen in between the finger webs, but also can be found along the sides of fingers, flexor aspects of wrist, elbows, axilla, buttocks, and genitalia.

## Treatment

Permethrin 5% cream is effective and safe when applied to the whole body from chin downward and washed off after 8–12 hours, with reapplication recommended after 2 weeks. Oral ivermectin is shown to be effective treatment when topical treatment is not effective or disease is severe and widespread. The whole family or contacts should also be treated regardless of their symptoms.

## ■ FOCAL HYPERHIDROSIS

A study reported that up to 1.6% of children and adolescents younger than 18 years of age had primary focal hyperhidrosis. Although the cause of this disorder is unknown, one suggestion is that it could be an abnormal or exaggerated central response to normal emotional stress. Palmar hyperhidrosis can interfere with shaking hands when one meets people and also with school work and activities that require dry hands. Plantar and craniofacial hyperhidrosis can cause physical and social discomfort. Axillary hyperhidrosis can produce skin maceration and wet clothing, leading to frequent clothing changes during the day.

## Treatment

Most treatment options, except surgical sympathectomy, bring about remissions that last only for a few months and therefore patients should be counseled accordingly. Topical therapy with antiperspirants helps in controlling axillary hyperhidrosis. The mechanism of action is thought to be physical blockage of the eccrine sweat gland leading to structural and functional degeneration of the sweat glands. Iontophoresis, a method in which an electric current is passed through tissue is effective, but needs multiple sittings. If topical therapy fails to control, botulinum toxin A can be used.

## ■ PLANTAR WARTS

Plantar warts, or verruca plantaris, are cutaneous lesions on the plantar aspect of the foot that are caused by the infection of keratinocytes with the human papillomavirus (HPV). Plantar warts exhibit an annual incidence of 14%. The majority of cases occur in children and adolescents. Once a plantar wart is established, it sheds HPV via desquamated epithelial cells. The viral particles can subsequently infect other sites and hosts.

Once infection occurs, three outcomes are possible: clearance of the infection with resultant immunity to that particular HPV type, latent infection, or clinically manifested infection as a plantar wart.

Young children experience a steady increase in warts as they age until a peak incidence between 12 and 16 years of age. Athletes have been observed to have higher rates of warts, including plantar warts, compared with the general population. Hyperhidrosis of the feet is associated with increased risk of plantar warts. Patients with plantar warts most commonly present with pain or the sensation of a stone or swelling under their foot. Pain most commonly occurs with activities that exert pressure on the soles of the feet. Physicians may choose to initially pursue a wait-and-see approach for immunocompetent patients, with most plantar warts resolving within 2 years. The two most common treatments for plantar warts are topical salicylic acid and cryotherapy with liquid nitrogen.

## ■ SEXUALLY TRANSMITTED INFECTION

Although not very frequently seen, sexually transmitted infections (STIs) are a rapidly emerging group of illnesses in the adolescent age group. More so because of the lower age having sexual contact at present times. The skin manifestations are myriad which can lead to a lot of stress and therefore proper counseling, sexual education, and need for protection like vaccination with HPV needs to be stressed and made available to this group of individuals who form a huge dividend of the society.

## HAIR AND HIRSUTISM

Hair abnormalities can have tremendous psychosocial impacts on adolescents, leading to a great amount of anxiety regarding physical appearance and potential clinical course. The pathophysiology varies from congenital, infectious, autoimmune, nutritional, or environmental. An abnormal increase in hair is present in hypertrichosis and hirsutism. Many hair disorders may have no cure, where pediatricians can have a positive impact by identifying the abnormality and educating the patient regarding disease course. Hirsutism is defined as male-pattern growth of terminal body hair in women in androgen-stimulated locations such as face, chest, and areolae. It can be classified broadly into two groups, viz., androgen induced and nonandrogen induced. Androgen induced can either be due to excessive endogenous androgen production (ovarian/adrenal) or exogenous due to drugs. It can mainly be treated by two approaches: (1) Cosmetically—electrolysis and photoepilation (laser and intense pulsed light) which are effective in reducing hair and (2) Pharmacologically—targeting the androgen production and action to minimize hair regrowth. These can be used concomitantly.

## TATTOOING

Recently, tattooing has gained increasing popularity worldwide especially among adolescents. In Western society, tattooing have become mainstream activity among adolescents and young adults. Prevalence of tattooing in these age groups vary, ranging from 1–24%. Evidence showed that tattooed individuals have a higher risk of being infected by blood-borne viruses, including hepatitis B and C and HIV. Information about their knowledge and practices could help in effective planning for health promotion strategies and appropriate preventive measures by healthcare providers and parents who are in contact with adolescents to help them make informed choices. Furthermore, collaborative educational programs could be developed between healthcare providers and schools, sharing information about body art in general, including the inherent risks associated with it, and encouraging adolescents to contemplate their decisions carefully in advance.

## COSMETOLOGY AND ADOLESCENTS

As a child enters teenage, they become more preoccupied by his or her appearance as a communication of identity and attractiveness to others. Teenagers seek remedies to their skin conditions with toiletries, including cleansers, photoprotective products, and hydrating agents. Teenagers are fans of hair conditioners and hair cosmetics, including gels, mousses, or foams, temporary colors in bold shades, bleaching products, and waving products. Protein hydrolysates (collagen, keratin, elastin, milk, wheat, almond, and silk) are frequently added to hair care products and can cause contact urticaria. Cosmetics claiming to be natural usually attract adolescents, they believe that the products referred to as natural have special effectiveness and are more compatible with human physiology. As such teenagers tend to incline more for such cosmetic items to enhance their outward appearance either under peer pressure or to be more appealing to others in their social group.

## COUNSELING

Of importance in this discussion remains the core of the adolescent to identify oneself and understand that a strong inner self is far more appealing to the society at large and gives one the boost to transition into a confident and independent adult. Therefore a detailed HEEADSSS history and a detailed counseling of the teen along with his/her parents is important to enable them to accommodate better with their environment and surroundings.

## CONCLUSION

Adolescence is a period of rapid changes. The young adolescent is already burdened with dealing with a myriad of problems as their body transitions through a whole spectrum of changes. Having a skin condition, even if only of cosmetic importance, has an impact on their psychological functioning and self-esteem.

## POINTS TO REMEMBER

- Adolescence is a very sensitive phase of life.
- The problems of adolescents are unique to each and needs individual care and attention.
- Skin and complexion play an important role in the appearance of an adolescent and therefore their issues should be addressed patiently and genuinely.
- Proper redressal of their issues can enable them to grow into healthy adults socially and emotionally as well.
- Early recognition and timely management of their problems can avert long-term treatments.

## ACKNOWLEDGMENT

I would like to thank all my adolescent patients who gave me this opportunity and encouragement to work on various aspects of adolescent pediatrics.

## SUGGESTED READING

1. Akram S, Zaman H. Warts and verrucas: assessment and treatment. Pharm J. 2015; 294(7867).
2. Ash K, Lord J, Zukowskl M, McDaniel DH. Comparison of topical therapy for striae alba (20% glycolic acid/0.05% tretinoin versus 20% glycolic acid/10% L-ascorbic acid). Dermatol Surg. 1998;24(8):849-56.
3. Bacelieri R, Johnson SM. Cutaneous warts: an evidence-based approach to therapy. Am Fam Physician. 2005;72(4):647-52.
4. Bellet JS. Diagnosis and treatment of primary focal hyperhidrosis in children and adolescents. Semin Cutan Med Surg. 2010;29(2):121-6).
5. Bruggink SC, Eekhof JA, Egberts PF, van Blijswijk SC, Assendelft WJ, Gussekloo J. Warts transmitted in families and schools: a prospective cohort. Pediatrics. 2013;131(5):928-34.
6. Bruggink SC, Gussekloo J, de Koning MN, Feltkamp MC, Bavinck JN, Quint WG, et al. HPV type in plantar warts influences natural course and treatment response: secondary analysis of a randomised controlled trial. J Clin Virol. 2013;57(3):227-32.
7. Burns T, Breathnach SM, Cox N, Griffiths C. Rook's Textbook of Dermatology. New York, United States: John Wiley & Sons; 2008.
8. Chosidow O. Scabies and pediculosis. Lancet. 2000;355(9206):819-26.
9. Faergemann J. Pityrosporum infections. J Am Acad Dermatol. 1994;31(3):S18-20.
10. Feinberg AN, Shwayder TA, Tereen R, Tempark T. Dermatology: Pediatric and adolescent medicine. Int J Child Health Human Develop. 2015;8(3):257.
11. Ghadgepatil SS, Gupta S, Sharma YK. Clinicoepidemiological study of different types of warts. Dermatol Res Pract. 2016;2016:7989817.
12. Gieler U, Gieler T, Kupfer JP. Acne and quality of life-impact and management. J Eur Acad Dermatol Venereol. 2015;29:12-4.
13. Harper J, Oranje AP. Harper's Textbook of Pediatric Dermatology. New York, United States: John Wiley & Sons; 2019.
14. Heller D. Lesson of the week: lumbar physiological striae in adolescence suspected to be non-accidental injury. BMJ. 1995;311(7007):738.
15. Heng AH, Chew FT. Systematic review of the epidemiology of acne vulgaris. Sci Rep. 2020;10:5754.
16. Hwang S, Schwartz RA. Keratosis pilaris: a common follicular hyperkeratosis. Cutis. 2008;82(3):177-80.
17. Kang S. Topical tretinoin therapy for management of early striae. J Am Acad Dermatol. 1998;39(2):S90-2.
18. Krishna SK, Jethwa AS. Human papillomavirus infections in adults and children. Am J Epidemiol Infect Dis. 2013;1(2):11-9.
19. Kubba R, Bajaj AK, Thappa DM, Sharma R, Vedamurthy M, Dhar S, et al. Cosmetics and skin care in acne. Indian J Dermatol Venereol Leprol. 2009; 75(S1):55-6.
20. Levit F. Simple device for treatment of hyperhidrosis by iontophoresis. Arch Dermatol. 1968;98(5):505-7.
21. Lipke MM. An armamentarium of wart treatments. Clin Med Res. 2006;4(4): 273-93.
22. Lonsdale-Eccles A, Leonard N, Lawrence C. Axillary hyperhidrosis: eccrine or apocrine? Clin Exp Dermatol. 2003;28(1):2-7.

23. Lowe NJ, Glaser DA, Eadie N, Daggett S, Kowalski JW, Lai PY, et al. Botulinum toxin type A in the treatment of primary axillary hyperhidrosis: a 52-week multicenter double-blind, randomized, placebo-controlled study of efficacy and safety. J Am Acad Dermatol. 2007;56(4):604-11.
24. Marcoux D. Appearance, cosmetics, and body art in adolescents. Dermatol Clin. 2000;18(4):667-73.
25. McDaniel DH, Ash K, Zukowski M. Treatment of stretch marks with the 585-nm flash lamp-pumped pulsed dye laser. Dermatol Surg. 1996;22(4):332-7.
26. Meixiong J, Ricco C, Vasavda C, Ho BK. Diet and acne: A systematic review. JAAD international. 2022;7:95-112.
27. Oinam J, Singh AB, Singh YN. Prevalence of tattooing and knowledge about health risk associated with it among adolescent school students in Manipur, North-eastern India: a cross-sectional study. Int J Community Med Public Health, 2019;6(2):774-9.
28. Rai R, Natarajan K. Laser and light based treatments of acne. Indian J Dermatol Venereol Leprol. 2013;79(3):300-9.
29. Ricci G, Bellini F, Dondi A, Patrizi A, Pession A. Atopic dermatitis in adolescence. Dermatol Reports. 2012;4(1):e1.
30. Rubenstein RM, Malerich SA. Malassezia (pityrosporum) folliculitis. J Clin Aesthet Dermatol. 2014;7(3):37-41.
31. Sanclemente G, Gill DK. Human papillomavirus molecular biology and pathogenesis. J Eur Acad Dermatol Venereol. 2002;16(3):231-40.
32. Sharma NL, Mahajan VK, Jindal R, Gupta M, Lath A. Hirsutism: Clinico-investigative profile of 50 Indian patients. Indian J Dermatol. 2008;53(3):111.
33. Sheu HM, Yu HS, Chang CH. Mast cell degranulation and elastolysis in the early stage of striae distensae. J Cutan Pathol. 1991;18(6):410-6.
34. Singh S, Chouhan K, Gupta S. Intralesional immunotherapy with killed Mycobacterium indicus pranii vaccine for the treatment of extensive cutaneous warts. Indian J Dermatol Venereol Leprol. 2014;80(6):509.
35. Sisson WR. Colored striae in adolescent children. J Pediatr. 1954;45(5):520-30.
36. Sladden MJ, Johnston GA. Common skin infections in children. BMJ. 2004;329(7457):95-9.
37. Sterling JC, Gibbs S, Haque Hussain SS, Mohd Mustapa MF, Handfield-Jones SE, Hughes JR, et al. British Association of Dermatologists' guidelines for the management of cutaneous warts 2014. Br J Dermatol. 2014;171(4):696-712.
38. Strutton DR, Kowalski JW, Glaser DA, Stang PE. US prevalence of hyperhidrosis and impact on individuals with axillary hyperhidrosis: results from a national survey. J Am Acad Dermatol. 2004;51(2):241-8.
39. Sudhakar GK, Pai V, Pai A, Kamath V. Therapeutic approaches in the management of plantar warts by human papillomaviruses: a review. Asian J Biomed Pharma Sci. 2013;3(26):1-4.
40. Turgeon EW. Adolescent skin: How to keep it healthy. Can Fam Physician. 1986;32:2427-33.
41. Watkins P. Identifying and treating plantar warts. Nurs Stand. 2006;20(42):50-4.
42. Witchey DJ, Witchey NB, Roth-Kauffman MM, Kauffman MK. Plantar warts: epidemiology, pathophysiology, and clinical management. J Osteopath Med. 2018;118(2):92-105.

# CHAPTER 16

# Irritable Bowel Syndrome in Children and Adolescents

*Ramaswamy Ganesh, Suresh Natarajan, Malathi Sathiyasekaran*

## ■ INTRODUCTION

Irritable bowel syndrome (IBS) is a common functional gastrointestinal disorder (FGID) seen in adults and children characterized by abdominal discomfort, abdominal pain, bloating, and altered bowel pattern (form or frequency) of defecation in the absence of an identifiable organic cause on routine investigations. Manning's criteria introduced in 1978 reiterated that IBS was a positive diagnosis and not one of exclusion. The drawbacks with Manning's criteria paved the way for the introduction of Rome criteria which over the last three decades underwent several iterations through Rome I, II, III, and the last one Rome IV in 2016.

Rome IV includes an exhaustive coverage of all FGIDs. IBS is categorized under functional abdominal pain disorders (FAPDs) which include functional dyspepsia, abdominal migraine, functional abdominal pain not otherwise specified (NOS), and IBS. This is a symptom-based diagnosis as shown in **Box 1**.

## ■ SUBTYPES OF IRRITABLE BOWEL SYNDROME

Irritable bowel syndrome can be classified into the four subtypes **(Table 1)** based upon the stool consistency, using the Bristol stool chart **(Table 2)**.

**BOX 1:** Rome IV criteria for pediatric irritable bowel syndrome (IBS).

> Diagnostic criteria for irritable bowel syndrome fulfilled for at least 2 months before diagnosis must include all of the following:
> - Abdominal pain at least 4 days per month associated with one or more of the following:
>   – Related to defecation
>   – A change in frequency of stool
>   – A change in form (appearance) of stool
> - In children with constipation, the pain does not resolve with resolution of the constipation (children in whom the pain resolves have functional constipation, not irritable bowel syndrome)
> - After appropriate evaluation, the symptoms cannot be fully explained by another medical condition

**TABLE 1:** Subtypes of irritable bowel syndrome IBS.

| Subtypes | Definition |
|---|---|
| Constipation-predominant IBS (IBS-C) | >25% of bowel movements with Bristol stool form types 1 or 2 and <25% bowel movements with types 6 or 7 |
| Diarrhea-predominant IBS (IBS-D) | >25% of bowel movements with Bristol stool form types 6 or 7 and <25% bowel movements with types 1 or 2 |
| Mixed type IBS (IBS-M) | >25% of bowel movements with Bristol stool form types 1 or 2 and >25% bowel movements with types 6 or 7 |
| Unclassified IBS (IBS-U) | Patients who meet criteria for IBS but whose bowel habits cannot be categorized into 1 of the 3 groups above |

**TABLE 2:** Bristol stool form scale.

| Types | Diagrammatic representation | Description |
|---|---|---|
| Type I | | Separate hard lumps like nuts (hard to pass) |
| Type II | | Sausage shaped but lumpy |
| Type III | | Like a sausage but with cracks on the surface |
| Type IV | | Like a sausage or snake, smooth and soft |
| Type V | | Soft blobs with clear cut edges |
| Type VI | | Fluffy pieces with rugged edges, a mushy stool |
| Type VII | | Watery no solid pieces entirely liquid |

These subtype classification helps in therapy since drugs useful in diarrhea-predominant IBS (IBS-D) may aggravate symptoms if used in IBS type C.

## ■ EPIDEMIOLOGY

Prevalence of IBS in childhood is reported between 1.2 and 5.4% with a worldwide pooled prevalence of 13.8%. The prevalence in India is 7.5% in school children aged 10–17 years. The varying prevalence among countries is probably due to different Rome criteria used in their study. It is difficult to diagnose IBS in young children who cannot verbally express their problems. In the West, IBS constitutes 50% of functional abdominal pain in children. The prevalence of subtypes of IBS also differs with constipation-predominant IBS (IBS-C) being more common in Italy whereas in Greece and Nigeria nearly 50% are type mixed type IBS (IBS-M). The reported prevalence of the subtypes in Asia is uniform—30% among each in IBS-C, IBS-D, and IBS-M. The utility of these subtypes is however debatable as within 1 year, many are reported to change subtypes, and a third may switch between IBS-C and IBS-D.

## ■ PREDISPOSING RISK FACTORS

### Sex
Some studies have shown a higher prevalence in girls. However, this preponderance in girls is not universal.

### Age
The role of age in FAPD has been inconclusive probably because of the different age groups analyzed. The peak prevalence of IBS is 11 years in children and adolescents.

### Psychosocial Factors
Children with IBS have higher levels of anxiety and/or depression and/or emotional problems, higher stress levels or experienced stressful events such as physical, emotional, or sexual abuse, and have lower quality of life than healthy children. It has also been noted that children of mothers with IBS report disturbing gastrointestinal (GI) symptoms, have higher school absence with increase in hospital visits compared to children in control families.

### Early Life Events
Several early life events such as neonatal intensive care unit (NICU) hospitalizations, pyloric stenosis, and cow's milk protein allergy have been associated with IBS but not proven.

### Gastrointestinal Infections
Irritable bowel syndrome following GI infections is well recognized and is seen in nearly 10%. Postinfectious IBS (PI-IBS) has been reported more often with bacteria such as *Campylobacter* species, *Escherichia coli*, and *Salmonella* species and rarely following viral infection.

### Genetic Factors

A family history of IBS has been reported as an epidemiological risk factor. The overall concordance rate of IBS in twins is low though significantly higher in monozygotic twins (17.2%) than in dizygotic twins (8.4%) indicating that other factors social and environmental are at play.

### Other Factors

Atopy, spicy diet, and affluent socioeconomic status have been linked with IBS but more studies are required to prove this association.

## CLINICAL FEATURES

The clinical manifestations may be both intestinal and extraintestinal. The two main GI symptoms include chronic abdominal pain and alteration in bowel habits.

### Chronic Abdominal Pain

The pain in IBS is usually dull, crampy, colicky, or sharp in nature situated in the left iliac fossa, lower abdomen, or less often periumbilical. The child may also complain of discomfort and less often bloat. It has no specific pattern and can be aggravated by stress or food. These abdominal symptoms though associated with defecation are not relieved by passing stools unlike in functional constipation. The Asian study of IBS in adults has also reported dyspeptic symptoms in IBS.

### Defecation and Stools Pattern

Depending on the subtype, the stools may vary in form and consistency. Other features not included in the definition such as straining, urgency, and mucorrhea are also encountered in IBS. A sense of incomplete bowel emptying is a common symptom.

### Extraintestinal Symptoms

Non-GI symptoms such as headache, fatigue, back pain, myalgia, urinary frequency, and dizziness are more common in adult patients with IBS than controls. Children with IBS also suffer from somatic complaints and psychological issues such as maladjustment, depression, and anxiety.

## ALARM FEATURES

The presence of alarm features as shown in **(Box 2)** helps to consider the possibility of an organic disease necessitating investigations. On the contrary, the absence of red flag signs helps avoid unnecessary tests to some extent.

**BOX 2:** Alarm features indicating an organic disease.

- Family history of inflammatory bowel disease, celiac disease, or peptic ulcer disease
- Persistent right upper or lower abdominal pain
- Dysphagia
- Odynophagia
- Persistent vomiting
- Gastrointestinal blood loss
- Nocturnal diarrhea
- Arthritis
- Perirectal disease
- Involuntary weight loss
- Deceleration of linear growth
- Delayed puberty
- Unexplained fever

## ■ PATHOPHYSIOLOGY OF IRRITABLE BOWEL SYNDROME

It is now well recognized that the pathogenesis of IBS is multifactorial and in simple terms is considered as a gut-brain dysfunction. Two models have been proposed to explain the pathophysiology of IBS. In the "top-down model", the main pathophysiological changes are initiated in the brain whereas it is vice versa in the bottom up model. The FGIDs in the Rome IV system have been designated "disorders of gut-brain interaction" and this term is preferred to that of "brain-gut interaction" since the problem is initiated in the intestine rather than the brain. Several peripheral factors, such as low-grade inflammation, motility changes, and alteration of gut microbiota, and central factors have been identified in etiopathogenesis of IBS. The intestinal factors cause various changes in the "little brain" (enteric nervous system) of the gut which in turn conveys messages by the bidirectional connections to the "big brain" through the spinal cord. This results in the different symptoms experienced by the individuals. Specialists on FGID from Asia have designated the FGIDs as "microorganic disorders".

### Peripheral Factors

The peripheral factors are as follows.

#### *Visceral Hypersensitivity*

Visceral hypersensitivity plays a major role in IBS. This is a heightened perception of the bowel to mechanical triggers that present as pain and discomfort. Two main types of visceral hypersensitivity have been identified so far. They are hyperalgesia and allodynia. Hyperalgesia is defined as in intensified pain sensation in response to normal stimuli which usually do not provoke pain, while allodynia is the elevated nociceptive sensation in response to normal stimuli. In pediatric IBS, a decreased rectal sensory threshold for pain has been documented. Several factors, both peripheral and central, may induce visceral hypersensitivity.

### Altered Gut Motility

Alteration in gut motility has been observed in IBS. IBS-C has slower motility, especially colonic transit, whereas IBS-D patients have faster motility. Stress can also alter the aminergic network and therefore result in altered motility. However, whether the altered motility as the cause or effect of IBS still remains a debate.

### Gut Microbiota Dysbiosis

Gut microbiota may have a different pattern with increased Firmicutes/Bacteroidetes ratio in patients with IBS compared to healthy individuals. Patients with IBS are reported to have lower levels of genera *Lactobacillus* and *Bifidobacterium* and marginally higher levels of *Enterobacter* compared with the controls. It has also been observed that children with IBS have significantly greater percentage of *Haemophilus parainfluenzae* in their gut. This gut microbiota in patients with IBS may be the cause of increasing visceral sensitivity and permeability of the intestine and altered GI transit of the intestine. Methanogenic microbes, *Methanobrevibacter smithii*, slow gut transit causing constipation because of the methane produced by them. A significant link between small intestinal bacterial overgrowth (SIBO) and IBS, especially in IBS-D, has been documented.

### Low-grade Inflammation

Increase in the mononuclear inflammatory cells including mast cells which are indicators of low-grade inflammation have been reported in the intestinal mucosa of patients with IBS-D. Serotonin may be released by the mast cells which increase visceral sensitivity by stimulating the peripheral nerves in the submucosa.

### Immune Activation

Increase in mucosal T cells is suggestive of an adaptive immune response to luminal antigens including microbes and has been reported in the intestinal mucosa of IBS patients. There is a cytokine imbalance with a decrease in the proinflammatory cytokines such as interleukin-6 (IL-6) and IL-8 and an increase in the anti-inflammatory cytokines such as IL-10. These findings indicate a low-grade inflammation of the intestine.

## Abnormal Gut Permeability
Abnormal intestinal permeability "leaky gut" has been observed in patients with IBS-D and postinfective IBS.

## Bile Acid Malabsorption
Bile acid malabsorption is well recognized to cause chronic diarrhea and IBS-D. The probable explanation is a decrease in feedback inhibition of bile acid synthesis in liver because of the downregulation of the ileal fibroblast growth factor 19. This results in increased production of bile acid which in turn is delivered to the colon.

## High FODMAP Diet
Fermentable oligo-, di-, and monosaccharides and polyols (FODMAPs) foods which constitute a group of poorly absorbed short-chain carbohydrates such as fructose and lactose, fructans, galacto-oligosaccharides, and polyols or sugar alcohols have been considered to cause some of the symptoms of IBS. They are abdominal distension, bloating, flatulence, pain, and loose motion. The two postulated mechanisms are: (1) increased osmotic activity of these substances which drag fluid to the lumen causing abdominal distension and (2) FODMAPs are fermented by the colonic microflora resulting in increased gas production and colonic distention.

## Post-infection Irritable Bowel Syndrome
This entity post-infection IBS (PI-IBS) is reported in 7–9% of adults who have symptoms of IBS or functional dyspepsia (not present earlier) following a GI infection. The plausible explanation for development of PI-IBS includes a change in gut microbiota, immune activation, low-grade inflammation, increase in mucosal permeability, and neurohormonal and GI motility dysfunction.

## Alteration in Neurotransmitters and Receptors
Serotonin (5-hydrodytryptamine; 5-HT) is secreted by enterochromaffin (EC) cells in the intestinal mucosa. 5-HT is a vital neurotransmitter which is present in enteric neurons and paracrine signaling substance. It is in charge of mediating communication between the brain and the gut and is causative agent for symptoms like bloating, nausea, and vomiting in IBS. Serotonin transporter (SERT) is a highly selective transporter which removes serotonin. Genetic mutations of SERT receptors may be seen in patients with IBS.

## Genetics

The genetic association with IBS has been controversial. *SERT* gene polymorphisms have been studied in detail. Environmental and central factors along with epigenetic changes in the genome may play an indirect role in the pathogenesis of IBS.

## Central Factors

The three important central factors are psychological issues, cognitive function, and neurohormonal dysregulation. These play a significant role in the severe form of IBS. The peripheral factors are however more common and may cause the milder forms of IBS.

## Autonomic Nervous System

Autonomic nervous system is one of the main communicators between the brain and the gut. A correlation between vagal response and postprandial abdominal symptoms of IBS-D and IBS-C has been documented in adults.

## Hypothalamic-Pituitary-Adrenal Axis

The hypothalamic-pituitary-adrenal axis (HPA axis) is an important communicator in the brain-gut axis. Activation of HPA axis results in increased release of corticotropin-releasing hormone (CRH), which promotes central sensitization. Whereas peripheral sensitization is a result of release of adrenocorticotropic hormone (ACTH). Cortisol activates resident immune cells and extrinsic primary afferents in the GI tract. Corticotropin-releasing factor (CRF) is as an important factor in the development of FGIDs including IBS.

# ■ DIAGNOSIS

The diagnosis of IBS is mainly symptom-based since there are no diagnostic markers. Rome IV criteria are used to diagnose IBS.

# ■ HISTORY AND EXAMINATION

- A detailed and accurate history and complete physical examination help in the diagnosis of IBS. The history should include details of the presenting complaints (abdominal pain, stool and defecation pattern, and extra-GI symptoms) social events, school performance, extracurricular activities, and family relationships.
- It is useful to classify the various subtypes of IBS such as IBS-C, IBS-D, IBS-M, and unclassified IBS (IBS-U) based on the stool characteristics using the standard Bristol stool chart.

- The main point in history is to ascertain the presence of the red flag signs or warning signs to identify organic disease.
- The physical examination is usually normal and therefore more time should be allotted for observing child's behavior, body language, communication skills, eye contact, and socializing abilities. The concept that IBS is a diagnosis of exclusion is not acceptable in this era.

## ▪ DIFFERENTIAL DIAGNOSIS

The differential diagnosis (DD) of IBS will depend on the subtype of IBS and also the associated symptoms. Celiac disease, food intolerance, lactose intolerance, inflammatory bowel disease, eosinophilic GI disorders, giardiasis, SIBO, and microscopic colitis are causes to be considered in the presence of abdominal pain, bloat, and features of IBS-D. Functional constipation, solitary rectal ulcer syndrome, and pediatric intestinal pseudo-obstruction (PIPO) are the DD for IBS-C.

## ▪ INVESTIGATION

Since IBS is a symptom-based diagnosis in the majority of children and adolescents with IBS, clinical examination and evaluation of available past medical records and investigations will suffice. The investigations are done for two main reasons: (1) to exclude organic disease with similar symptoms of IBS and (2) to identify the pathophysiology in a small subset.

### Tests to Exclude Organic Disease

When there is a suspicion of IBS, basic investigations such as complete blood count, inflammatory markers [C-reactive protein (CRP) and erythrocyte sedimentation rate (ESR)], and stool and urine examination are suggested for those without any warning signals. The presence of low hemoglobin, elevated ESR and CRP, and stool occult blood positivity are pointers toward an organic disease. A more detailed evaluation including total serum protein, albumin, creatinine, and thyroid function tests are done when there is suggestion of an organic cause.

The following tests have their own benefits and limitations but should be included on an individualized basis.

### *Celiac Screening*

It is recommended to screen children with IBS, especially IBS-D, for celiac disease in areas with a high prevalence of celiac disease. Since the prevalence of celiac disease is 1% in North India, screening children with IBS helps early identification of the disease.

### Fecal Calprotectin

This fecal test is a sensitive noninvasive marker of intestinal inflammation that may help in differentiating between IBS and IBD. A normal or low fecal calprotectin <50 µg/g may help to defer colonoscopy.

### Endoscopy

Upper GI and ileocolonoscopy are not indicated to diagnose IBS. They are done if there are some alarm features (growth failure, blood in stools, chronic diarrhea, and hematemesis) suggesting an organic disease. These individuals should undergo both upper and lower GI endoscopy with segmental biopsy and histopathology even if they fulfill criteria for IBS.

### Imaging

*Ultrasound of abdomen:* Though it is simple and noninvasive, it has no role in the evaluation of IBS. However, if there are some alarm features, such as fever, jaundice, and weight loss, it will help in identifying lymphadenopathy, thickened bowel loops, and biliary disease. Similarly, contrast-enhanced computerized tomography (CECT) abdomen has no role and should not be done unless definitely indicated.

## Tests to Identify the Pathophysiology

Since a subset of IBS may have a microorganic basis for their symptoms, it is essential that some of these pathophysiological changes are identified to assist therapy. Hence, investigations may be necessary to identify the pathophysiology.

### Motility Studies

These studies, if available, play a role in understanding the pathophysiology and improving the management in some children with IBS. Delayed gastric emptying and low rectal threshold to pain have been reported in children with IBS.

### Upper Gut Aspirate Culture and Hydrogen Breath Tests

Since SIBO explains some of the symptoms of IBS, quantitative culture of upper small bowel bacteria is done for confirmation. High-grade SIBO is when the count is $\geq 10^5$ colony-forming unit/mL of aspirate and low-grade SIBO $\geq 10^3$ but $\leq 10^5$ colony-forming unit/mL. Qualitative change in microbiota (relative proportion of healthy and pathogenic microbes) is performed by next-generation sequencing.

*Hydrogen breath tests (HBTs):* Glucose and lactulose HBTs are noninvasive but not sensitive and specific tests for diagnosis of SIBO. Patients with SIBO and IBS may be responsive to antibiotic treatment than those without SIBO.

## NATURAL HISTORY

All children or adolescents with IBS will not outgrow their symptoms with increasing age as assumed earlier. It has been reported that 40% of children with FAPDs will continue to present as IBS or other FGIDs in adults. Children with psychological factors tend to have a more severe and longer duration of illness.

## PRACTICAL MANAGEMENT OF IRRITABLE BOWEL SYNDROME

Since the pathophysiology is complex, the management of IBS involves a multidisciplinary approach. It is very imperative that the treating pediatrician should first understand the pathophysiological basis of symptoms.

The Rome IV has therefore introduced the *Multidimensional Clinical Profile (MDCP)* which should form the background of treatment. MDCP includes five issues: (1) Diagnosis of IBS using Rome criteria, (2) Classification into types of IBS, (3) Assessment of severity: Quality of life of the patient and his/her family may be as seriously impacted in children, just as in adults; hence it is advisable to assess the severity of IBS by health-related quality of life (HRQoL), (4) Physiological abnormalities or biomarkers, and (5) Psychological influences of the disorder.

### Counseling of Parents and Patients

This is very essential in the management of IBS in children and adolescents with IBS. The multifactorial causes, gut-brain-gut communication, the vicious circle of pain leading to inactivity, lack of sleep, low energy and effect on mood, and the impact of the disease on the child/adolescent and his family on different levels: physical, functional, emotional, and social should be all explained clearly in age-appropriated words. They should be taught self-management strategies to decrease pain, fear, and anxiety and improve functionality and clear out negative cognitions. Healthy food habits, school attendance, regular exercise, and extracurricular activities should be encouraged.

### Medication

According to the predominant symptom, constipation, diarrhea, bloat, and pain drugs have been recommended in adults with IBS.

### Constipation-predominant Irritable Bowel Syndrome

The first-line drugs are fiber, osmotic laxative including polyethylene glycol, and lactulose/lactitol. Fiber as well as osmotic laxatives may increase the bloat symptom. The second-line drugs are bisacodyl, sodium picosulfate, lubiprostone, linaclotide (act on ion channels present in the intestinal enterocytes resulting in water efflux thereby accelerating the intestinal transit), and prucalopride (5-HT4 agonist that has less cardiovascular side effects). There are no pediatric studies on the use of prucalopride, linaclotide, and lubiprostone in IBS-C.

### Diarrhea-predominant Irritable Bowel Syndrome

The first-line drug is loperamide diphenoxylate (0.05–0.1 mg/kg, maximum 4 mg) that is very effective in decreasing diarrhea but has no effect on bloat and pain. The second-line drugs are ondansetron, bile acid sequestrant (cholestyramine and colestipol), and rifaximin. There are no pediatric studies with cholestyramine and loperamide in children with IBS-D.

### Pain

Antispasmodics are effective when pain is the predominant symptom. Antispasmodics include the antimuscarinics, smooth-muscle relaxants, and anticholinergics. Peppermint oil (0.1–0.2 mL capsule three times daily, taken 1 hour before food) has shown limited evidence in children with IBS. Drotaverine (1–5 years, 20 mg tid; 6–12 years, 40 mg tid) and Mebeverine 25–200 mg tid are often prescribed. Since constipation is a common side effect of antispasmodics, it is not preferred in IBS-C.

### Centrally-acting Medications

Centrally-acting medications such as antidepressants [tricyclic antidepressants and selective serotonin reuptake inhibitor (SSRI)] are equally effective in IBS even in absence of any psychiatric illness. They act by altering pain perception, improving sleep, and alleviating any associated psychological illness. Tricyclic and SSRI antidepressant in pediatric IBS are nonconclusive. Tricyclic antidepressant (amitriptyline 0.5–1 mg/kg/day at night, maximum: 30 mg) can be considered when there is diarrhea and pain with some features of depression.

### Bloat

Usually constipation is associated with bloat so this should be treated. Rifaximin and probiotics have been prescribed. Rifaximin is a broad-spectrum antibiotic poorly absorbed from the gut. It is active against gram-negative bacteria, gram-positive bacteria, and anaerobes. The beneficial effect of rifaximin emphasizes the fact that in a subset IBS may be due to altered gut microbiota. Rifaximin is also used in IBS-D and IBS-M.

## Probiotics

Since altered gut microbiota have been considered in the pathophysiology of IBS, the role of probiotics has been studied extensively in adults. However, no single strain has been proved consistently effective. Some benefit of *Lactobacillus rhamnosus* GG and *Lactobacillus reuteri* DSM17938 have been shown in pediatric IBS, but evidence is considered insufficient for a recommendation.

## Psychological Therapies

Cognitive behavioral therapy, gut-directed hypnotherapy, relaxation therapy, multicomponent psychological therapy, and dynamic psychotherapies not only exert their central effects on mood but also exerts their effects on peripheral pain perception, visceral hypersensitivity, and GI motility. Psychotherapy clinical trials have methodological limitations and there lack of wide spread availability can be a problem in most primary care practices. Despite these limitations, psychotherapy is recommended for IBS patients who do not respond to standard pharmacological treatment.

## Dietary Therapy

Various dietary modifications have been recommended in patients with IBS. They are generally advised to increase soluble dietary fiber (psyllium and ispaghula) in their diet, avoid insoluble fiber (wheat bran), eat small meals, and avoid known triggers (high fat diet, caffeine, spicy food, milk, and dairy products) though its efficacy in controlling the symptoms remains variable. Lactose intolerance is equally prevalent in IBS and healthy controls but patients with IBS are more symptomatic following a lactose load. Randomized control trials have shown that low-FODMAP diet as a second-line diet might be effective in older children with bloat IBS, but its implementation must be supervised by a dietician. Dietary FODMAPs have prolonged intestinal hydrogen production more in individuals with IBS. FODMAPs also influence the amount of methane production, and in addition may induce GI and systemic symptoms in patients with IBS. Neither food elimination diets based on immunoglobulin G (IgG) antibodies nor are gluten-free diets recommended in IBS.

## ■ CONCLUSION

The management of IBS still remains a challenge throughout the world since no consensus is available. It becomes more complex in a country like ours where psychological therapies are available only in select centers. The success in managing pediatric IBS depends upon forming a multidisciplinary team involving the pediatrician, pediatric gastroenterologist, dietician, child psychologist, and a psychiatrist. Quality time spent at explaining the pathophysiology and reassuring the child and parents helps the child with IBS to a great extent.

## KEY MESSAGES

- IBS is a common FAPD in children and adolescents and needs to be recognized.
- IBS, though included as a functional disorder, is considered as a gut-brain-gut disorder which has several triggers.
- The diagnosis of IBS is symptom based and should fulfil the Rome IV criteria.
- There are four types of IBS depending on the predominant symptom, i.e., constipation, diarrhea, mixed, and unclassified.
- In children and adolescents suspected as IBS, the well-recognized red flag signs and symptoms should be checked to exclude organic disease.
- Investigations are necessary only for those where red flag signs and symptoms are present.
- Management is multidisciplinary and includes pharmacological, psychological, and dietary therapy.

## SUGGESTED READING

1. Barrett JS, Gearry RB, Muir JG, Irving PM, Rose R, Rosella O, et al. Dietary poorly absorbed, short-chain carbohydrates increase delivery of water and fermentable substrates to the proximal colon. Aliment Pharmacol Ther. 2010;31:874-82.
2. Card T, Enck P, Barbara G, Boeckxstaens GE, Santos J, Azpiroz F, et al. Post-infectious IBS: Defining its clinical features and prognosis using an internet-based survey. United European Gastroenterol J. 2018;6(8):1245-53.
3. Devanarayana NM, Rajindrajith S. Irritable bowel syndrome in children: Current knowledge, challenges and opportunities. World J Gastroenterol. 2018;24(21):2211-35.
4. Drossman DA, Hasler WL. Rome IV-Functional GI Disorders: Disorders of Gut-Brain Interaction. Gastroenterology. 2016;150(6):1257-61.
5. Drossman DA. Guidelines for use of the multi-dimensional clinical profile. In: Drossman DA (Ed). Multi-Dimensional Clinical Profile (MDCP): For the Functional Gastrointestinal Disorders, 1st edition. North Carolina; Rome Foundation; 2015. pp. 7-14.
6. Farzaei MH, Bahramsoltani R, Abdollahi M, Rahimi R. The role of visceral hypersensitivity in irritable bowel syndrome: pharmacological targets and novel treatments. J Neurogastroenterol Motil. 2016;22:558-74.
7. Ford AC, Lacy BE, Harris LA, Quigley EMM, Moayyedi P. Effect of antidepressants and psychological therapies in irritable bowel syndrome: an updated systematic review and meta-analysis. Am J Gastroenterol. 2019;114(1):21-39.

8. Ford AC, Sperber AD, Corsetti M, Camilleri M. Irritable bowel syndrome. Lancet. 2020;396(10263):1675-88.
9. Ghoshal UC. Marshall and Warren Lecture 2019: a paradigm shift in pathophysiological basis of irritable bowel syndrome and its implication on treatment. J Gastroenterol Hepatol. 2020;35:712-21.
10. Levy RL, Jones KR, Whitehead WE, Feld SI, Talley NJ, Corey LA. Irritable bowel syndrome in twins: heredity and social learning both contribute to etiology. Gastroenterology. 2001;121(4):799-804.
11. Mahler T, Hoffman I, Smets F, Vandenplas Y The Belgian consensus on irritable bowel syndrome: the paediatric gastroenterologist view. Acta Gastro-Enterologica Belgica. 2022;85:384-6.
12. Rajindrajith S, Devanarayana NM. Subtypes and symptomatology of irritable bowel syndrome in children and adolescents: a school-based survey using rome III criteria. J Neurogastroenterol Motil. 2012;18:298-304.
13. Saulnier DM, Riehle K, Mistretta TA, Diaz MA, Mandal D, Raza S, et al. Gastrointestinal microbiome signatures of pediatric patients with irritable bowel syndrome. Gastroenterology. 2011;141:1782-91.
14. Scarpellini E, Giorgio V, Gabrielli M, Filoni S, Vitale G, Tortora A, et al. Rifaximin treatment for small intestinal bacterial overgrowth in children with irritable bowel syndrome. Eur Rev Med Pharmacol Sci. 2013;17:1314-20.
15. Vincenzi M, Del Ciondolo I, Pasquini E, Gennai K, Paolini B. Effects of a low FODMAP diet and specific carbohydrate diet on symptoms and nutritional adequacy of patients with irritable bowel syndrome: preliminary results of a single-blinded randomized trial. J Transl Int Med. 2017;5(2):120-6.

# CHAPTER 17

# Adolescent Obesity

*Viji Thirugnanam, Hemchand K Prasad*

## ■ INTRODUCTION

Prevalence of adolescent overweight and obesity in adolescents is on the rise across our country. A systematic analysis on 52 studies from 16 states on the trend of childhood obesity in India identified a significant increase in prevalence from 16.3% reported previously to 19.3%, after 2010. The increased prevalence is seen maximally in urban-affluent adolescents. However, studies on adolescents from the lower socioeconomic classes, as well as rural settings, have identified a significant prevalence of overweight and obesity. Thus, it becomes pivotal for pediatricians to be sensitized to early identification and appropriate evaluation and management of this important public health issue to optimize the short-term and long-term health of these adolescents. Authors' group have previously described simple approach to tackle adolescent obesity. However, many new guidelines and recommendations have emerged to combat adolescent obesity in the past 8 years (2014–2022). The Indian Academy of Pediatrics (IAP) has published numerous guidelines to help pediatricians crush the tide of obesity in adolescents with an iron hand. Also, the pandemic of COVID-19 and related lockdown has paved the way to a new pandemic of adolescent obesity, which has to be tackled by the pediatricians. This article summarizes the current recommendations to facilitate early identification and evidence-based rational management of adolescents with obesity, in the perspective of available Indian data.

## ■ EARLY IDENTIFICATION OF OVERWEIGHT AND OBESE ADOLESCENTS

Body mass index (BMI) is the most accepted anthropometric measure to identify excess nutritional state. To stem the tide of obesity, IAP came up with the revised charts in 2015. A significant 646 children with weight for height Z-score above +2 were excluded from the study sample to avoid "normalization" of obesity. Also, the new percentile lines to identify overweight and obesity were added, which were equivalent of 23 kg/m² and 27 kg/m² adult equivalent BMI. This resulted in lowering of BMI cut off for overweight from conventional 85th percentile to 71st and 75th percentile in boys and girls, respectively. Thus, use of BMI charts of IAP remains the most valuable tool to identify overweight and obese adolescents, early. The IAP in its "growth monitoring guidelines—2007" recommended that all adolescents have an annual assessment of BMI. Proper measurement of height with a stadiometer and weight (in kg) using a calibrated digital weighing scale should be done annually in all adolescents. BMI is calculated using the formula:

$$BMI = \frac{Weight\ (in\ kg)}{Height\ (in\ m)^2}$$

The calculated BMI is plotted on the IAP 2015 BMI charts. Any BMI above the 23rd adult equivalent is considered as overweight and BMI above the 27th adult equivalent is considered as obesity **(Fig. 1)**.

Body mass index assessment involves meticulous calculation, which is often challenging in busy office practice. The IAP has recently come up with a gender-specific graphic tool called as a "BMI look-up tool", without the need to calculate BMI It involves measurement of height and weight as per the standard techniques and plotting the point of intersection of height and weight on the graph. Any measurement above the OB line indicates obesity and OW line indicates overweight **(Fig. 1)**. The BMI look-up tool complements the conventional BMI calculation and plot on IAP 2015 BMI charts.

## ETIOLOGY OF OBESITY IN ADOLESCENTS

The most common cause for adolescent obesity is nutritional. A mismatch between calories consumed and burnt results in accumulation of excess calories and elevated BMI. The other secondary causes for adolescent obesity include:
- *Endocrine etiology:* Hypothyroidism, Cushing's disease, pseudohypoparathyroidism and growth hormone deficiency
- *Genetic syndromes:* Prader-Willi syndrome, Bardet-Biedl syndrome, and Alstrom syndrome
- *Monogenic causes:* Leptin deficiency, leptin receptor defects
- *Drug induced:* Corticosteroid therapy, antiepileptic drugs such as sodium valproate, psychotropic drugs such as risperidone and antidepressants
- *Central causes:* Hypothalamic dysfunction associated with tumors, irradiation, meningitis, and surgery.

    Pediatricians evaluating obese adolescents should consider secondary etiology based on clinical judgement.

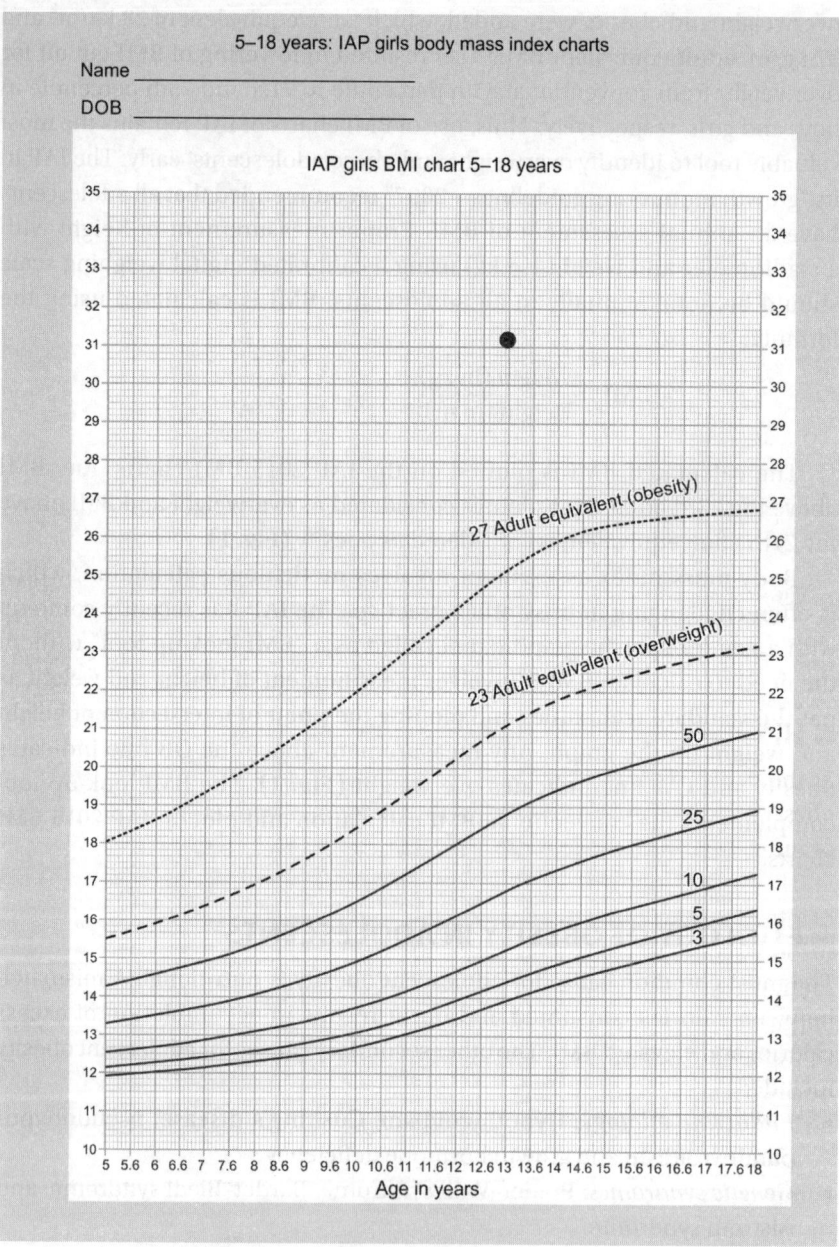

**Fig. 1:** *(Contd…)*
A 7-year-old child with height of 150 cm and weight of 70 kg. BMI is calculated as 31.1 kg/m².

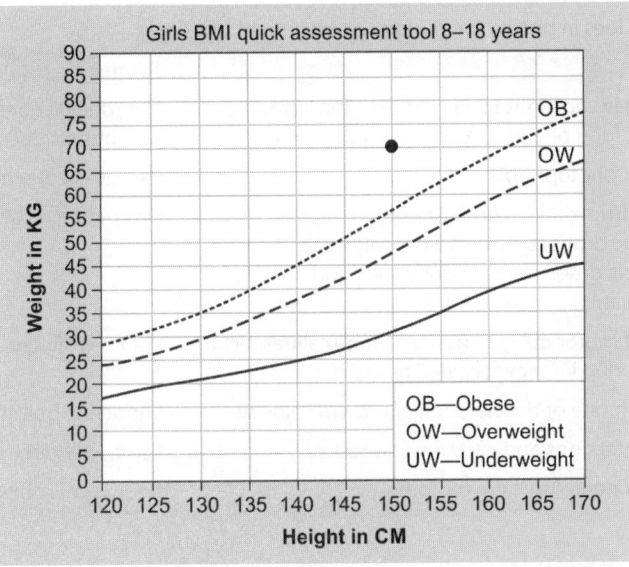

**Fig. 1:** Diagnosis of obesity in adolescents using the IAP 2015 BMI charts and BMI lookup tool. (BMI: body mass index; IAP: Indian Academy Pediatrics)

## ■ HISTORY AND PHYSICAL EXAMINATION

At the end of a proper history and a meticulous physical examination in an obese adolescent, the pediatrician should be able to ascertain the likelihood of nutritional versus secondary obesity, risk factors for nutritional obesity, and likely presence of comorbidities and complications of obesity. Frequency of intake of unhealthy calories, eating out, skipping breakfast, online ordering of food, screen time—during weekdays and weekends should be ascertained meticulously. The frequency and duration of physical activity should be enquired into. Behavioral pattern of physical activity in daily activities such as walking to school, taking stairs, and participation in daily chores should be determined. A history that reveals significant intake of unhealthy calories, lack of physical activity and significant screen time puts the adolescent at a high risk of nutritional obesity. The other risk factors for metabolic complications of obesity in adolescents should be enquired: Family history of type 2 diabetes mellitus (DM), hypertension, premature coronary artery disease, gestational diabetes, and birth as born as small for gestational age. The pointers to non-nutritional obesity and comorbidities of obesity in adolescents are shown in **Tables 1 and 2**, respectively. Adolescents with elevated BMI have low self-esteem, tend to be bullied, teased, tend to skip meals and tend to binge eat. Hence, they are prone to develop psychological distress and other psychiatric disorders (such as depression and eating disorders), which should be carefully screened for, with a proper history.

**TABLE 1:** Clues in history for etiology of adolescent obesity.

| History | Pointer |
|---|---|
| Awakening in the night to eat, extreme food craving (stealing of food or eating food left over by others) | Neurogenic obesity or monogenic obesity |
| Presence of photophobia | Bardet–Biedl syndrome |
| History of drug intake (corticosteroid therapy, antiepileptic drugs such as sodium valproate, psychotropic drugs such as risperidone and antidepressants) | Drug-induced obesity |
| Presence of motor delay or genital abnormalities; failure to thrive during infancy followed by rapid weight gain | Prader–Willi syndrome |
| Poor growth rate or deceleration of growth velocity | Endocrine obesity |
| Frequent infections and early onset obesity | Leptin deficiency |
| Presence of neurological symptoms | Neurogenic obesity |

**TABLE 2:** Comorbidities of obesity.

| Clinical clue | Possible comorbidity | Screening tool/action plan |
|---|---|---|
| Polydipsia, polyuria, weight loss, nonhealing ulcer, recurrent vaginal fungal infections | Type 2 DM | Glucose tolerance test, HbA1C |
| Gastrointestinal discomfort, right upper quadrant pain, hepatomegaly | NAFLD | SGPT, USG abdomen, fibroscan |
| Headaches, presence of elevated blood pressure | Hypertension | Ambulatory BP monitoring |
| Menstrual irregularities, hirsutism, acne | PCOD | USG abdomen, hormone evaluation |
| Abnormal behavior, daytime sleepiness, headaches, snoring, restless sleep | OSAS | Overnight pulse oximetry, sleep study |
| Hip pain, knee pain | SCFE | Radiological evaluation |
| School refusal, school absenteeism, teasing by peers, self-harm, anger outbursts, anxiety | Psychological disturbance | Psychiatrist referral |
| Headache and numbness; fundus showing papilledema | Pseudotumor cerebri | CT scan |

(BP: blood; CT: computed tomography; DM: diabetes mellitus; NFALD: nonalcoholic fatty liver disease; OSAS: obstructive sleep apnea syndrome; PCOD: polycystic ovarian syndrome; SCFE: slipped capital femoral epiphysis; SGPT: serum glutamic pyruvic transaminase; USG: ultrasonography)

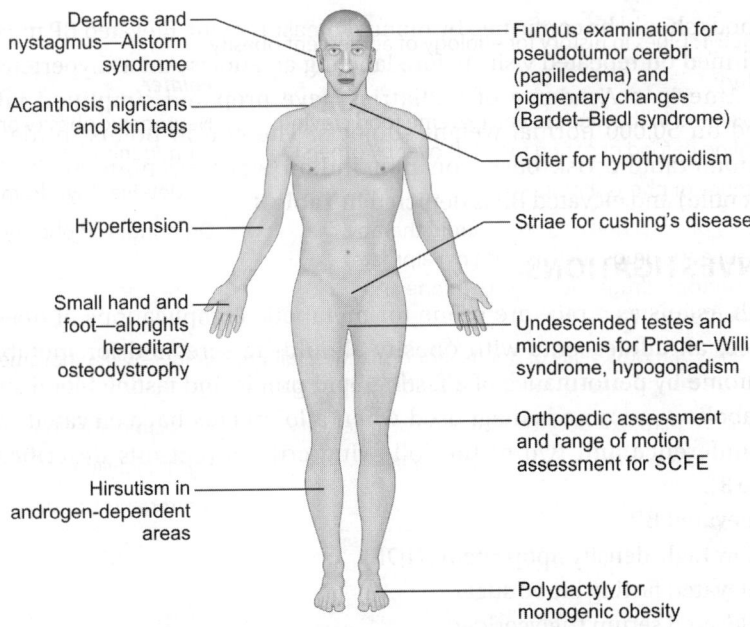

**Fig. 2:** Head-to-foot examination in adolescent obesity.
(SCFE: slipped capital femoral epiphysis)

Proper measurement of height, weight, and arriving at BMI as described above and plotting on the IAP charts give valuable clues to the etiology. Elevated BMI with tall stature and normal growth velocity suggests nutritional obesity in adolescents. Elevated BMI with short stature and faltering of growth suggests non-nutritional obesity. Height and weight on two different sides of the median, often suggests a pathological cause for obesity.

A proper head-to-foot examination should be done in every obese adolescent for clues for secondary obesity and comorbidities of nutritional obesity **(Fig. 2)**. It is pivotal to perform sexual maturity rating (SMR) and progress of SMR in all obese adolescents.

To ascertain the metabolic risk in obese adolescents, two valuable clinical assessments should be performed in every adolescent: Measurement of waist circumference and blood pressure. Waist circumference should be measured in the standing position to the nearest 0.1 cm at the mid-point between the lowest rib and the iliac crest in the mid-axillary line. Measurement should be done at the end of normal expiration using a non-elastic tape. Pan Indian charts to interpret measured waist circumference are available. Any value above the 70th percentile is considered as elevated and put the adolescent at metabolic risk. BP should be measured using auscultatory or automated methods. BP measurement should be performed after a rest of 5 minutes with the adolescent seated with the back supported, feet on floor, cubital fossa at heart level and using the right arm. Elevated values using automated methods should be confirmed by manual measurement. Elevated BP must be confirmed on repeated visits before labeling an adolescent as hypertensive. The American Academy of Pediatrics have prepared simplified tables based on 50,000 normal weight subjects. The cut-off points to identify cardiometabolic risk based on pan Indian waist circumference (70th percentile) and elevated BP is depicted in **Table 3**.

## ■ INVESTIGATIONS

South Asians as a race are prone for metabolic complications of obesity. Hence, all adolescents with obesity should be screened for metabolic syndrome by performance of a fasting lipid profile and fasting blood sugar. Metabolic syndrome is diagnosed when adolescents have elevated waist circumference and two of the following criteria (cut-offs described in **Table 3**).

- Elevated BP
- Low high-density lipoprotein (HDL)
- Elevated fasting blood sugar
- Elevated serum triglycerides.

There is no "one rule fits all" on screening for secondary causes and comorbid states, every adolescent should be individualized. In the presence of normal stature and normal growth velocity, secondary causes are less likely. Hence, endocrine society recommends screening for endocrine causes if there is short stature (height <3rd percentile) or growth velocity below the 25th percentile. When an endocrine cause is thought of, investigations to be performed include: Free T4, TSH, Prolactin, insulin-like growth factor-1 (for growth hormone deficiency), bone age measurement and overnight dexamethasone suppression test (ONDST—for cortisol excess state). ONDST is done by administration of 30 µg/kg of oral dexamethasone at bedtime (previous night) and measurement of 8 am serum cortisol next day morning. Appropriately suppressed serum cortisol levels <1.8 µg/dL rules out cortisol excess state. One should be careful while interpretation of thyroid functions in an obese adolescent. Often obese adolescents tend to have marginally raised TSH levels and normal Free T4 because of an adaptive state, which often only requires masterly inactivity. Thyroxine replacement is indicated only if there is low Free T4, TSH showing a rising trend above 10 µIU/mL or positive thyroid peroxidase antibody.

Evaluation for comorbid states should be performed as depicted in **Table 2**. Hormone evaluation for polycystic ovarian syndrome (PCOD) should be performed in the follicular phase (day 5 after menses) including: Total testosterone, luteinizing hormone, follicle-stimulating hormone, 17-hydroxy progesterone and prolactin. PCOD is diagnosed in the presence of polycystic ovaries (12 or more follicles, 2–9 mm and ovarian volume ≥10 cm$^3$), clinical or biochemical hyperandrogenism and oligoanovulation.

**TABLE 3:** Diagnosis of metabolic syndrome in adolescents.

| | Boys | | | | | | Girls | | | | | |
|---|---|---|---|---|---|---|---|---|---|---|---|---|
| | Systolic BP (mm Hg) | Diastolic BP (mm Hg) | 70th percentile of waist circumference (cm) | Fasting blood glucose (mg/dL) | Serum Triglycerides | HDL (in mg/dL) | Systolic BP (mm Hg) | Diastolic BP (mm Hg) | 70th percentile of waist circumference (cm) | Fasting blood glucose (mg/dl) | Serum Triglycerides | HDL (in mg/dL) |
| 11 years | 110 | 74 | 74.9 | 100 | 150 | 40 | 111 | 74 | 74.8 | 100 | 150 | 40 |
| 12 years | 113 | 75 | 78 | 100 | 150 | 40 | 114 | 75 | 78.1 | 100 | 150 | 40 |
| 13 years | 120 | 80 | 80.7 | 100 | 150 | 40 | 120 | 80 | 80.8 | 100 | 150 | 40 |
| 14 years | 120 | 80 | 83 | 100 | 150 | 40 | 120 | 80 | 82.7 | 100 | 150 | 40 |
| 15 years | 120 | 80 | 84.9 | 100 | 150 | 40 | 120 | 80 | 84.1 | 100 | 150 | 40 |
| 16 years | 120 | 80 | 86.5 | 100 | 150 | 40 | 120 | 80 | 85.1 | 100 | 150 | 50 |
| 17 years | 120 | 80 | 90 | 100 | 150 | 40 | 120 | 80 | 85.9 | 100 | 150 | 50 |
| 18 years | 120 | 80 | 90 | 100 | 150 | 40 | 120 | 80 | 85.9 | 100 | 150 | 50 |

Metabolic syndrome diagnosed if waist circumference elevated along with two criteria: elevated BP, low HDL, elevated Fasting BS, and high triglyceride level.
(BP: blood pressure; BS: blood sugar; HDL: high-density lipoprotein)

One should be cautious that polycystic ovaries and menstrual irregularities may be physiological in the first 18 months after onset of menarche. Ambulatory blood pressure recording or repeated home monitoring of BP is helpful to avoid white coat hypertension in obese adolescents. One should screen for end-organ complications such as echocardiography, urine protein estimation, and retinal screening in persistent hypertension.

Symptoms of nonalcoholic fatty liver disease (NAFLD) are nonspecific. Measurement of serum glutamic pyruvic transaminase (SGPT) (lowered cut-off of 22 IU/L in girls and 25 IU/L in boys) is helpful to diagnose NAFLD early. Often, concerns are raised about penile size which is buried in fat and gives a perception of being small for age. Appropriate size of testes, measurement and plotting of penile length on penile length charts may be needed to reassure adolescents with a significant anxiety. Hormone measurement should be done only if hypogonadism is clinically suspected. In the presence of symptoms or elevated fasting blood sugar, evaluate for type 2 DM Measurement of Anti-GAD (glutamic acid decarboxylase antibody), C-peptide and glycosylated hemoglobin should be done for a proper diagnosis. Diagnosis of diabetes is made if Fasting BS, postprandial BS and HBA1C are ≥125 mg/dL, ≥200 mg/dL and ≥6.5%, respectively. Adolescents with Type 2 DM should be screened for retinopathy (by indirect ophthalmoscopy) and nephropathy (spot urine albumin creatinine ratio measurement) at diagnosis.

## ■ MANAGEMENT

Management of adolescent obesity is often challenging. A four-step approach in combating adolescent obesity is recommended by experts **(Box 1)**. The principles of healthy eating, regular exercise, and minimization of screen time are escalated with every higher step. Steps 1 and 2 are managed by the pediatrician, whereas steps 3 and 4 involve multidisciplinary team including pediatrician, endocrinologist, dietician, physiotherapist, and psychiatrist. Step 2 involves monthly follow-up during intensive phase, whereas steps 3 and 4 require weekly follow-up during the active phase (either direct or telephonic). Adolescents with elevated BMI and no comorbidity begin with step 2 intervention, elevated BMI, and at least one comorbidity usually begin with step 3 intervention. Adolescents with morbid obesity or those with established complications are managed in a tertiary care center.

**BOX 1:** Stepwise approach to combating adolescent obesity.

*Step-1:* Prevention of adolescent obesity
*Step-2:* Structured weight management of adolescents
*Step-3:* Multidisciplinary intervention
*Step-4:* Tertiary care intervention

**BOX 2:** Ten commandments of lifestyle advice for obese Indian adolescents.

- Portion control of food resulting in a 500 kcal deficit in adolescents
- Freshly cooked home-based foods
- Restrict to ontime three meals and one to two snacks
- Never skip breakfast
- Avoid JUNCS
- Family eating
- Traffic light approach to food
- 20–30 minutes of moderate-to-vigorous physical activity for 5 days/week
- Bare minimum nonacademic screen time
- 8–11 hours of good quality sleep without electronic media

*Lifestyle measures* form the cornerstone of the management of adolescent obesity. Weight loss by lifestyle measures such as diet resulting in a reduction of 1.5 kg/m$^2$ of BMI improves metabolic parameters, delays onset of complications, and prevents the progress of complications in adolescent obesity. Thus, pediatricians caring for adolescents with obesity should suggest family-centric, age-appropriate and intensive lifestyle measures, individualized on a case-to-case basis. The four pillars of lifestyle measures include: (1) Diet, (2) exercise, (3) reduction in screen time, and (4) adequate sleep. The key lifestyle advices to be given to adolescents are summarized in **Box 2** as ten commandments by every pediatrician who encounters adolescent obesity.

*Dietary advice* should be individualized for every obese adolescent. A diet chart that is prepared and advised to follow is often challenging for the adolescents to practice and sustain. Challenges faced by Indian adolescents include higher liberty in choice of foods, higher craving for high-salt and sugar foods. Portion control (reduction in the caloric intake by around 30%) that results in a 500 kcal deficit should be advised. One should remember that RDA is recommended based on an active lifestyle, not a sedentary lifestyle, which is a part of many obese adolescents. Sugar intake should be <5–10% of total dietary intake, and <30% caloric intake from fat is advised.

One should stress on consuming three properly timed meals (including an adequate balanced breakfast) and one to two snacks. Freshly cooked home foods and home-prepared snacks are encouraged. Five servings of fruits and vegetables should be consumed through the day. Adequate fiber intake (age in years + 5 g/day) should be advised. Encourage intake of whole grains (brown rice and whole wheat) and avoid refined grains (maida, suji, and white rice). The IAP in 2019 coined the term "JUNCS" food to cover: Junk foods, ultraprocessed foods, nutritionally inappropriate foods, caffeinated and colored drinks, sugar-sweetened beverages—which are best avoided by all adolescents.

Meals should be prepared from whole grains, dals, and seasonal vegetables. Ingredients such as fruits, peanuts, and seeds, can be used to prepare healthy snack options. Beverages in the form of fruit shakes, smoothies with skimmed milk, rasam, lassi, butter milk, and lime water can be consumed by adolescents. A traffic light approach to foods can be explained to the adolescents: high-salt, sweet, and fat foods as red light (best avoided), whole grains in yellow light (eaten with moderation), fruits and vegetables as green light (consumed ad lib).

Eating together as a family, eating slowly with proper chewing, and mindful eating (with awareness and focus on food eaten) should be encouraged in obese adolescents. The following practices of eating that is highly prevalent in today's adolescents is strongly discouraged: skipping breakfast, grazing and frequent snacking, online ordering of foods, eating out, fast foods, very rigorous dieting, resorting to unbalanced unsupervised hypocaloric diets. Adolescents who are technology savvy should be encouraged to use mobile applications to track and share their progress as a positive reinforcement. The IAP JUNCS 2019 guidelines advise to limit to 250 mL of fresh juices, one cup (200 mL) per day of caffeinated drinks such as coffee in adolescents.

### Exercise

A goal of 60 minutes of moderate-to-vigorous physical activity is recommended for at least 5 days a week in adolescents. In adolescents who are very sedentary, begin with 20 min/day of exercise that is spread through the day. Gym can be considered in adolescents above 16 years of age. Choice of activity can be made as per the inclination of the adolescent from a range of activities including baseball, dancing, cycling, running, martial arts, etc. Enjoyable exercise such as joining a sports academy along with peers is more likely to have a better adherence and positive outcome. Use of mobile applications to track activity can be considered in adolescents with an inclination for technology. Each metabolic equivalent hour of exercise results in a BMI reduction of 0.13 $kg/m^2$ per week. Simple changes in lifestyle made by adolescents such as walking or cycling to school, taking staircase instead of the elevator, helping in household chores and gardening often complements the benefits of regular exercise.

### Screen Time

Nonacademic screen time should be bare minimum in all adolescents. The IAP 2021 guidelines on screen time recommended balancing screen time with effective physical activity, sleep, and other day-to-day activities. The government of India advised not more than 30–45 minutes for four sessions for adolescents studying in class 9–12 for online education during

COVID Pandemic. The IAP recommends minimal permissible age for Facebook, Twitter, Instagram, Whatsapp, and Youtube platforms as 13 years, 13 years, 13 years, 16 years, and 18 years, respectively. Use of screen time during eating and bedroom is strongly discouraged. Parental role modeling by using bare minimum screen time is often of added value. Even during commercial breaks during television programs, adolescents may be advised simple exercises such as jumping, aerobics, and pushups.

## Sleep

Adolescents should receive at least 8-11 hours of good sleep in a quiet surrounding. No electronic media usage should be permitted in the sleeping area. Reduction in the leptin levels, increase in ghrelin levels and improved glucose utilization are documented with good quality of sleep in the adolescent age group.

## Pharmacotherapy (Table 4)

The indications for use and auxological response of drug therapy in isolated adolescent obesity for weight loss in adolescents are not well established. Three drugs: (1) Orlistat, (2) liraglutide, and (3) phentermine are approved by regulatory authorities for use in adolescents aged above 12 years, 12 years, and 16 years, respectively. Pharmacotherapy is embarked upon in adolescents in the presence of weight-related comorbidity only after lifestyle measures have failed in combination with the lifestyle measures. Metformin can be considered in adolescents with type 2 diabetes mellitus or polycystic ovary syndrome. Recently, regulatory authorities have approved the use of a fixed combination of phentermine and topiramate extended release (7.5/46 mg) for weight reduction in adolescents above 12 years with BMI in the obese range targeting 4.8-7% reduction in BMI. Indian data on utility of pharmacotherapy in adolescent obesity is very scarce. Adolescents with monogenic obesity due to Prader-Willi syndrome should be initiated on growth hormone therapy for improved growth and BMI reduction.

## Comorbid Conditions

Aggressive lifestyle measures remain the most useful tool to combat and prevent progression of most obesity-related comorbid states in adolescents. Specific pharmacotherapy may be considered in adolescents with severe dyslipidemia, persistent hypertension, PCOD, and type 2 DM as described in **Table 2**. Laser therapy for cosmetic reasons in hirsutism in adolescent PCOD can be considered after hormonal improvement. Respiratory support may be indicated in those with severe obstructive sleep apnea syndrome (OSAS); no specific therapy is established for adolescents with NAFLD.

**TABLE 4:** Pharmacotherapy for adolescent obesity and associated complications.

| Drug | Indication | Mechanism of action | Dose | Side effect | Precaution/note of caution |
|---|---|---|---|---|---|
| Orlistat | Significant obesity with weight related comorbidity and failed lifestyle measure (above 12 years) | Reduced gastrointestinal lipase inhibitor | 120 mg TDS | Oily stools | Screen for fat-soluble vitamin deficiency |
| Phentermine | Significant obesity with weight related comorbidity and failed lifestyle measure (above 16 years) | Reduced reuptake of norepinephrine | 15–30 mg/day | Irritability and insomnia | Very limited pediatric experience. Monitor for cardiovascular side effects |
| Liraglutide | BMI >30 kg/m$^2$ or above 27 kg/m$^2$ with a comorbidity | GLP-1 analog | 0.6–3 mg/day SC injection | Gastrointestinal side effects | Avoided in individuals with medullary thyroid carcinoma |
| Metformin | Adolescents with type 2 diabetes mellitus or established polycystic ovary syndrome | Reduced hepatic glucose production and increased peripheral insulin sensitivity | 500–1,800 mg/day | Gastrointestinal side effects and lactic acidosis | Extended release preparation can be considered to avoid hypoglycemia |
| Growth hormone | Genetically proven Prader–Willi syndrome | Improved auxology and muscle tone | 0.5–1 mg/m$^2$ | Obstructive sleep apnea, carpal tunnel syndrome, adrenal hypofunction | Sleep study mandatory prior to commencement |

*Contd...*

**CHAPTER 17:** Adolescent Obesity

*Contd...*

| Drug | Indication | Mechanism of action | Dose | Side effect | Precaution/ note of caution |
|---|---|---|---|---|---|
| Hypolipidemic agents | Baseline LDL ≥250 mg/dL or persistent elevated LDL ≥190 mg/dL or persistent elevated LDL ≥160 mg/dL with comorbid states like type 2 Diabetes mellitus and hypertension | • Atorvastatin<br>• Lovastatin<br>• Simvastatin<br>• Rosuvastatin | • 10–20 mg/day<br>• 10–40 mg/day<br>• 10–40 mg/day<br>• 5–20 mg/day | Monitor CPK and liver functions | Adjust doses based on LDL levels |
| Hypolipidemic agents | Persistent triglycerides ≥500 mg/dL | • Fenofibrate | 160 mg/day | | Adjust doses based on Triglyceride levels |
| Antihypertensives | Persistent elevation of BP, despite lifestyle measures or presence of end-organ damage | • Enalapril<br>• Losartan<br>• Hydrochlorothiazide<br>• Amlodipine | 0.1–0.6 mg/kg/day<br>0.7–1.4 mg/kg/day<br>1–2 mg/kg/day<br>Amlodipine 0.1–0.6 mg/kg/day | Hypotension dizziness | BP monitoring pivotal |
| PCOD | Antiandrogens | Spironolactone | 25–100 mg/day | Electrolyte disturbances | Combine with OC pills |
| | Progestins | • Drospirenone<br>• Cyproterone | • 4 mg/day<br>• 2 mg/day | Thromboembolism | Given with estrogen as cyclical pills |

(BMI: body mass index; CPK: creatine phosphokinase; GLP-1: glucagon-like peptide-1; LDL: low-density lipoprotein; OC: oral contraceptive; PCOD: polycystic ovarian syndrome; SC: subcutaneous)

## Surgery

The endocrine society recommends that adolescents who are in Tanner 4 or 5, who have completed growth and have a BMI >40 kg/m$^2$ or BMI >35 kg/m$^2$ with a significant comorbidity and the obesity persists despite all medical measures, bariatric surgery can be contemplated. Prerequisites for surgery include assent from the adolescent, demonstration of adherence to lifestyle measures, and psychiatrist assessment to rule out eating disorders. Options that are available include malabsorptive procedures that alter food path to reduce absorption, restrictive procedures that reduce gastric volume like vertical sleeve gastrectomy and combination procedures like Roux-en-Y bypass. Significant improvement in metabolic parameters and comorbid pathologies has been described. Clinicians should screen for long-term complications such as iron deficiency, vitamin D deficiency, low bone mineral density, vitamin B12 deficiency, and other micronutrient deficiency. There is very minimal published data on efficacy of bariatric surgery in Indian adolescents.

## Target

A gradual sustained weight loss should be aimed in all obese adolescents. Weight loss can be divided into two phases: Active phase and maintenance phase. One should aim for 1 kg/week reduction in weight till about 10% weight reduction in achieved in the first active phase. A demonstration of the reduction in BMI in the color-coded IAP BMI charts will motivate them to adhere to lifestyle measures. Reduction of 4% of BMI in 3 months of full dose of pharmacological agent replacement is a prerequisite for continuation of medications. Frequent self-weighing should be encouraged in all obese adolescents.

Approach to adolescent obesity is summarized in **Flowchart 1**. Prevention of the onset of obesity in adolescents by healthy lifestyle and early recognition using growth monitoring with the IAP 2015 BMI charts and BMI look-up tool is the most powerful weapon to combat the rising tide of adolescent obesity and its associated complications.

## ■ CONFLICT OF INTEREST

Nil.

## ■ ACKNOWLEDGMENT

Prof K Nedunchelian, Head Research, Mehta Hospital for reading and comments to improvise the manuscript.

**Flowchart 1:** Approach to obesity in adolescents.

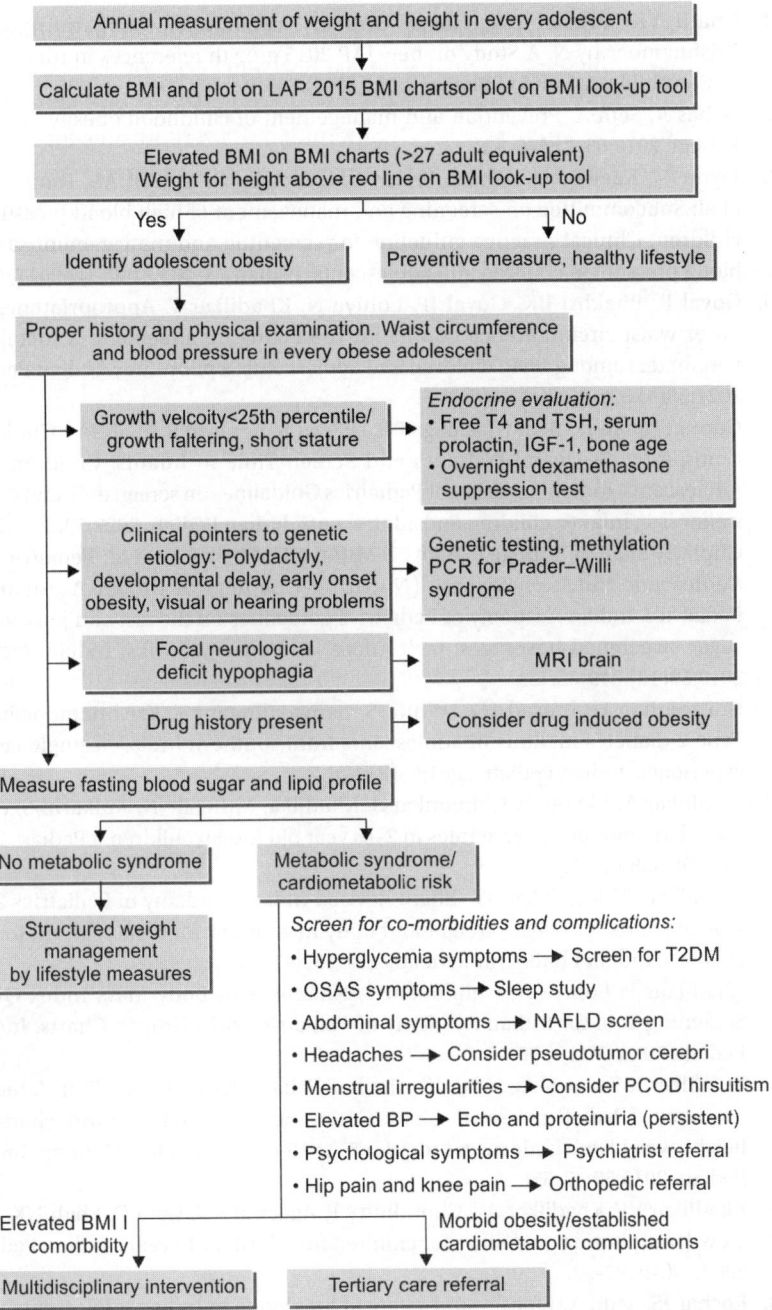

(BMI: body mass index; BP; blood pressure; Echo: echocardiography; IAP: Indian Academy Pediatrics; IGF: insulin-like growth factor; MRI: magnetic resonance imaging; NAFLD: nonalcoholic fatty liver disease; OSAS: obstructive sleep apnea syndrome; PCOD: polycystic ovarian syndrome; PCR: polymerase chain reaction; TSH: thyroid-stimulating hormone; T2DM: type 2 diabetes mellitus; T4: thyroxine)

## SUGGESTED READING

1. Chalil VK, Prasad HK, Nassir SAMA, Arulalan KV, Sangaralingam T, Krishnamoorthy N. A Study on new IAP 2015 growth references in rural South Indian children. Indian J Pediatr. 2021;88(7):645-9.
2. Dabas A, Seth A. Prevention and management of childhood obesity. Indian J Pediatr. 2018;85(7):546-53.
3. Flynn JT, Kaelber DC, Baker-Smith CM, Blowey D, Carroll AE, Daniels SR, et al; Subcommittee on screening and management of high blood pressure in children. Clinical practice guideline for screening and management of high blood pressure in children and adolescents. Pediatrics. 2017;140(3):e20171904.
4. Goyal R, Bhakhri BK, Goyal JP, Lohiya N, Khadilkar V. Appropriateness of lower waist circumference cutoffs for predicting derangement in metabolic parameters among asian children and adolescents: a pilot study. Indian Pediatr. 2021;58(4):392-4.
5. Gupta P, Shah D, Bedi N, Galagali P, Dalwai S, Agrawal S, et al; IAP Guideline Committee on Digital Wellness and Screen Time in Infants, Children, and Adolescents. Indian Academy of Pediatrics Guidelines on screen time and digital wellness in infants, children and adolescents. Indian Pediatr. 2022;59(3):235-44.
6. Gupta P, Shah D, Kumar P, Bedi N, Mittal HG, Mishra K, et al; Pediatric and Adolescent Nutrition Society (Nutrition Chapter) of Indian Academy of Pediatrics. Indian Academy of Pediatrics guidelines on the fast and junk foods, sugar sweetened beverages, fruit juices, and energy drinks. Indian Pediatr. 2019;56(10):849-63.
7. Gurunathan U, Prasad HK, White S, Sangalalingam T, Krishnamoorthy N. Type 2 diabetes mellitus in adolescents from southern India—a single center experience. Indian Pediatr. 2021;58(2):176-7.
8. Khadilkar A, Ekbote V, Chiplonkar S, Khadilkar V, Kajale N, Kulkarni S, et al. Waist circumference percentiles in 2-18 year old Indian children. J Pediatr. 2014 164(6):1358-62.e2.
9. Khadilkar VV, Khadilkar AV. Share Revised Indian Academy of Pediatrics 2015 growth charts for height, weight and body mass index for 5-18-year-old Indian children. Indian J Endocrinol Metab. 2015;52:47-55.
10. Khadilkar V, Lohiya N, Chiplonkar S, Khadilkar A. Body Mass Index Quick Screening Tool for Indian Academy of Pediatrics 2015 Growth Charts. Indian Pediatr. 2020; 57(10):904-6.
11. Khadilkar V, Yadav S, Agrawal KK, Tamboli S, Banerjee M, Goyal JP, et al. Indian Academy of Pediatrics Growth Charts Committee. Revised IAP growth charts for height, weight and body mass index for 5- to 18-year-old Indian children. Indian Pediatr. 2015;52:47-55.
12. Khadilkar VV, Khadilkar AV, Choudhury P, Agarwal KN, Ugra D, Shah NK. IAP growth monitoring guidelines for children from birth to 18 years. Indian Pediatr. 2007;44(3):187-97.
13. Kochar IS, Sethi A. Efficacy and safety of liraglutide in Indian adolescents with obesity. Obes Sci Pract. 2019;5(3):251-7.
14. Kumar K, Prasad HK. Adolescent obesity. Indian J Pract Ped. 2015;17(2):97-108.
15. Lohiya N, Khadilkar V, Pawar S, Khadilkar A, Chiplonkar S, Jahagirdar R. Field testing of IAP2015 Charts. Indian J Pediatr. 2018;85(9):723-8.

16. Mittal M, Jain V. Management of obesity and its complications in children and adolescents. Indian J Pediatr. 2021;88(12):1222-34.
17. Muthukumar A, Krishna VG, Prasad HK, Narayanaswamy K, Ravisekar CV, Krishnamoorthy M. Clinical, biochemical, and radiological profile of polycystic ovary syndrome in adolescents attending an obesity clinic. Indian J Child Health. 2021;8(1):20-5.
18. Premkumar S, Venkatramanan P, Dhivyalakshmi J, Gayathri T. Comparison of nutrition status as assessed by revised IAP 2015 growth charts and CDC 2000 growth charts in lower socioeconomic class school children. Indian J Pediatr. 2019;86(12):1136-8.
19. Ranjani H, Mehreen TS, Pradeepa R, Anjana RM, Garg R, Anand K, et al. Epidemiology of childhood overweight & obesity in India: a systematic review. Indian J Med Res. 2016;143(2):160-74.
20. Seth A, Sharma R. Childhood obesity. Indian J Pediatr. 2013;80(4):309-17.
21. Styne DM, Arslanian SA, Connor EL, Farooqi IS, Murad MH, Silverstein JH, Yanovski JA. Pediatric obesity-assessment, treatment, and prevention: An Endocrine Society Clinical Practice Guideline. J Clin Endocrinol Metab. 2017;102(3):709-57.

# Adolescent Polycystic Ovary Syndrome

*MKC Nair, Sheila Balakrishnan, Varsha Bharti*

## ■ INTRODUCTION

Polycystic ovary syndrome (PCOS) is now being increasingly seen among adolescents. The prevalence of PCOS has been shown to be 5–10% in women of reproductive age. The disorder was initially described by Stein and Leventhal in 1935. PCOS, traditionally thought of as a triad of oligomenorrhea, hirsutism, and obesity, is now recognized as a heterogeneous disorder that results in overproduction of androgens, primarily from the ovary and is associated with insulin resistance.

## ■ DEFINITION

### Rotterdam Criteria

According to the Rotterdam consensus it has been recommended that PCOS be defined when at least two of the following three features are present; irregular menses, clinical and/or biochemical signs of hyperandrogenism, and polycystic ovarian morphology on ultrasound in the absence of another etiology for the above symptoms. Using menstrual irregularity to diagnose PCOS in the adolescent age group is difficult as menstrual irregularity is considered normal in the first few years following menarche. Transabdominal ultrasound, the only option available in young girls, is technically difficult in obese girls. Also, multicystic ovaries are usual in adolescence.

### Recommendations of International Guidelines for Polycystic Ovary Syndrome

The International Guidelines for the assessment and management of PCOS brought out recently, endorse the Rotterdam criteria in adults with specific recommendations to diagnose PCOS in adolescence. Adolescent PCOS should only be diagnosed >2 years after menarche and if both irregular periods and hyperandrogenism are present. Irregular periods are defined as cycles >35 days or <21 days. Androgen excess can be assessed clinically and when required biochemically. Polycystic ovaries on ultrasound are not required for the diagnosis.

The recent guidelines among adolescents suggest the following diagnostic approach to improve the accuracy and avoid over diagnosis:
- Irregular menstrual cycles defined according to years' postmenarche; >90 days for any one cycle (>1 year postmenarche), cycles <21 or >45 days (>1 to <3 years postmenarche); cycles <21 or >35 days (>3 years postmenarche) and primary amenorrhea by age 15 or >3 years postthelarche. Irregular menstrual cycles (<1-year postmenarche) represent normal pubertal transition.
- Hyperandrogenism defined as hirsutism, severe acne, and/or biochemical hyperandrogenemia confirmed using validated high-quality assays.
- Pelvic ultrasound is not recommended for diagnosis of PCOS within 8 years postmenarche.
- Anti-Müllerian hormone levels are not recommended for PCOS diagnosis.
- Exclusion of other disorders that mimic PCOS.

For adolescents who have features of PCOS but do not meet diagnostic criteria an "at risk" label can be considered with appropriate symptomatic treatment and regular reevaluations. Menstrual cycle reevaluation can occur over 3 years postmenarche and where only menstrual irregularity or hyperandrogenism are present initially, evaluation with ultrasound can occur after 8 years postmenarche. Screening for anxiety and depression is required and assessment of eating disorders warrants consideration.

## PATHOGENESIS

Insulin resistance and compensatory hyperinsulinemia are seen in most cases of PCOS. Hyperinsulinemia is responsible for the hyperandrogenism, which in turn causes dyslipidemia with an increase in triglycerides and low-density lipoprotein (LDL) and a decrease in high-density lipoprotein (HDL). The theca cells of the ovaries have a generalized overactive steroidogenesis in PCOS. There is excess of estradiol also in addition to the excess androgens. In the ovary, inhibin is increased, which causes low follicle-stimulating hormone (FSH) concentrations compared with luteinizing hormone (LH), in girls with PCOS. Since inhibin stimulates androgen production which in turn stimulate inhibin secretion, the result is a vicious cycle in the ovary that inhibits follicular development and ovulation. There is a genetic component as most cases of PCOS show a familial clustering in female siblings and there may be a family history of diabetes. A defect in the insulin receptor gene has been demonstrated. Both X linked and autosomal genes are thought to be responsible.

## CLINICAL PRESENTATION

Polycystic ovary syndrome usually presents for the first time at puberty along with weight gain. Menstrual disorders along with hirsutism are the most common presentation.

### Menstrual Disorders

The menstrual disorder may be anovulation or oligo-ovulation and ranges from amenorrhea to oligomenorrhea. Amenorrhea is usually secondary but may rarely be primary. Irregular or infrequent menstrual cycles are common in the first few years following menarche but are usually self-limiting once ovulation is established. If it persists or is associated with signs of hyperandrogenism like hirsutism, evaluation is necessary. The current recommendations are that the diagnosis of PCOS should be made when irregular periods/amenorrhea persists for 2 years after menarche.

### Hyperandrogenism

Progressive hirsutism is a manifestation of hyperandrogenism and should be assessed by the Ferriman–Gallwey scale. Acne is common in adolescence and hence not to be used as a marker of hyperandrogenism in adolescence. In the absence of clinical hyperandrogenism, biochemical evaluation is recommended to confirm the diagnosis of adolescent PCOS. Free testosterone or free androgen index should be used. Overt signs of virilization such as male pattern baldness, increased muscle mass, clitoromegaly and deepening of voice, and very high androgen levels usually indicate the presence of an androgen producing tumor.

### Obesity

It is seen in 50–70% of girls with PCOS. The South Asian guidelines consider a body mass index (BMI) of 23 or more as overweight and 25 or more as obese. A waist circumference >80 cm is considered significant in the South Asian context. Obesity is not essential for the diagnosis of PCOS but should be considered as "at risk" for the metabolic syndrome.

### Acanthosis Nigricans

This is the presence of dark, velvety patches in the armpits, nape of neck, and under the breasts. This is a definite sign of insulin resistance.

## ▪ DIFFERENTIAL DIAGNOSIS

The differential diagnosis includes hypothyroidism, hyperprolactinemia, androgen-secreting tumors of ovary and adrenal, late onset congenital adrenal hyperplasia, and Cushing's syndrome.

## ▪ INVESTIGATIONS

### Ultrasound Abdomen

It may show the presence of polycystic ovaries. However, in adolescence ultrasound evidence of PCOS is not necessary as multifollicular ovaries are common in adolescence. Ultrasound helps to rule out androgen-secreting tumors in cases of severe hyperandrogenism.

## Hormonal Investigations

It includes thyroid function tests and prolactin. Free testosterone or free androgen index is the best marker of ovarian androgen production. Dehydroepiandrosterone (DHEA) is increased if there is an adrenal tumor. 17-OH progesterone is increased in late onset congenital adrenal hyperplasia.

## ■ TESTS TO DETECT METABOLIC PROBLEMS

Fasting blood glucose and a 75 g oral glucose tolerance test (OGTT) may reveal overt diabetes or impaired glucose tolerance while lipid profile may show increased total cholesterol, triglycerides and LDL and low levels of HDL. At present there is no reliable test to detect insulin resistance. Routine testing of insulin level is not mandatory for detecting insulin resistance. The best markers of insulin resistance are BMI, waist circumference >80 cm, acanthosis nigricans, and impaired glucose tolerance on OGTT.

## ■ WHY DIAGNOSE POLYCYSTIC OVARY SYNDROME IN ADOLESCENCE?

The problems in adolescent PCOS are menstrual disorders, cosmetic problems, obesity, and psychosocial problems. Menstrual problems include irregular or excessive bleeding and amenorrhea. Cosmetic problems are hirsutism and acne which are very distressing to the adolescent. Psychological problems such as anxiety and depressive symptoms are common in adolescent PCOS. Obesity and hirsutism may have a negative impact on body image, which will contribute to loss of self-esteem resulting in psychological problems. The natural history of PCOS suggest that after a gap of 2 years, among adolescent girls with confirmed menstrual irregularity with or without ultrasound diagnosed polycystic ovaries, percentage of those with menstrual irregularities have reduced but those with hirsutism have increased.

Detecting PCOS in the late adolescence or early adulthood is essential to identify a target population at risk of infertility and metabolic syndrome and institute preventive measures like lifestyle changes. This is of public health importance in preventing the metabolic and cardiovascular sequelae of PCOS and the disease burden.

## ■ LONG-TERM PROBLEMS

### Pregnancy-related Problems

The most widely known long-term problem is infertility. PCOS is responsible for about 30–40% of the overall infertility. Even if the woman becomes pregnant, there is increased morbidity due to an increased chance of miscarriage, gestational diabetes, preeclampsia, and all the associated problems of obesity.

## Long-term Sequelae

Polycystic ovary syndrome is a forerunner of the metabolic syndrome. Indeed, many adolescent girls with PCOS already exhibit features of the metabolic syndrome. This is even more relevant as the prevalence of the metabolic syndrome, especially type 2 diabetes is much more in India compared to the West. The metabolic syndrome is a constellation of cardiovascular disease risk factors associated with insulin resistance; glucose intolerance, dyslipidemia, hypertension, and central obesity. Analogous to the situation in adults, the prevalence of the metabolic syndrome increases with obesity, reaching as high as 50% among morbidly obese adolescents. There is intriguing evidence that this increased risk may be conferred not only by insulin resistance but also by hyperandrogenemia. There is an increased risk of the metabolic syndrome in girls and women with PCOS associated with increased androgen levels and independent of obesity. PCOS also predisposes to endometrial cancer, due to unopposed estrogenic stimulation of the endometrium.

Pediatricians are increasingly concerned about the long-term health effects of childhood and adolescent metabolic syndrome, and they rightly believe that it may be associated with early cardiovascular disease in adulthood. Cardiovascular event endpoints are difficult to target because of the long latency period between the onset of atherosclerosis and the first cardiovascular event. However, there is evidence from autopsy studies that atherosclerosis starts in childhood.

## ■ MANAGEMENT

This includes management of presenting complaint and prevention of long-term sequelae. The presenting complaint may be menstrual problems such as menorrhagia, irregular periods, or amenorrhea and cosmetic problems like hirsutism. Adolescents with these symptoms should not be denied treatment.

## Prevention of the Metabolic Syndrome

### *Lifestyle Modification*

Lifestyle modification by diet and regular moderate intensity aerobic exercise for a minimum of 30 minutes 5 days a week remains the first line of treatment, especially in obese PCOS. Weight loss can cause spontaneous resumption of menstrual cycle and lower androgen levels. Even a 5% reduction in weight can result in these changes. Weight loss results in lowered insulin levels leading to an increased sex hormone binding globulin and thereby a decrease in the free testosterone levels. This approach is ideal in the adolescent group as this is the period when lifestyle modification is easiest to achieve.

## Insulin Sensitizers

Association of overweight and insulin resistance with PCOS has been clearly demonstrated. Insulin sensitizers help the body to utilize insulin in a more efficient manner. Metformin is the drug, which has been most widely used in adolescents. Metformin acts by decreasing glucose production by the liver. It produces improvement in insulin resistance, reduction in androgens, and in many cases, spontaneous resumption of periods has been observed. The initial dose of 500 mg OD can be increased to 1,000–1,500 mg daily in divided doses. Side effects are nausea, vomiting, and dyspepsia. Lactic acidosis is a rare side effect. It should be avoided in girls and women with altered renal or hepatic function. Long-acting preparations are also available with fewer side effects. The use of metformin is best restricted to those with definite evidence of insulin resistance such as obesity, acanthosis nigricans, or impaired glucose tolerance. At the moment, lifestyle modification remains the best option in preventing long-term sequelae. Further research is awaited regarding long-term use of metformin in preventing the metabolic syndrome.

## Menstrual Problems and Hyperandrogenism

### Combination Pills

The low dose oral contraceptive pill (OCP) containing ethinylestradiol and the third-generation progestin desogestrel is given to regularize menstrual cycle and will also combat hirsutism. 6–12 cycles are needed for a demonstrable effect on hirsutism. The best effects are seen in young girls and are found to have beneficial effects on future fertility as well, by normalizing the hormonal milieu. The drug prevents unopposed estrogenic stimulation of endometrium and future endometrial cancer.

### Role of Myo-inositol

Administration of myo-inositol is a safe and effective method to prevent and correct metabolic disorders in teenagers affected by PCOS. With combination of myo-inositol and OCPs antiandrogenic effects are enhanced, negative impact of OCPs on weight gain is balanced, and metabolic profile is improved. A simultaneous treatment with both these drugs along with lifestyle modification can be considered as a highly effective approach in teenagers affected by PCOS.

### Cyclical Progesterone

Medroxyprogesterone acetate 10 mg twice daily for 5 days in a month will regularize periods if hirsutism is not a problem. It is important to remember that the young women to get endometrial cancer are those with PCOS or estrogen-secreting tumors. Hence, it is imperative that girls or women with PCOS should get withdrawal bleeds at least once in 2–3 months.

## Antiandrogens

Antiandrogens are only recommended when the low dose combined pill has no effect on the hyperandrogenism. Spironolactone, an aldosterone antagonist, in the dose of 50–100 mg daily twice daily is very effective in combating hirsutism. Electrolyte disturbances like hypokalemia should be monitored. Cyproterone acetate is associated with liver toxicity. Hence, assessment of liver function is advisable before commencing treatment, at 3 months and thereafter every 6 months. Other antiandrogens in clinical use are flutamide, finasteride, and ketoconazole. Antiandrogens if used should be in combination with the combined pill.

## Acne Therapy

Antibiotics such as tetracycline, erythromycin, and minocycline are the mainstay of treatment for acne and can be used in conjunction with antiandrogen therapy. Retinoic acid is indicated in intractable acne with severe scarring but such drugs are best administered by a dermatologist, because of potential teratogenic effects.

## Cosmetic Procedures

Cosmetic procedures, primarily for improving body image, can be combined with the low dose combined pill or antiandrogens for tackling hirsutism to provide an immediate effect, while the impact of long-term hormonal treatment is awaited. Electrolysis and laser are acceptable if done in good centers and are especially useful in removing hair, which has been present for a long time.

### ■ POINTS TO REMEMBER

- Adolescent PCOS is diagnosed 2 years after menarche, if both irregular periods and hyperandrogenism (clinical and/or biochemical) are present.
- Polycystic ovaries on ultrasound are not necessary for the diagnosis of adolescent PCOS.
- Screening is recommended in adolescence to prevent long-term sequelae.
- Management should include measures to prevent the metabolic syndrome.

### ■ SUGGESTED READING

1. Avvad CK, Holeuwerger R, Silva VC, Bordallo MA, Breitenbach MM. Menstrual irregularity in the first postmenarchal years: an early clinical sign of polycystic ovary syndrome in adolescence. Gynecol Endocrinol. 2001;15:170-7.
2. Azziz R, Woods KS, Reyna R, Key TJ, Knochenhauer ES, Yildiz BO. The prevalence and features of the polycystic ovary syndrome in an unselected population. J Clin Endocrinol Metab. 2004;89:2745-9.

3. Balen AH, Laven JS, Tan SL, Dewailly D. Ultrasound assessment of the polycystic ovary: international consensus definition. Hum Reprod Update. 2003;9(6):505-14.
4. Chang JR, Coffler MS. Polycystic ovary syndrome: early detection in the adolescent. Clin Obstet Gynecol. 2007;50:178-87.
5. Cook S. The metabolic syndrome: Antecedent of adult cardiovascular disease in pediatrics. J Pediatr. 2004;145:427-30.
6. Coviello AD, Legro RS, Dunaif A. Adolescent girls with PCOS have an increased risk of the metabolic syndrome associated with increasing androgen levels independent of obesity and insulin resistance. J Clin Endocrinol Metab. 2006;91(2):492-7.
7. Dunaif A. Insulin resistance and the polycystic ovary syndrome: mechanisms and implications for pathogenesis. Endocr Rev. 1997;18:774-800.
8. Fauser B, Tarlatzis BC, Rebar RW, Legro RS, Balen AH, Lobo R, et al. Consensus on women's health aspects of polycystic ovary syndrome (PCOS): the Amsterdam ESHRE/ASRM-Sponsored 3rd PCOS Consensus Workshop Group. Fertil Steril. 2012;97(1):28-38.
9. Ferriman D, Gallwey JD. Clinical assessment of body hair growth in women. J Clin Endocrinol Metab. 1961;21:1440-7.
10. Hoeger K, Davidson K, Kochman L, Cherry T, Kopin L, Guzick DS. The impact of metformin, oral contraceptives and lifestyle modification on polycystic ovary syndrome in obese adolescent women in two randomized, placebo-controlled clinical trials. J Clin Endocrinol Metab. 2008;93(11):4299-306.
11. Legro RS, Arslanian SA, Ehrmann DA, Hoeger KM, Hassan Murad M, Pasquali R, et al. Diagnosis and treatment of polycystic ovary syndrome: An Endocrine Society clinical practice guideline. J Clin Endocrinol Metab. 2013;98(12):4565-92.
12. Lord JM, Flight IH, Norman RJ. Metformin in polycystic ovary syndrome: systematic review and meta analysis. BMJ. 2003;327:951-3.
13. Nair MKC, Pappachan P, Balakrishnan S, Leena ML, George B, Russell PS. Menstrual irregularity and poly cystic ovarian syndrome among adolescent girls-a 2 year follow-up study. Indian J Pediatr. 2012;79 Suppl1:S69-73.
14. Peña AS, Witchel SF, Hoeger KM, Oberfield SE, Vogiatzi MG, Misso M, et al. Adolescent polycystic ovary syndrome according to the international evidence-based guideline. BMC Med. 2020;18:72.
15. Pkhaladze L, Barbakadze L, Kvashilava N. Myo-Inositol in the Treatment of Teenagers Affected by PCOS. Int J Endocrinol. 2016;2016:1473612.
16. Sreekumari R, Nair MKC, Nirmala C. Association of overweight and insulin resistance with polycystic ovary syndrome (PCOS). Health Sci J. 2016;1(2):17-22.
17. Stein I, Leventhal M. Amenorrhoea associated with bilateral polycysticovaries. Am J Obstet Gynecol. 1935;29:181-5.
18. Teede HJ, Misso ML, Costello MF, Dokras A, Laven J, Moran L, et al. Recommendations from the international evidence-based guidelines for the assessment and management of polycystic ovary syndrome. Hum Reprod. 2018;33(9):1602-18.
19. The Rotterdam ESHRE/ASRM-Sponsored PCOS consensus workshop group. Revised 2003 consensus on diagnostic criteria and long-term health risks related to polycystic ovary syndrome (PCOS). Hum Reprod. 2004;19:41-7.
20. Weiss R, Dziura J, Burgert TS, Tamborlane WV, Taksali SE, Yeckel CW, et al. Obesity and the metabolic syndrome in children and adolescents. N Engl J Med. 2004;350:2362-74.

# CHAPTER 19

# Coping Strategies in Adolescents: Developmental Issues

*Shashi Kiran, Shekhar Seshadri*

*"If you are faced with a mountain, you have several options.*
*You can climb it and cross to the other side.*
*You can go around it.*
*You can dig under it.*
*You can fly over it.*
*You can blow it up.*
*You can ignore it and pretend it's not there.*
*You can turn around and go back the way you came.*
*Or you can stay on the mountain and make it your home."*

—**Vera Nazarian, The Perpetual Calendar of Inspiration**

## ■ INTRODUCTION

Adolescence is a time of uncertainty, growth, and change. This was the crux of the stance adopted by these authors over two decades ago. We described adolescence as *"a time of great contrast, which are not only difficult for others to understand but also of great confusion to the adolescents themselves"*. These contrasts were posited as leading to experiences of tension, conflict, and contradictory behaviors.

The stance at that point in time was that while adolescence had been mentioned over a long period of time. The study of adolescence itself was a relatively recent one. Even these studies were conceived as "rooted in poorly studied concepts and badly formulated hypothesis".

## ■ HYPOTHESES OF ADOLESCENCE

One of the most popular and compelling of such hypothesis has been one of a tumultuous adolescence filled with storm and stress.

Originating in classical Greece, this theory became lost in the concept of children as small adults. It arose again in the period of European Renaissance with Rousseau describing adolescence as *"a change in humor, frequent anger, a mind in constant agitation, makes the child almost unmanageable.*

*His feverishness turns him into a lion. He disregards his guide; he no longer wishes to be governed".* This hypothesis found its high point in the concept of adolescence as a period of storm and stress, a time of universal and of inevitable upheaval. While interesting and even compelling, these notions were not really based on rigorous study and could be seen as tainted ontologies of adolescence. These taints made adolescent a contested contrast from the anthropological perspective.

The hypothesis of adolescence as a phase of storm and stress has not however stood the test of time. Many large community-based studies have demonstrated adolescence as a period of constant development and change with no persistent or significant tumultuous or conflictual crises and that adolescence is no different from other developmental phases in individual's life. Despite this evidence, the stigmatizing and pathologizing view of a "tumultuous adolescence" continues to inform and influence public perception of adolescence. Despite ontological taints, these theories of adolescence are strong enough to create a developmental construct of adolescence that has been very helpful to understand cognitive, physical, and social development in the adolescent phase of childhood.

The most accepted legal formulation of childhood and the child occurs in the United Nations Conventions on the Rights of the Child (UNCRC) which has been ratified well most all countries in the world. The UNCRC defines a child as a person under the age of biological age of 18 years and within this framework defines adolescence to be the teenage years (13-19 years) and youth as 15-24 years age.

## ■ BIOLOGICAL FRAMEWORK OF ADOLESCENCE

The milestone defining the onset of adolescence is generally considered to be the onset of puberty. This biological approach embedded in endocrinology and hormonal physiology argues for a universal adolescent process with not much scope to consider the influence of social and cultural factors on the development of teenagers. There is a fair degree of evidence to suggest that underlying physiological processes, especially in the domain of endocrinology, do have a significant influence on emotional expression, expression of mood, and emotional regulation. It is during puberty that the individual achieves what is likely to be that individual's adult size and appearance.

Puberty is also the time that marks the culmination of brain development in the form of neuronal myelination, neuronal pathways, and hemispheric integration. Recent evidence however shows that while these neuronal processes reached their peak during adolescence, cognitive development itself continues to occur across the life span. Physiological and neurological processes during puberty certainly do influence how the young person views his/her own identity and perceives the external world.

There is also evidence to suggest that relationships outside of the family become increasingly important during adolescence, to the potential exclusion of relationships within the family. This evidence is however quite limited and seems to have focused on specific outcomes such as academic achievement and delinquency rather than on overall trajectory of adolescence. Relationships during adolescence have been largely studied as predictors of the above outcomes and not been seen as the primary objects of study and inquiry.

The physiological and neurological definition of adolescence has an advantage in that it has a benchmark for the beginning from the time of onset of puberty. There is however difficulty in identifying the end of this biological process. The endocrinal and neurological processes initiated during puberty are known to continue for the rest of their life span. It is therefore a psychological and social parameter that is more likely to servicer closure milestone for adolescence. The parameter most often used in this sense is that the formation of an identity. This is not to say that identity is in anyway easier to define than any biological delimitation for adolescence. What the study of identity is more likely to yield is an understanding regarding the passage of the teenager into adult life.

Thus, it might be useful to consider adolescence as a phase of childhood influenced by physiological processes of puberty, social factors of relationships outside of the family as well as an internal process of development of identity. It would also be extremely important to consider these processes as interacting with each other rather than as strictly independent streams of influence.

There is, for example, evidence on the biological aspects of puberty with not a significant body of evidence to understand the influence of social and cultural expectations of desirable behavior from the teenager during puberty. Similarly, there is a fairly good understanding of the physiology of menarche which is not much understood around the formal puberty rites practiced in different cultures and whether it has any educational and expectational value for the teenager.

## ■ TRAJECTORIES OF ADOLESCENCE

Emerging evidence strongly suggests that adolescence is a phase in life when future patterns of adult health are established, and study of adolescence gives scope for understanding how these patterns are established and creates opportunities for health and help seeking patterns. The dynamic interaction between physiological processes, social expectations of behaviors, and development of mature social roles is crucial to developing healthy help seeking patterns. Thus, it is extremely important to understand adolescence from a public health perspective since the success of public health agendas including global ones such as the Sustainable Development Goals might depend on such understanding.

Despite evidence suggesting otherwise, negative perceptions regarding adolescence continued to influence social and parental expectations and perceptions regarding behavior of adolescence. Evidence also suggests that negative parental perception and attitudes can indicate negative parent-adolescent relations as well as higher levels of behavioral difficulties in the adolescent. Further these parental beliefs and attitudes could be even stronger predictors of the kind of behaviors that parents expect from their adolescent offspring than the behaviors of the teenagers themselves.

These parental attitudes and beliefs could also be negatively related to parental well-being as well as have an impairing effect on communication between parents and their teenage children. The concept of tumultuous adolescence also tends to lead to stereotyped perception of teenagers which in turn could lead to parents becoming either overinvolved or restrictive toward that offspring during the teenage phase. The biological model of adolescence when viewed from this concept represents the adolescent brain as "under construction" leading to the perception that teenagers are extraordinarily vulnerable to risk taking and impulsive behavior. This stereotyped and stigmatizing perception of teenagers by itself could be potentially the biggest stress faced by teenagers.

The stress experienced by adolescents needs to be emphasized as normative stress that is the natural outcome of new and changing experiences in the life of a teenager. As described earlier a large part of the stress is likely to be related to misconception and misperception in parental attitudes which in turn could be impacting on parent child relationships. There is also stress related to expectations of achievement, acquisition of social and interpersonal competencies, the need to take decisions, and work toward forming one's own identity. While these issues are seen across every phase of an individual's life, they seem to take on new dimensions and new meaning over the course of adolescence.

The most prominent focus when studying coping behaviors in adolescents has been academic achievements and delinquent behaviors. More recently there has been an enlargement in this scope of study and now includes achievements in domains outside of the academic domain, especially in social interpersonal and emotional domains. There has also been an increase in looking at schools as socializing and cultural influences in addition to their conventional role of influencing academic and scholastic competencies.

## ADOLESCENCE AND COMPETENCE DEVELOPMENT

There has also been increasing interest in understanding how young people gain skills and competence in subjects of intrinsic interest and factors that motivate them in this process. Achievements are also seen as reflections of aspirations as well as sources of disappointment. It is the process of dynamic interaction between aspirations, disappointments, and anticipation of achievement which influences development of identity and self-esteem and could also pose as a potential source of stress.

Achievements could be in the academic and extracurricular activities which place them in the individual domain, and they could also be in the social and interpersonal dimensions which would place them in the public domain. The influence of intrinsic interests, parental attitudes, and peer influences are known to have a significant influence on development of competencies as well as attainment of achievements. Achievements and gaining of competences are an ongoing and dynamic process. Those who achieve success in these domains during adolescence are more likely to have higher levels of motivation to succeed in adult life as well.

One of the domains that has been studied well in relation to the exploration of adolescence is that of risk-taking behaviors in teenagers. While it is accepted that adolescents tend to have higher levels of risk-taking behaviors, the mechanisms and processes that lead to such heightened risk taking is not well understood. Hormonal, neurophysiological, and psychological causes have been studied as putative causes for such risk-taking behaviors.

While trying to understand the intensity and reasons for high risk-taking behaviors by teenagers it would be useful to attempt a definition of the risk-taking behaviors themselves. Rebellion against prescribed and conventional norms as well as behaviors with detrimental outcomes have been two streams in which this risk-taking behavior has been studied in the past. In more recent studies, risk-taking is perceived as the process of making choices and taking decisions when outcomes are more diverse and variable. A wide range of issues including optimization of benefit and a personalized perception of what constitutes the benefit in dynamic interaction with social and interpersonal expectations is thought to go into the decision leading to risk-taking behaviors.

Neurodevelopmental and endocrinal models give a certain insight into the process of risk taking by teenagers. The risk-taking process itself could be based on explicit and well understood risk factors or on ambiguous and internally perceived factors with an interaction between these factors influencing the nature of the risk-taking behaviour. Some of the well-known areas of risk-taking behaviors of adolescence are higher frequency of unintentional injuries and motor vehicle accidents, especially in male adolescents, onset of substance abuse in adolescence, and increase likelihood of onset of emotional and affective difficulties.

Some of the significant consequences of high frequency risk-taking behaviors in teenagers include academic underachievement, disaffection with the educational system as well as higher potential for feeling frustrated and engaging in self-harming behaviors. These consequences can unfortunately set up a vicious spiral of further high-risk behaviors including a predisposition for reduced self-esteem and emotional ill-health. This would sometimes result in self-harming behaviors and suicidal intent emotional difficulties that invariably go unrecognized.

## COPING STRATEGIES DEVELOPED IN ADOLESCENCE

Thus, while it seems to be reasonable to describe adolescence as a period of significant change and adaptation in an individual's life, it is also important to understand misperception and stereotyped attitude as having a significant degree of stressful impact on the life of teenagers. It would therefore be important to try and understand how the teenager tries to cope with situations that are likely to be engendered by these changes and what should constitute the adaptation. To understand the coping strategies that adolescents might adopt; it is extremely important to examine the definitions of coping.

"Coping is a multidimensional process which involves cognitive and behavioral strategies directed at eliminating or reducing demands, redefining demands so as to make them more manageable, increasing resources for dealing with demands, and/or managing the tension which is felt as a result of experiencing demands". This is essentially a definition of the strand of abilities common to all individuals interweaving with the strand of unique situatedness of individuals. Coping therefore could be a simple or a multidimensional response toward what an individual perceives as stressful.

The philosophy of coping posits that in the face of stress an individual can either cope with what is perceived as stressful or can rebel against the stress. Both responses imply an acknowledgment by the individual, of the systems that have triggered the stressful perception. The former implies making improvements in an existing system while the latter attempts at reconstruction of the system. Both however imagine the creation of a superior alternative.

The concept of perception of stress leads to the stance of subjectiveness in the domain of coping. Subjective well-being is defined as an individual's cognitive and affective positive evaluation of one's own life. The emphasis in this stance is the internal derivation of one's own sense of wellness. This subjective well-being forms the matrix of how individuals tried to manage what they perceive as stressful which in turn could be intense trauma or daily hassles. While coping strategies are diverse with outcome of these strategies depending upon the competence of the individual and nature of stress.

One of the earliest categorizations of coping strategies distinguished between predominantly problem focused coping strategies and emotion focused coping strategies. More recent categorization has included five broad dimensions of avoidance strategies, seeking social support, developing positive attitude, problem orientation, and transcendent orientation. As mentioned earlier, individuals tend to use a variety of coping strategies depending upon that understanding of the stress and the assurance they have in their own competence as well as the availability of social support systems.

Developmental changes during adolescence and parental attitudes toward the adolescent constitute the major source of stress for teenagers. Developmental change demands that the teenager develops new behavioral and cognitive strategies to cope with the change as well as redefine previously learnt strategies. The dynamic interaction of the various coping strategies used and the implicit need for either changing the system or improving the system influences the outcomes of these coping strategies.

Adolescents are known to share emotional and cognitive experiences with parents and with peers. There is some suggestion that exposure of adolescents to conflictual situations might be beneficial in that it could promote the development of individual identity and motivate the need for autonomy. There has however been very little understanding of the threshold when the conflict could turn from being beneficial to being a disadvantage.

The focal theory indicates that adolescents are likely to manage what they perceive as stressful by dealing with one stress at a time and accumulate a number of adaptive strategies overtime. This suggests why some adolescents cope and while others fail despite having similar exposure to stress and trauma. Adolescence is a period of opportunities and a period when future patterns of adult behaviors are established. It is therefore important that teenagers can develop the essential life skills they will need as adults.

Understanding of adolescence has grown but at a slow pace over the past two decades. However, there has been a substantial change in the systems which influence the motivation and ability of adolescents to develop coping strategies. There has been an explosion in access and availability of information in different domains without a concomitant increase in resources that can safely explained the information to the teenager. At the same time there has been exposure of the teenager to different dogmas and ideologies without a reassuring and credible method to critically analyze these dogmas and ideologies.

The most recent instance where adolescents were subjected to what could have been perceived as significant stress was the coronavirus disease (COVID) pandemic. In addition to the stress relating to the COVID infections themselves, there was also a significant degree of social isolation, uncertainty, and removal of structure from the life of adolescents. The losses in health as well as loss due to bereavement as well as the ensuing social and financial stress are likely to have led to heightened experience of anxiety and depression in children and adolescents. There is evidence to suggest that systemic restrictions that were put in place to contain the spread of the virus such as lockdowns were a greater source of concern for teenagers than the virus itself.

There is a clear need for systems themselves to adapt and facilitate coping with stress and gaining of competencies by adolescents. This adaptation by the system itself could ensure that the teenagers have adequate experiential learning of essential life skills and competences.

## ■ SUGGESTED READING

1. Bjork JM, Pardini DA. Who are those "risk-taking adolescents?" Individual differences in developmental neuroimaging research. Dev Cogn Neurosci. 2015;11:56-64.
2. Coleman JC. The focal theory of adolescence: A psychological perspective. In Hurrelmann K, Engel U (Eds). The Social World of Adolescents: International Perspectives. Berlin, Germany: Walter De Gruyter; 1989. pp. 43-56.
3. Coleman L, Coleman J. The measurement of puberty: a review. J Adolesc. 2002;25(5):535-50.
4. Diener E. Subjective well-being. In: Diener E (Ed). The Science of Well-being. Berlin, Germany: Springer Science+Business Media; 2009. pp. 11-58.
5. Figner B, Weber EU. Who takes risks when and why? Determinants of risk taking. Curr Dir Psychol Sci. 2011;20(4):211-6.
6. Giordano PC. Relationships in adolescence. Annu Rev Sociol. 2003;29:257-81.
7. Hadiwijaya H, Klimstra T, Vermunt JK, Branje SJT, Meeus WHJ. On the development of harmony, turbulence, and independence in parent–adolescent relationships: a five-wave longitudinal study. J Youth Adolesc. 2017;46:1772-88.
8. Hall GS. Adolescence: Its Psychology and Its Relations to Physiology, Anthropology, Sociology, Sex, Crime, Religion, and Education. New York: D. Appleton & Company; 1904.
9. Jacobs JE, Chhin CS, Shaver K. Longitudinal links between perceptions of adolescence and the social beliefs of adolescents: are parents' stereotypes related to beliefs held about and by their children? J Youth Adolesc. 2005;34:61-72.
10. Jenks C. Historical perspectives on childhood. In: Lindstrom B, Spencer N (Eds). Social Paediatrics. Oxford: Oxford University Press; 1995. pp. 195-209.
11. Kiran S, Seshadri S. (2001). Coping strategies in adolescents: developmental issues. Indian J Pract Paediatr. 2001;3(2):127-34.

12. Lazarus RS, Folkman S. Stress, Appraisal, and Coping. New York: Springer Publishing Company; 1984.
13. Magson NR, Freeman JYA, Rapee RM, Richardson CE, Oar El, Fardouly J. Risk and protective factors for prospective changes in adolescent mental health during the COVID-19 pandemic. J Youth Adolesc. 2021;50:44-57.
14. Marcia JE. Identity in adolescence. In: Adelson J (Ed). Handbook of Adolescent Psychology, 2nd edition. New York: Wiley; 1980. pp. 159-87.
15. Patterson JM, McCubbin HI. Adolescent coping style and behaviors: conceptualization and measurement. J Adolesc. 1987;10(2):163-86.
16. Rousseau JJ. Emile on Education. London: Nourse & Vaillant; 1763.
17. Sawyer S, Afifi RA, Bearinger LH, Blakemore S-J, Dick B, Ezeh AC, et al. Adolescence: a foundation for future health. Lancet. 2012;379(9826):1630-40.
18. Sawyer SM, Ambresin AE, Bennett KE, Patton GC. A measurement framework for quality health care for adolescents in hospital. J Adolesc Health. 2014;55(4):484-90.
19. Sercombe H. Risk, adaptation and the functional teenage brain. Brain Cogn. 2014;89:61-9.
20. Sica C, Novara C, Dorz S, Sanavio E. Coping strategies: Evidence for cross-cultural differences? A preliminary study with the Italian version of coping orientations to problems experienced (COPE). Pers Individ Differ. 1997;23(6):1025-9.
21. Silva K, Robles RJ, Friedrich E, Thiel MF, Ford CA, MillerVA. Stereotyped beliefs about adolescents and parent and teen well-being: the role of parent-teen communication. J Early Adolesc. 2021;41(6):886-904.
22. Steinberg L. A dual systems model of adolescent risk-taking. Dev Psychobiol. 2010;52(3):216-24.
23. Tesar M, Rodriguez S, Kupferman DW. Philosophy and pedagogy of childhood, adolescence and youth. Glob Stud Child. 2016;6(2):169-76.
24. United Nations. (1989). Convention on the Rights of the Child. [online] Available from https://www.unicef.org/child-rights-convention. [Last accessed January, 2023].

# CHAPTER 20

# School Performance in Adolescence

*Preeti M Galagali, Newton Luiz*

## ■ INTRODUCTION

Academic achievement in adolescence is an important determinant of high self-esteem and peer, teacher, family, and social approval. It has an impact on overall well-being, quality of life, and career prospects in adulthood. Scholastic underachievement commonly presents in clinical settings with mental distress. It is one of the most common causes of school dropout and suicide in adolescence. It can be a pointer toward an emerging mental disorder. Gifted adolescents need a creative and stimulating learning environment that nurtures their advanced learning abilities and avoids boredom.

During entry into middle and high school, adolescents encounter many academic challenges. There is an increase in academic input in terms of volume and complexity of the subject matter. High-level cerebral processing, increased working memory, and metacognitive abilities are required to cope with these demands. Also an efficient retrieval of stored information is required for doing well in scholastic tests and exams. To excel in academics, physical, emotional, and psychosocial well-being of students is essential along with family and school connectedness.

## ■ POOR SCHOOL PERFORMANCE

The prevalence of poor school performance (PSP) and specific learning disability (SLD) in India varies from 5 to 15%. The common causes of PSP include poor home environment and inefficient study strategies. In India, rote learning is the norm and there is an intensely competitive examination system. High parental expectations also increase the academic stress on adolescents.

## ■ DEFINITION

The precise definition of PSP is controversial. An adolescent may be considered as scholastically backward if his/her academic performance in one or more subjects is markedly below the average performance of adolescents of his/her age or grade. A practical definition in clinical practice is, "adolescents are said to be performing poorly in academics if they fail in one or more subject or class or if their marks are below 10th percentile in a particular class or subject or if they are identified by the parent or teacher as 'difficult' to teach".

## ■ CAUSES

Causes of poor academic performance are usually multifactorial. They can be broadly divided into factors in the school, family, or the adolescent **(Table 1)**. PSP in childhood can continue in adolescence from childhood or may present for the first time in this age group **(Flowchart 1)**. Disorders

**TABLE 1:** Causes of poor school performance in adolescence.

| Family factors | School factors | Adolescent factors |
|---|---|---|
| • Low socioeconomic status<br>• Low maternal education<br>• Illiteracy<br>• Marital discord<br>• Divorce<br>• Single parent<br>• Authoritarian or permissive parenting<br>• Punitive parenting<br>• High parental expectations<br>• Domestic violence<br>• Parental ill health and substance use disorder | • Change of school<br>• Change in medium of instruction<br>• Poor teaching methodology<br>• Crowded classrooms<br>• High student teacher ratio<br>• Overexpectations of teachers<br>• Abusive teachers<br>• Bullying<br>• Disruptive peer group | • Poor study skills<br>• Poor motivation<br>• Learning disability<br>• Intellectual disability<br>• Autism spectrum disorder<br>• Attention deficit hyperactivity disorder (ADHD), oppositional defiant disorder, and conduct disorder<br>• Prematurity<br>• Low birth weight<br>• Speech/language impairment<br>• Anemia<br>• Hearing impairment<br>• Visual impairment<br>• Mental disorders<br>• Abuse<br>• Chronic medical diseases<br>• Head injury |

**Flowchart 1:** Clinical presentation of PSP in adolescence.

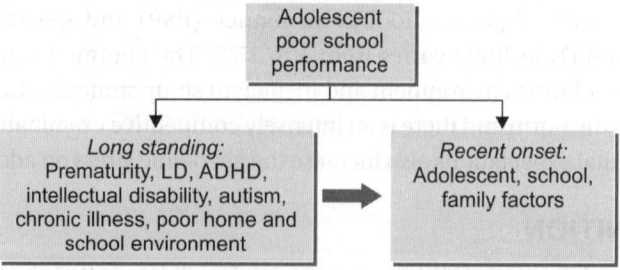

Due to increased academic load, mild LD, borderline intellectual disability, ADHD can present as recent onset PSP in adolescence

(ADHD: attention deficit hyperactivity disorder; LD: learning disability; PSP: poor school performance)

presenting in early childhood, such as mild attention deficit hyperactivity disorder (ADHD), SLD, intellectual disability (ID), autism, and cognitive defects due to prematurity or low birth weight may be compensated in nursery and primary school, due to relatively low academic load. These may present as PSP for the first time in adolescence when the academic load increases.

### ■ FAMILY FACTORS

A stable, nurturing, and stimulating home environment helps the adolescents to perform to their potential. Low socioeconomic status and low maternal education is associated with PSP at all ages. A recent study from India elucidated on chronic physical illness among family members and parental substance abuse as being important contributory factors to PSP. Appropriate parental expectations, authoritative parenting style, parental involvement in school activities, and a high investment by parents in social capital in terms of encouraging creative arts, hobbies, and sports play an important role in improving scholastic performance. Parental role modeling of a healthy lifestyle by adequate sleep, proper time management, following a balanced diet, adequate physical activity, and appropriate use of life skills is known to enhance school performance.

### ■ SCHOOL FACTORS

The school should provide an encouraging atmosphere that develops the all-round personality of the students. Teachers should accept the fact that not all adolescents are "hardwired" to excel in academics. They should avoid comparisons and rebuking students in public. Emotional abuse hurts their self-esteem and may result in school refusal, school dropout, and even suicide. Uncomfortable classrooms with poor and boring teaching methodologies can result in low academic performance.

Recent systematic reviews have suggested that school closures during coronavirus disease-2019 (COVID-19) pandemic have adversely affected the academic achievements of students, especially those belonging to low socioeconomic status. During this period, many students did not have access to online mode of education and had difficulty in grasping concepts. Increase in psychosocial stressors also resulted in a drop in learning.

Peer groups that give importance to academics help the adolescents to excel. Bullying and "ragging" can result in PSP.

### ■ ADOLESCENT FACTORS

Adolescents with low "intrinsic" motivation may do poorly in academics. Right from childhood the feeling of "joy in learning", faith in one's abilities, putting in hard work, and use of efficient study strategies has to be instilled by parents and teachers. Overzealous emphasis on academics can result in burnout and academic failure. Poor time management with excessive and inappropriate media usage impairs learning. Sexuality-related issues such as excessive viewing of pornography, love affairs, and promiscuity can also result in distractions from academics and PSP.

Specific learning disability is a neurodevelopmental disorder characterized by persistent impairment in reading (dyslexia), written expression (dysgraphia), and mathematics (dyscalculia) despite normal intelligence, conventional schooling, intact hearing and vision, adequate motivation, and sociocultural opportunity. Dyslexia is the most common SLD. Intrauterine growth restriction (IUGR), preterm birth, developmental delay, and family history of PSP have been associated with SLD. In most cases, the subtle signs of SLD and borderline ID [slow learners with intelligence quotient (IQ) between 71 and 84] are missed in early childhood and are recognized only in middle and high school that delays remedial measures and results in poor outcomes. In 60–80% cases, childhood ADHD persists into adolescence. In adolescence, the hyperactivity decreases while inattention and poor peer and social relationships persist. Comorbid mental disorders and emotional problems are commonly seen in adolescence with SLD, ADHD, autism, and ID.

Mental disorders such as depression, anxiety, substance addiction, bipolar disorders, conduct disorders, internet gaming disorders, problematic internet use, and schizophrenia may clinically present with a fall in academic performance as the only symptom. "Cyberloafing" is a new educational phenomenon and is defined as deviation from academic-related pursuits toward recreational media use during time allocated for studies. Adolescents with poor self-control are known to indulge in "cyberloafing" which can impact academic performance.

In a study from rural India, a positive association between personal hygiene and academic performance was reported, probably due to a decrease in prevalence of infectious diseases among students and thereby reduced school absenteeism. Anemia affects both physical and mental growth and is an important contributor to poor academic performance in adolescence. Adolescents with poorly controlled chronic disorders (e.g., diabetes mellitus and asthma) have increase school absenteeism and poor performance. Also, in diseases like epilepsy, side effects of medications (e.g., phenobarbitone) may contribute to cognitive defects. Head injuries, obstructive sleep apnea syndrome (OSAS), and visual and hearing impairment can also result in PSP.

A recently published longitudinal study from low- and middle-income countries revealed that linear growth in the first 1,000 days of life determines school performance and even IQ in adulthood. Changes in weight over the life span and linear growth in later periods of life was not associated with these outcomes. Hence to ensure academic achievement, it is essential to invest in early childhood development programs. Genetic disorders such as

**BOX 1:** Impact of poor school performance in adolescence.

- Psychosomatic problems
- Low self-esteem
- Mental distress
- Social isolation
- Aggressive behavior
- Anxiety
- Depression
- Suicide
- School absenteeism
- Dropping out of school
- Drug abuse
- Sexual promiscuity
- Parental distress, anxiety, and economic strain

Fragile X and Klinefelter syndrome may present with PSP for the first time in adolescence.

## IMPACT AND CONSEQUENCES

Poor school performance can lead to immediate, short-term, and long-term repercussions **(Box 1)**. The adolescent can clinically present with these problems in the backdrop of PSP. It has been reported that students with SLD face academic and social discrimination and feel socially isolated and develop emotional issues of anxieties and aggression. Even their parents suffer from anxiety-related issues. Remedial education, tuitions, assessments, and counseling for children with PSP, ID, ADHD, and SLD can lead to high economic burden and strain on families.

## CLINICAL APPROACH

A thorough clinical evaluation is essential to delineate the causes of poor academic performance to identify strengths and to plan further management. A clinical approach is outlined here.

### History Taking

A detailed history is taken from the parents and adolescent regarding:
- Presenting complaints such as aches and pains (psychosomatic disorder) or change in school performance and behavior
- Onset and duration of learning difficulty, namely problems in completing notes, concentration, spelling mistakes, memory lapses, and number of failures in a class or a subject
- Chronic diseases such as diabetes mellitus and asthma; current status; and disease severity along with adherence to medication is assessed

**TABLE 2:** HEEADSSS psychosocial history in poor school performance (PSP) in adolescence.

| Item | Key points |
|---|---|
| **H**ome | Relationship with parents and family members, type of parenting, marital discord, abuse, drug use, and mental disorder |
| **E**ducation | Details of scholastic problems, study habits, ambition, recent change in academic performance, peer group, relationship with teachers, and bullying |
| **E**ating habits | Caloric and green leafy vegetable intake and body image concerns |
| **A**ctivities | Sleep duration and time of onset, type and duration of media usage, time spent with peers, hobbies, and any recent loss of interest in activities |
| **D**epression | Any change in mood, behavior, and interest, duration of such change, and suicide ideation or attempt |
| **S**ubstance use | Attitude toward drug use, drug use among peers, and type and frequency of drug use |
| **S**exuality | Details regarding sexual health, intimate partners, sexual encounters, pregnancy, abortion, and abuse |
| **S**afety | Indulgence in violent acts and run-away behavior |

- Symptoms suggestive of OSAS, hypothyroidism, anemia, and head injury and meningitis in the past
- Birth and developmental history including history of prematurity, low birth weight, and delayed milestones may be suggestive of SLD, ADHD, and autism in childhood. Family history of SLD, ADHD, autism, and mental disorders is also taken as these are heritable.

Psychosocial history is taken from parents and adolescent. History is taken in privacy maintaining confidentiality. One of the practical methods of eliciting a psychosocial history is by using the HEEADSSS tool. HEEADSSS is an acronym that stands for home, education, eating habits, activities, depression, substance use, sexuality, and safety. Important points to be noted under various headings are given in **Table 2**. Apart from identifying weaknesses and various adolescent, family, and school factors contributing to PSP, HEEADSSS is an excellent tool to delineate strengths of the adolescents like nonacademic achievements that can be used in strength-based counseling for motivating an improvement in academic performance.

A report from the teacher regarding current school performance and behavior and changes if any, in the recent past is also beneficial in assessment.

## Examination

Physical, systemic, and mental status examinations are essential. On physical examination, signs of undernutrition, nutrient deficiency, anemia, goiter, visual and hearing impairment, stigmata of Fragile X syndrome (large testes), and Klinefelter syndrome (small testes and tall stature) are carefully looked for. Systemic and mental status examinations are done for clinical assessment of chronic diseases and mental disorders. An informal academic assessment can be done by reviewing current and previous classwork notebooks, exam papers, and report cards that may give pointers to long-standing learning problems like SLD. A brief assessment of reading, writing, analytical, and mathematical ability and skills can be carried out by giving age-appropriate tasks and short assignments.

## Investigations

Investigations vary according to the provisional diagnosis that is made after history and examination. Hemogram and thyroid function tests may be done routinely in recent-onset PSP. Audiometry, refraction, and karyotyping may be required in select cases. The DSM-5 criteria for mental disorders, Connors scale for ADHD, and Beck's inventory for depression are examples of clinically useful screening and diagnostic tools. Psychoeducational testing that includes standardized tests for IQ and learning disability assessments are required in most cases of PSP. These tests should be carried out by a trained clinical psychologist. A simple algorithmic approach to a case of PSP in adolescence is shown in **Flowchart 2**.

## ■ MANAGEMENT

Management of a case of PSP in adolescence requires a multidisciplinary approach and team work. The team leader is usually the pediatrician/

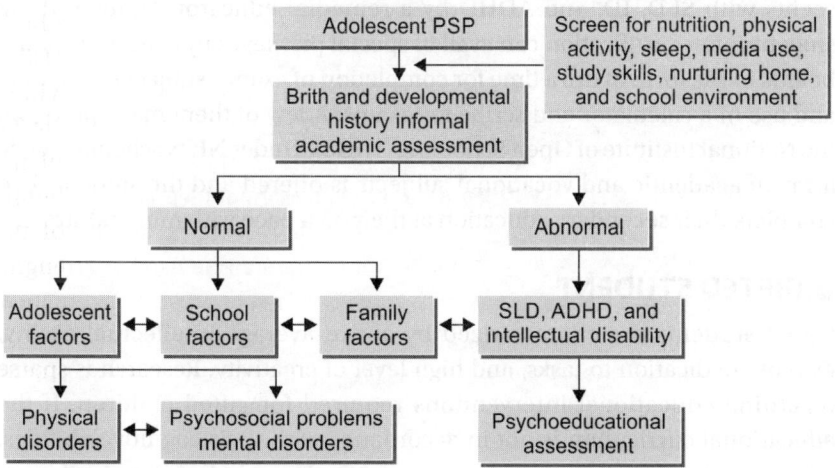

Flowchart 2: Approach of PSP in adolescence.

Note: Multiple factors may coexist and contribute to PSP
(ADHD: attention deficit hyperactivity disorder; SLD: specific learning disability; PSP: poor school performance)

adolescent specialist who shares a good rapport with the adolescent and family. The pediatrician makes the provisional diagnosis, does appropriate investigations and referrals, and coordinates with other team members. According to the final diagnosis, the team members may vary but essentially include a psychologist, the class teacher, and in most cases a remedial educator and psychiatrist.

The treating pediatrician must inform the adolescent and parents about the different factors contributing to PSP and discuss with them various treatment options. The pediatrician should help them to set realistic scholastic and career goals. Multiple counseling sessions may be required. At each session, strengths of the adolescent such as participation in sports, music, and dance are appreciated and encouraged. Medical problems such as anemia and chronic disorders should be managed appropriately emphasizing on importance of adherence. Mental disorders such as depression, anxiety, and ADHD may need psychotherapy in the form of cognitive behavior therapy and a few cases may require specific drugs such as fluoxetine (selective serotonin reuptake inhibitors) and methylphenidate, respectively.

Adolescents, parents, and teachers are counseled about the importance of ensuring age-appropriate sleep, nutrition, physical activity, healthy media use, study skills, annual wellness visits, completing age appropriate vaccination, and a nurturing school and family environment. A few important study skills that can be discussed with the adolescent include time management, active listening skills, methodology of taking notes, use of mnemonics, mind maps, flash cards, and repeated rehearsals for improving memory abilities and efficient exam-taking techniques.

An individualized education plan (IEP) may be charted out for adolescents with SLD, ID, and ADHD by a remedial educator. Many of these students after certification can avail of special privileges by state and central boards in the form of extra time for completion of exams, subject exemption, and use of a calculator and scribe for exams. A few of them may opt to join the National Institute of Open Schooling (NIOS). Under NIOS scheme, a wide array of academic and vocational subjects is offered and the students can complete their secondary education at their own pace with minimal stress.

## ■ GIFTED STUDENT

Gifted students are characterized by above-average intellectual ability, extreme dedication to tasks, and high level of creativity. Research is sparse regarding educational interventions required for gifted children. If the educational curriculum is not in accordance with their cognitive abilities, gifted children are known to get into a negative spiral of boredom, poor motivation, extreme perfectionism, depression, anxiety, and even academic failure. In adolescence, a lot of importance is given to self-image and "fitting in" with the peer group, some gifted students may perform badly on purpose lest they may be branded as "nerds" by their friends. Hence gifted students need family, social, and educational support that acknowledge their superior abilities and helps them to achieve their innate potential. They too need an IEP that is engaging and challenging and goes beyond the basic curriculum. Twice-exceptional (2e) learners have both exceptional ability and a disability in developmental, learning, emotional, physical, or sensory domains. These children need specialized educational and psychological interventions. Parents of gifted children often get stressed while meeting their exceptional needs and may require frequent reassurance and counseling by healthcare professionals.

# GOVERNMENT EDUCATIONAL SCHEMES AND PROGRAMS

Apart from the mid-day meal scheme launched in 1995 to improve nutritional status of school students, pediatricians should be aware about the provisions under Right to Education Act 2009, the inclusion of SLD as a disability under the Rights of Persons with Disability Act 2016, School Health Program 2018, and the recent launch of the landmark National Education Policy 2020 **(Table 3)**.

# CONCLUSION

During annual wellness visits, pediatricians should screen for academic and school problems and give anticipatory guidance regarding study skills. They can play a major role in managing cases of academic difficulties in adolescence as they enjoy the trust and faith of both the adolescent and parents. They should screen for physical, mental, and psychosocial causes, give initial counseling and treatment for the disorders contributing to scholastic concerns and make appropriate referrals. They can assist mental health professionals and partner with parents, teachers, and adolescents themselves in formulating a case-specific management plan. They can also assess response to treatment during follow-up sessions. Hence, pediatricians can ensure that adolescents perform to their potential and lead healthy and productive lives.

# POINTS TO REMEMBER

- Academic performance in adolescence is an important determinant of self-esteem and overall well-being.
- PSP in adolescence may indicate an emerging mental disorder.
- Detailed clinical evaluation of multiple contributory factors in the adolescent, family, or school is the key to appropriate management.

**TABLE 3:** Key educational programs and schemes of Government of India.

| Educational program/scheme/Act/policy | Salient features |
|---|---|
| Right of Children to Free and Compulsory Education (RTE) Act, 2009 | All children from 6 to 14 years age group, including those with disabilities should have access to free and compulsory education |
| Rights of Persons with Disabilities (RPwD) Act, 2016 | All students to be screened for SLD on completion of 8 years of age, establish resource rooms for imparting remedial education and provisions in examinations for students with disability. Students with SLD to get reservations in higher education and government jobs |
| School Health Program under Ayushman Bharat, 2018 | All schools to ensure health education sessions, screen for diseases, provide weekly tablets of iron and biannual tablets of albendazole and sanitary napkins, maintain electronic health records, and train teachers in first aid |
| National Education Policy, 2020 | The policy is based on the principles of universal access, equity, quality, affordability, and accountability to increase gross enrolment ratio to 50%. It aims to provide infrastructure support, encourage enrolment of school drop outs, establish innovative digital education centers, track learning levels, facilitate learning by creative formal and nonformal modes, formulate school, vocational courses, and life-enrichment programs |

- Gifted students need adequate psychoeducational and family support to cater to their exceptional needs.
- A multidisciplinary team that essentially includes a pediatrician and mental health professional in collaboration with parents and teachers should manage issues related to academic performance.

## SUGGESTED READING

1. Arasu S, Fathima FN, Raghu N, Vasnaik M, Mishael T, D'Souza R, et al. Nutritional status, hygiene level, morbidity profile, and their effect on scholastic performance among school children in two subcenter areas of a PHC in Anekal Taluk, Karnataka, India. Indian J Community Med. 2019;44:125-8.
2. Chacko D, Vidhukumar K. The Prevalence of Specific Learning Disorder among School-going Children in Ernakulam District, Kerala, India: Ernakulam Learning Disorder (ELD) Study. Indian J Psychol Med. 2020;42:250-5.
3. Galagali PM, Rao C, Dinakar C, Gupta P, Shah D, Chandrashekaraiah S, et al. Indian Academy of Pediatrics Consensus Guidelines for Adolescent Friendly Health Services. Indian Pediatr. 2022;59:477-84.
4. Galagali PM. Study Skills. In: Choudhry J (Ed). Behavioral Problems in Children and Adolescents. New Delhi: Jaypee Brothers Medical Publishers (P) Ltd.; 2014. pp. 203-14.

5. García-Martínez I, Gutiérrez Cáceres R, de la Rosa AL, León SP. Analysing Educational Interventions with Gifted Students. Systematic Review. Children (Basel). 2021;8:365.
6. Hammerstein S, König C, Dreisörner T, Frey A. Effects of COVID-19-Related School Closures on Student Achievement-A Systematic Review. Front Psychol. 2021;12:746289.
7. Karande S, Doshi B, Thadhani A, Sholapurwala R. Profile of children with poor school performance in Mumbai. Indian Pediatr. 2013;50:427.
8. Karande S, Kulkarni M. Poor School Performance. Indian J Pediatr. 2005;72:961-7.
9. Karande S, Ramadoss D, Gogtay N. Economic burden of slow learners: a prevalence-based cost of illness study of its direct, indirect, and intangible costs. J Postgrad Med. 2019;65:219-26.
10. Karande S. Specific Learning Disabilities in India: Current Situation and the Path Ahead. Indian Pediatr. 2022;59:367-70.
11. Kelly PD. Learning disorders in adolescence: The role of the primary care physician. Adolesc Med. 2008;19:229-41.
12. Lowenson PR, Schubiner H, Robin AL, Neinstein LS. School problems and ADHD. In: Neinstein LS (Ed). Adolescent Health Care: A Practical Guide. 5th edition. Philadelphia: Lippincot Williams & Wilkins; 2008. pp. 1027-41.
13. Ministry of Health and Family Welfare. Operational Guidelines on School Health Programme under Ayushman Bharat Health and Wellness Ambassadors partnering to build a stronger future. Government of India: Ministry of Health and Family Welfare; 2018. Accessed on 30 January 2023. Available from: https://nhm.gov.in/New_Updates_2018/NHM_Components/RMNCHA/AH/guidelines/Operational_guidelines_on_School_Health_Programme_under_Ayushman_Bharat.pdf
14. Ministry of Human Resource Development. (2020). National Education Policy 2020. [online] Available from: https://www.education.gov.in/sites/upload_files/mhrd/files/NEP_Final_English_0.pdf. [Last accessed February, 2023].
15. Panagouli E, Stavridou A, Savvidi C, Kourti A, Psaltopoulou T, Sergentanis TN, et al. School Performance among Children and Adolescents during COVID-19 Pandemic: A Systematic Review. Children. 2021;8:1134.
16. Papadopoulos D. Parenting the Exceptional Social-Emotional Needs of Gifted and Talented Children: What Do We Know? Children (Basel). 2021;8:953.
17. Poveda NE, Hartwig FP, Victora CG, Adair LS, Barros FC, Bhargava SK, et al. Patterns of Growth in Childhood in Relation to Adult Schooling Attainment and Intelligence Quotient in 6 Birth Cohorts in Low- and Middle-Income Countries: Evidence from the Consortium of Health-Oriented Research in Transitioning Societies (COHORTS). J Nutr. 2021;151:2342-52.
18. Sharma N, Das RC, Srivastava K, Upasani R. A study of family-related factors associated with scholastic backwardness in urban lower middle class school children. Ind Psychiatry. 2022;31(1):98-103.
19. Shashidhar S, Rao C, Hegde R. Factors affecting Scholastic Problems. Indian J Pediatr. 2009;76:495-9.
20. Steinberg L. Achievement. In: Steinberg L (Ed). Adolescence. 5th edition. New York: McGraw Hill; 2011. pp. 371-400.
21. Sukumaran TU. Poor Scholastic Performance in Children and Adolescents. Mumbai, India: Indian Academy of Pediatrics; 2011.

22. Thacker N. Poor scholastic performance in children and adolescents. Indian Pediatr. 2007;44:411-2.
23. Tobias SE, Sudler NC. Academic overachievement and underachievement. In: Fisher MM (Ed). Textbook of Adolescent Health Care. United States: American Academy of Pediatrics; 2011. pp. 1907-11.
24. Unni JC, Galagali PM. Academic backwardness in adolescent children. In: Nair MKC (Ed). Trainers Module Adolescent Care in Office Practice. Mumbai, India: Indian Academy of Pediatrics; 2011. pp. 89-104.
25. Zhou B, Li Y, Tang Y, Cao W. An Experience-Sampling Study on Academic Stressors and Cyberloafing in College Students: The Moderating Role of Trait Self-Control. Front Psychol. 2021;12:514252.

# CHAPTER 21

# Adolescent Anxiety and Depression

*MKC Nair, Shyamal Kumar*

## ■ INTRODUCTION

The life between childhood and adulthood, i.e., from 10 to 19 years of age is the adolescence phase. It is a unique phase of human development as well as an important time for laying the foundations of good health. They experience rapid cognitive physical and psychosocial growth and this affects how they feel, think, make decisions, and interact with the world around them.

Despite being thought of as a healthy stage of life, it is associated with significant death, illness, and injury, much of which is preventable or treatable. During this phase, adolescents establish specific patterns of behavior—for instance, related to diet, physical activity, substance use, and sexual activity—that can protect their health and the health of others around them, or put their health at risk now and in the future. Adolescents need information to grow and develop in good health, which includes age-appropriate comprehensive sexuality education, opportunities to develop life skills, health services that are acceptable, equitable, appropriate, and effective, and safe and supportive environments. They also need opportunities to meaningfully participate in the design and delivery of interventions to improve and maintain their health. Expanding such opportunities is key to responding to adolescents' specific needs and rights.

## ■ ADOLESCENT ANXIETY AND DEPRESSION

The mental health of child, adolescent, and youth is probably a continuum from a child's development perspective—normal and abnormal, evolution of problems, causative and risk factors, and ultimately the outcome. Any retrospective search for cause is likely to be biased. It is said that many of the adult psychiatric disorders have their onset in adolescence. Mental health issues of adolescents have to be addressed in the primary care setup itself because there are far too many children and adolescents with behavioral, emotional, and mental health problems in the community and only limited number of psychiatrists, clinical psychologists, and trained counsellors are available. Yet in India, trends in adolescent health in priority mental health areas have uniformly been static or adverse, in contrast to gains made in other countries.

Hence, what we need in India is a team approach with a referral line starting with parents/teachers/community health workers who may suspect a problem, which may be diagnosed and managed at the primary care setting itself. Referral services to higher centers are needed only for a few selected cases, primarily to confirm the diagnosis, rule out comorbid conditions and chalk out a management strategy, implementation of which can be done by the primary care team, if only they could suspect and diagnose early. We need to remember that although the Diagnostic and Statistical Manual of Mental Disorders, Fifth Edition (DSM-5)/the International Classification of Diseases, Tenth Edition (ICD-10) criteria is the gold standard for diagnosing mental health disorders including anxiety disorders and depression, what is more important, for a primary care physician is to remember that the symptom complex per se do not make a diagnosis, unless it is (1) more than explainable by the apparent cause, (2) have significant bodily symptoms, and (3) symptoms are severe enough to cause impairment in daily functions.

## ■ CORONAVIRUS DISEASE AND MENTAL HEALTH

The WHO defines mental health as "a state of well-being in which an individual realizes his or her own abilities, can cope with the normal stresses of life, can work productively, and is able to contribute to his or her community". The peak age of onset of mental illness occurs during adolescence and early adulthood. Around 20% of the world's children and adolescents have a mental health condition. The coronavirus disease-2019 (COVID-19) pandemic (and subsequent consequences) has been hard on everyone, but recent research suggests no age group has been hit harder than young adults. A recent service-oriented study for mental health issues among B.Ed college students conducted in Kerala highlighted the need for early screening and providing early counseling support during the COVID era.

## ■ ANXIETY DISORDERS

Anxiety disorders are a group of mental health disorders, characterized by excessive feelings of anxiety and fear, the anxiety directed towards worries about future events and fear, a reaction to current events causing physical symptoms such as a racing heart and shakiness. Fear and anxiety are in the same continuum, fear is the reaction to a present danger, an adaptive and evolutionary refined process and anxiety is the response to a potential threat. Anxiety is a disproportionately intense, chronic, and potentially irreversible reaction to an imagined threat, operated through brain-body-emotion-cognitive-changes and their interaction with the environment. The anxiety disorders may be grouped as follows.

## Generalized Anxiety Disorder

Generalized anxiety disorder (GAD) is a common and chronic disorder characterized by long-lasting anxiety that is not focused on any one object or situation. Those suffering from GAD experience nonspecific persistent fear and worry and become overly concerned with everyday matters. In children, GAD may be associated with headache, restlessness, abdominal pain, and palpitations. Typically, it begins around 8-9 years of age. If a child has GAD, they may worry about anything, even if it is seemingly minor. They long for attention, approval, and encouragement from others.

## Phobias

Phobic disorders include all cases in which fear and anxiety are triggered by a specific stimulus or situation. Sufferers typically anticipate terrifying consequences from encountering the object of their fear. Sufferers understand that their fear is not proportional to the actual potential danger but still are overwhelmed by the fear. School phobia is a common anxiety disorder in children, which in some cases can be a type of separation anxiety, with no obvious cause. School phobia may also be a form of social phobia, also known as social anxiety.

## Panic Disorder

With panic disorder, a person suffers from brief attacks of intense terror and apprehension, often marked by trembling, shaking, confusion, dizziness, nausea, and/or difficulty in breathing. These panic attacks are fear or discomfort that abruptly arise and peak in <10 minutes and can last for several hours. Attacks can be triggered by stress, fear, or even exercise; the specific cause is not always apparent.

## Social Anxiety Disorder

Social anxiety disorder (SAD) also known as social phobia describes an intense fear and avoidance of negative public scrutiny, public embarrassment, humiliation, or social interaction.

This fear can be specific to particular social situations (such as public speaking) or, more typically, is experienced in most (or all) social interactions.

## Obsessive-compulsive Disorder

Obsessive-compulsive disorder (OCD) is a type of anxiety disorder primarily characterized by repetitive obsession (distressing, persistent, and intrusive thoughts or images) and compulsion (urges to perform specific acts or rituals).

## Post-traumatic Stress Disorder

Post-traumatic stress disorder (PTSD) is an anxiety disorder that results from a traumatic experience. Adolescents would normally feel upset and anxious with any unusual event, but when there is (1) a history of real or perceived catastrophic trauma like death of parents, (2) an intrusive recollection of the traumatic event, (3) with autonomic arousal symptoms such as sweating and palpitation and altogether resulting in, (4) avoidance of the situation. It is called a post-traumatic stress syndrome.

## Separation Anxiety Disorder

Separation anxiety disorder (SepAD) is the feeling of excessive and inappropriate levels of anxiety over being separated from a person or place. Separation anxiety is a normal part of development in babies or children, and it is only when this feeling is excessive or inappropriate that it can be considered as a disorder.

## Situational Anxiety

Situational anxiety is caused by new situations or changing events. It can also be caused by various events that make that particular individual uncomfortable. Often, an individual will experience panic attacks or extreme anxiety in specific situations.

Although anxiety disorders are among the most common and functionally impairing mental health disorders to occur in adolescence, there is paucity of comprehensive data on adolescent anxiety disorders in India. Among the juvenile age group globally, the reported prevalence of anxiety disorders vary from 6.9 to 27% which is more than the most often seen morbidity of mood disorders (6.4%), disruptive disorders (6.4%), and substance abuse (5.3%).

The reported prevalence of GAD varies from 0.2 to 5.8%, SAD from 1.6 to 12.8%, panic disorder from 0.2 to 10% of those attending child psychiatry clinics, and SepAD (4.1%). The common symptoms among anxiety disorders in adolescents observed in India are anxious mood (12.6%), cognitive symptoms (9.9%), and physical symptoms (9.2%). The predominant symptoms among various subtypes anxious mood; (1) panic disorder (32%), (2) GAD (12.2%), (3) SepAD (5.3%), and (4) SAD (1%).

To screen for anxiety disorders among adolescents in primary care settings, many self rating measures exists; a recent meta-analysis has shown that the most commonly used one to evaluate anxiety disorder symptoms is "Screen for Child Anxiety Related Emotional Disorders (SCARED)". SCARED, a self-rated questionnaire has 41 items under the five subscales of panic/somatic, generalized anxiety, separation anxiety, social phobia, and school phobia. Adolescents are asked to rate the frequency with which they experience each symptom using a 3-point Likert scale (0 = almost never, 1 = sometimes, and 2 = often). As against the original cut-off score of 31, a recent community study in Kerala has suggested a cut-off score of 21 for screening anxiety disorders among adolescents with better diagnostic accuracy properties.

# ▪ DEPRESSION

Historically, children were not considered candidates for depression. Today, childhood depression is widely recognized and health professionals see depression as a serious condition affecting both adolescents and young children. Because adolescents are already moody and unpredictable due to other changes and pressures in their lives, parents must know how to differentiate between the normal struggles of adolescent growth and serious emotional problems. One of the factors that make depression so difficult to diagnose in adolescents is the common behavior change that are normally associated with the hormonal changes of this period. It has only been in recent years that the medical community has acknowledged childhood depression and viewed it as a condition, which requires intervention.

## Self-esteem

One of the chief differences between adult and adolescent depression is that depression in adolescents usually involves more social and interpersonal difficulties, which directly leads to self-esteem problems. The inability to relate positively in social situations may lead to low self-esteem which leads to depression. The depression then leads to further inability to relate with others or be fully accepted in social groups which then adds to the feelings of low self-esteem.

## Autonomy

Another factor associated with adolescent depression and negative behaviors is difficulty in establishing autonomy in the adolescent's relationship with parents. Adolescent depression is seen in higher frequency in families where the children have difficulty establishing their own identity because of negative communication patterns and other dysfunctional family attributes.

## Suicidal Ideation

Adolescents are also more likely to idealize suicide as a solution to feelings of helplessness. Adolescents may also socially isolate themselves when depressed out of feelings of guilt. Dramatic behaviors such as aggression and an obsession or fascination with death often accompany their depression.

Depressive disorders, which include major depressive disorder (unipolar depression), dysthymic disorder (chronic and mild depression), and bipolar disorder (manic depression), can have far reaching effects on the functioning and adjustment of young people. Among both children and adolescents, depressive disorders confer an increased risk for illness and interpersonal and psychosocial difficulties that persist long after the depressive episode is resolved; in adolescents there is also an increased risk for substance abuse and suicidal behavior.

## Diagnosis

Symptoms of major depressive disorder common to adults, children, and adolescents are: (1) persistent sad or irritable mood, (2) loss of interest in activities once enjoyed, (3) significant change in appetite or body weight, (4) difficulty in sleeping or oversleeping, (5) psychomotor agitation or retardation, (6) loss of energy, (7) feelings of worthlessness or inappropriate guilt, (8) difficulty concentrating, and (9) recurrent thoughts of death or suicide. Five or more of these symptoms must persist for 2 or more weeks before a diagnosis of major depression is indicated. Depression may often be seen in physical ailments such as digestive problems, sleep disorders, or persistent boredom (vegetative symptoms). Lamarine considers that in children, depression may often be mistaken for other conditions such as attention deficit disorder, aggressiveness, physical illness, sleep and eating disorders, and hyperactivity. Although depression in children may be confused with attention deficit hyperactivity disorder (ADHD), ADHD must begin before the age of 7. According to Fritz, about 5% of adolescents suffer from depression symptoms such as persistent sadness, falling academic performance, and a lack of interest in previously enjoyable tasks. In order to be considered major depression, symptoms such as suicidal thoughts, lack of appetite, and loss of interest in social activities must continue for a period of at least 2 weeks.

Community diagnosis, however, usually rely on a formal testing using Beck's Depression Inventory (BDI) or Children's Depression Rating Scale (Revised). Information provided by collaterals, including parents, teachers, and community advisors should also be taken into account. BDI is a mood measuring device developed by Dr Aaron T Beck (US). The device detects the presence of depression and accurately rates its severity. The multiple choice questionnaire has 21 groups of statement. The score ranges from 0 to 3 for each statement. The total score is 63.

The questionnaire is scored by adding up the score for each of the 21 items and obtaining the total. A score of 21 and above suggests moderate depression needing individual cognitive behavior therapy and score 31 and above suggests severe depression needing medication in addition to psychotherapy.

## Management

There are two main avenues to treatment: psychotherapy and medication. Often, both may be required. The majority of mild depression in adolescents responds to supportive psychotherapy with active listening, advice and encouragement. Issues of alcohol and substance abuse may have to be addressed by referral to relevant agencies. Formal family therapy may be required to deal with specific problems or issues. Comorbidity is not unusual in adolescents and possible pathology, including anxiety, OCD, learning disability, or attention deficit hyperactivity disorder, should be searched for and treated, if present.

For the more serious and persistent depression, particularly those with vegetative symptoms or suicidal ideation, medication is essential and may be lifesaving. Adolescents because of the common side effects, including sedation and anticholinergic action, generally poorly tolerate traditional antidepressant drugs. This leads to poor compliance. The advent of selective serotonin reuptake inhibitors (SSRIs) has largely put these worries to rest. SSRIs are well tolerated by adolescents because of their fairly rapid action and low tendency to cause side effects.

Low toxicity also makes them particularly helpful in an impulsive patient population. It is important that an adequate time period should be given to allow the medication to work (4-6 weeks) and an adequate dose to be used **(Table 1)**.

### Acute Phase

The drug is continued for 4-6 weeks.

Always target symptoms desired, the side effects, dose schedule, and delayed onset of antidepressant action should be discussed. Look for side effects and if response is inadequate, increase the dose or change the drug.

### Continuation Phase

Continue the same dose for 6-12 months along with psychological methods.

**TABLE 1**

| Disorder | Medication | Dose/day | Dosing | Evidence |
| --- | --- | --- | --- | --- |
| Psychoses | Risperidone | 2-4 mg | OD-TID | Level Ib |
| Depression | Fluoxetine | 10-20 mg | OD (breakfast) | Level Ia |
| Anxiety | Fluoxetine | 10-40 mg | OD (breakfast) | Level Ib |
| Conduct disorder | Valproate sodium | 20 mg/kg | OD (dinner) | Level Ib |
| Mania | • Risperidone<br>• Valproate | 2-4 mg<br>20 mg/kg | OD-TID<br>OD (dinner) | Level IIa |
| Tics | Risperidone | 0.25-2 mg | OD (dinner) | Level Ib |

*Maintenance:* This is to prevent recurrence of depression in the following situations which includes multiple severe episodes, family history of bipolar disorder or recurrent depressive disorder, comorbid psychotic symptoms, stressful/nonsupportive environment, and residual symptoms.

While the recovery rate from a single episode of major depression in children and adolescents is quite high, episodes are likely to recur. In addition, youth with dysthymic disorder are at risk for developing major depression. Prompt identification and treatment of depression can reduce its duration and severity and associated functional impairment.

In summary, mood disorders, particularly depression, are increasingly being recognized among adolescents. The adolescent may not look depressed always, instead may try to cover-up depression by showing over activity. The pediatrician must ask for evidence of a persistent feeling of (1) worthlessness, (2) hopelessness, (3) helplessness, (4) no future at all, and (5) suicidal ideation. In depression, the biopsychosocial model denotes that there are neurotransmitters involved and hence drug therapy is of prime importance. Cognition or the thought process as such, primarily affects mood and hence the primary defect is in the thought process called cognitive error-overgeneralization; minimization of positive and maximization of negative attributes, necessitating cognitive behavior therapy by trained clinical psychologists.

The pediatrician must ensure the support of family, teachers, and friends to maintain positive results of therapy. Psychiatrist consultation is necessary in case of non response after 6 weeks of drug therapy, in which case therapy may be extended for 6 months to 1 year.

## ■ POINTS TO REMEMBER

- Many of the mental health problems in adolescents can be effectively managed at the primary care setting itself.
- Anxiety disorders are the most common and functionally impairing mental health disorders in adolescents.
- Anxiety disorders are characterized by worry about future and current events and fear causing palpitations and tremors.
- Depression in adolescents manifests with problems in establishing self-esteem and autonomy and occurrence of suicidal ideas.
- Both psychotherapy and pharmacotherapy will be required in majority of adolescents with depression.
- Support of family, teenagers, and friends is essential to sustain the good results of treatment.
- In case of no response in 6 weeks or whenever the primary pediatrician feels the need, psychiatrist has to be consulted.

## SUGGESTED READING

1. Allen JP, Hauser ST, Bell KL, O'Connor TG. Autonomy and relatedness in family interactions as predictors of expressions of negative adolescent affect. J Res Adolesc. 1994;4:535-52.
2. American Psychiatric Association. Diagnostic and Statistical Manual of Mental Disorders, Fourth Edition (DSM-4). Washington, DC: American Psychiatric Press; 1994.
3. Arbetter S. Way beyond the blues. Current Health. 1993;20:4-11.
4. Birmaher B, Brent DA, Benson RS. Summary of the practice parameters for the assessment and treatment of children and adolescents with depressive disorders. American Academy of Child and Adolescent Psychiatry. J Am Acad Child and Adoles Psychiatry. 1998;37(11):1234-8.
5. Burford S. What's wrong with this 12-year-old boy? Patient Care. 1995;29:85-8.
6. Child, adolescent depression distinct from the adult version. The Brown University Child and Adolescent Behavior Letter. 1995;11:1-3.
7. Davila J, Hammen C, Burge D, Paley B, Daley S. Poor interpersonal problem solving as a mechanism of stress generation in depression among adolescent women. J Abnorm Psychol. 1995;104:592-601.
8. Felman A, Legg TJ. (2022). What is mental health? [online] Available from https://www.medicalnewstoday.com/articles/154543#early-signs. [Last accessed January, 2023].
9. Kessler RC, Berglund P, Demler O, Jin R, Merikangas KR, Walters EE. Lifetime prevalence and age-of-onset distributions of DSM-4 disorders in the National Comorbidity Survey Replication. Arch Gen Psychiatry. 2005;62(6):593-602.
10. Klein DN, Schwartz JE, Rose S, Leader JB. Five-year course and outcome of dysthymic disorder: a prospective, naturalistic follow-up study. Am J Psychiatry. 2000;157(6):931-9.
11. Kovacs M, Feinberg TL, Crouse-Novak MA, Paulauskas SL, Finkelstein R. Depressive disorders in childhood. I. A longitudinal prospective study of characteristics and recovery. Arch Gen Psych. 1984;41(3):229-37.
12. Kumar S, Lukose R, Nair MKC, Swapna S, Jyothi U, Anjana. Mental Health Screening Among Young Adults—A Comparative Study. Kerala: Pediatric Companion; 2021.
13. Lamarine R. Child and adolescent depression. J School Health. 1995;65:390-4.
14. Lewinsohn PM, Clarke GN, Seeley JR, Rohde P. Major depression in community adolescents: age at onset, episode duration, and time to recurrence. J Am Acad Child Adolesc Psychiatry. 1994;33(6):809-18.
15. Nair MKC, George B, Nair AB. Adolescent mental health counselling. In: Nair MKC, Russell P, George B, Bhaskaran D (Eds). Adolescent Pediatrics, 1st edition. Delhi: Noble Vision; 2017. pp. 75-86.
16. Nair MKC, Russell PS, Ellangovan K. Editorial: The fear factor and forbidden facts. Indian J Pediatr. 2013;80 Suppl 2:S129-31.
17. Nair MKC, Russell PS, Krishnan R, Russell S, Subramaniam VS, Nazeema S, et al. ADad 4: The symptomatology and clinical presentation of Anxiety Disorders among adolescents in a rural community population in India. Indian J Pediatr. 2013;80 Suppl 2:S149-54.
18. Nair MKC, Russell PS, Mammen P, Abhiram Chandran R, Krishnan R, Nazeema S, et al. ADad.3: The epidemiology of Anxiety Disorders among adolescents in a rural community population in India. Indian J Pediatr. 2013;80 Suppl 2:S144-8.

19. Nair MKC, Russell PS. Adolescent health care in India: progressive, regressive or at the cross-roads? Indian J Pediatr. 2012;79 Suppl 1:S1-5.
20. Russell PS, Nair MKC, MammenP, Shankar SR. Priority Mental Health Disorders of Children and Adolescents in Primary-care Pediatric Settings in India 2: Diagnosis, Pharmacological Treatment and Referral. Indian J Pediatr. 2012;79 Suppl 1:S14-9.
21. Russell PS, Nair MKC, Russell S, Subramaniam VS, Sequeira AZ, Nazeema S, et al. ADad 2: the validation of the Screen for Child Anxiety Related Emotional Disorders for Anxiety Disorders among adolescents in a rural community population in India. Indian J Pediatr. 2013;80 Suppl 2:S139-43.
22. Rutgers Institute for Translational Medicine and Science. (2021). More Young Adults Are Thinking About Suicide and Death, National Survey Finds. [online] Available from https://ritms.rutgers.edu/news/more-young-adults-are-thinking-about-suicide-and-death-national-survey-finds/. [Last accessed January, 2023].
23. Ryan ND, Puig-Antich J, Ambrosini P, Rabinovich H, Robinson D, Nelson B, et al. The clinical picture of major depression in children and adolescents. Arch Gen Psychiatry. 1987;44:854-61.
24. Trivedi JK, Gupta PK. An overview of Indian research in anxiety disorders. Indian J Psych. 2010;52:S210-8.
25. Weissman MM, Wolk S, Goldstein RB, Moreau D, Adams P, Greenwald S, et al. Depressed adolescents grown up. JAMA. 1999;281:1701-13.
26. Whitley G. The seductive diagnosis. Downtown Dallas: D Magazine; 1996. pp. 84-99.

# CHAPTER 22

# Disruptive Behavior Disorders in Adolescents: Management

*Harish K Pemde, Prerna Kukreti*

## ■ INTRODUCTION

Adolescence is a phase of changes and the changes occur not only in body but also in behavior. Adolescents' behavior develops from "child-like" to "adult-like" through behaviors known as "being an adolescent". The latter varies from family to family and from culture to culture and certain behaviors such as risk taking, thrill seeking, limit testing, challenging rules, and questioning authority are considered normal. But when it becomes a fixed pattern, repetitive, and influences the routine functioning of adolescent and/or the family and other close contacts, then it represents a trajectory toward disruptive behaviors. Such behaviors are often harmful to self and to others in family and society and hence need evaluation and treatment.

Disruptive behavior and dissocial disorders are characterized by persistent behavior problems that range from markedly and persistently defiant, disobedient, provocative, or spiteful (i.e., disruptive) behaviors to those that persistently violate the basic rights of others or major age-appropriate societal norms, rules, or laws (i.e., dissocial).

In diagnostic classificatory systems, "disruptive behavior disorder (DBD)" refers to two disorders, i.e., oppositional defiant disorder (ODD) and conduct disorder (CD) and the current article will focus on diagnosis and management of these two only. However, DBD as a symptom constellation can be a part of presentation of several other disorders also such as attention deficit hyperactive disorder (ADHD), mood disorders, disruptive mood dysregulation disorder, pervasive developmental disorder, etc.

## ■ DEVELOPMENT OF DISRUPTIVE BEHAVIORS

In every society, certain behaviors are acceptable and some behaviors are unacceptable as determined by societal norms or by law. Context defines behavior and it is important to understand ecological and systemic approach to study the disruptive behaviors in adolescents. These behaviors affect others more than the self and hence categorized as "externalizing (acting out) behaviors".

## EXTERNALIZING BEHAVIOR PROBLEMS

These refer to a constellation of behaviors characterized by noncompliance, aggression, destructiveness, attention problems, impulsivity, hyperactivity, and delinquent type of behaviors. "Conduct problems" (CD, antisocial behaviors, and ODD) and "hyperactivity (ADHD)" are the two main categories of externalizing disorders. The Diagnostic and Statistical Manual of Mental Disorders, 5th edition, Text Revision (DSM-5-TR) includes ODD, CD, antisocial personality disorder (ASPD), and DBDs not otherwise specified under DBD. These behaviors represent a trajectory from ODD in childhood, CD in adolescence, and ASPD in adult life. However, various interventions can break or modify this trajectory. These individuals are known to have high levels of past-traumatic experiences. Early recognition of these features and appropriate interventions can help these adolescents in avoiding the ill consequences of such behaviors and deviate from potential maladaptive patterns.

## DIAGNOSIS OF DISRUPTIVE BEHAVIOR DISORDER

Certain features **(Box 1)** suggest the presence of DBD. The features of DBD could be gauged early in life **(Table 1)** and such children and adolescents should be subjected to detailed history and evaluation.

## ELICITING HISTORY

After establishing a good rapport with adolescent and family, history can be elicited using the following questions. The history given by the informant should be given more importance for DBD. "YES" or "NO" answers should

**BOX 1:** Features often associated with disruptive behavior disorder (DBD).

*Child's behavior:*
- Oppositional defiance of authority
- Aggressive stealing vandalism
- Frequent anger outburst/irritability
- Argumentative
- Callous/unemotional
- No guilt/remorse/distress
- No concern about performance

*Family:*
Large size ineffective discipline

*Parental style:*
Parental rejection neglect

*Schooling:*
- Deviant role models
- Poor scholastic performance

# CHAPTER 22: Disruptive Behavior Disorders in Adolescents: Management

**TABLE 1:** Early indicators of disruptive behavior disorder (DBD).

| 5 years | 8 years | 11 years | 14 years | 17 years |
|---|---|---|---|---|
| Oppositional and defiant | Gets into fights | Hard to control | Stealing and truancy | Career offender |
| Blamed by parents | Rejected by peers | Poor school achievements | Deviant peer group | Unemployed |
| Disliked by siblings | Low self-esteem | Blames others | Antisocial attitude | Drug misuse |

be avoided and answers must be pursued to the fullest. History about most serious accidents or injuries, regardless of whether a negative response was given, especially about cars, bicycles, falls from high places, blows to heads, headache, dizziness, and blackout should be probed.

Detailed history about scars on face, arms, legs, and body should also be asked.

- Do you get frequently punished for doing wrong things?
- Have you ever bullied or threatened anybody?
- Have you ever got into physical fight with others?
- Have you ever injured anyone with bat, knife, or broken bottle or any similar objects?
- Have you ever been in trouble with the law?
- Have you ever stayed away from home because you were angry?
- Do you enjoy setting fire or enjoy playing with fire?
- Have you ever had sex with someone much younger or older than you? This can be asked to the parent/situational assessment to be done by the pediatrician. This history is important and relevant even in Indian context.
- Have you ever missed school without permission from teachers or parents?
- Do you face difficulty in understanding school subjects?
- Do you often lose temper or get easily annoyed and get into frequent arguments?

These questions can be the entry points for detailed history. The parents, teachers, and other significant adolescents or adults in the immediate environment of the "adolescent under evaluation" should also be included in the history taking as the children suffering from DBD may not actually realize the wrongdoings and may describe all these as "normal" or may not reveal the truth.

Please, remember that a detailed physical and neurological examination is important to find any physical comorbid condition.

Certain tools/scales can be used in the evaluation of an adolescent for DBD.

## Child Behavior Checklist

The Child Behavior Checklist (CBCL) is one of the most comprehensively studied of the child and adolescent rating scales available. It is designed to be completed by an independent rater, usually the parent. It can be used for the age range 4–16 years and provides information about a child's social functioning and behaviors. Eight subscales could be derived from the CBCL and each provides a measure of a unique but not totally independent category (aggression behavior, anxious depressed, attention problems, delinquent problems, social problems, somatic complaints, thought problems, and withdrawal). Detailed description is out of scope of this article.

## Conners Scale

This will yield a number of useful domains including conduct problems, learning problems, psychosomatic problems, impulsiveness, hyperactivity, and anxiety.

## ■ DIAGNOSING DISRUPTIVE BEHAVIOR DISORDER

The DSM-5-TR and the World Health Organization–Eleventh Revision of the International Classification of Diseases (WHO–ICD-11) provide diagnostic criteria for ODD and CD **(Boxes 2 and 3)**.

**BOX 2:** ICD-11 and DSM-5-TR criteria for ODD.

### DSM-5 criteria of ODD
Four symptoms of following three dimensions:
1. *Angry/irritable mood:*
    - Often loses temper
    - Is touchy/easily annoyed
    - Is often resentful

2. *Argumentative/defiant behavior:*
    - Argues with authority figures or peers
    - Active defiance or refusal to comply with rules/requests from authority
    - Deliberately annoys others
    - Blames others for own mistakes or misbehavior

3. *Vindictiveness:*
    - Has been spiteful or vindictive with no remorse
    - All the above behavior should compromise academic, social, and occupational functioning

### ICD-11 Criteria of ODD
Same features as DSM-5 and has following subtypes:
- ODD without chronic irritability-anger
- ODD with chronic irritability-anger

(DSM-5-TR: The Diagnostic and Statistical Manual of Mental Disorders, 5th edition, Text Revision; ICD-11: Eleventh Revision of the International Classification of Diseases; ODD: oppositional defiant disorder)

**BOX 3:** ICD-11 and DSM-5-TR criteria for CD.

**DSM-5 criteria for CD**
Presence of minimum three criteria listed under following four domains, present for minimum 12 months:
1. *Aggression to people and animals:*
   - Overpowering animals and people, either by aggression, threat, fighting, or intimidation
   - Forcing sexual activity with persons or animals
   - Cruelty toward animals or persons
2. *Destruction of property:*
   - Deliberately setting fire/destroying other's property
3. *Deceitfulness or theft:*
   - Breaking into someone's house
   - Lying to obtain favors
   - Stealing things of no material value
4. *Serious violations of rules:*
   - Staying out of house/running away/truancy

The disturbance in behavior should impair social, academic, or occupational functioning

**ICD-11 criteria of conduct disorder**
CD is named as "conduct dissocial disorder". It has same features as CD of DSM-5. It has following subtypes:
- Childhood onset
- Adolescent onset (with limited prosocial emotions/with typical prosocial emotions)

(DSM-5-TR: The Diagnostic and Statistical Manual of Mental Disorders, 5th edition, Text Revision; ICD-11: Eleventh Revision of the International Classification of Diseases; CD: conduct disorder)

# DIFFERENTIAL DIAGNOSIS FOR DISRUPTIVE BEHAVIOR DISORDERS

Assessment of other differential diagnosis for disruptive behavior is important such as ADHD, mood disorders, disruptive mood dysregulation disorder, and pervasive developmental disorder. In many children, increased negativity and hostility may occur in the context of a mood or psychotic disorder, and the diagnosis of ODD is not allowed when the symptoms occur exclusively during the course of one of these.

Many adolescents who meet the criteria for a diagnosis of CD or ODD have comorbid psychiatric disorders that may have led to their disruptive behavior and may influence their responsiveness to treatment and their long term.

# TREATMENT OF DISRUPTIVE BEHAVIORAL DISORDERS

Pediatricians are likely to manage any adolescent with ODD and CD and it is important to be familiar with various modalities of treatment so that the

**BOX 4:** When to refer to a psychiatrist or a psychotherapist.

- When the treating physician is unable to make an effective working relationship with the parent or the adolescent
- When adolescent engages in risky or illegal activities (substance abuse and reckless driving)
- When adolescent is severely depressed or has not responded to standard antidepressant therapy
- When adolescent has suicidal tendency
- When adolescent has lost touch with reality (feature of psychosis)

family could be counseled and a shared care could be continued. However, certain features indicate that a referral to psychiatrist would be necessary **(Box 4)**.

Individual and family therapy are most useful in treating ODD. Parents are educated about behavioral management techniques and parenting approaches. Interpersonal and cognitive behavioral psychotherapy are beneficial for children and adolescents. These treatment modalities help adolescents understand their own behaviors, their responses to situations, and the effects of their behaviors on others in their environment.

Following practices can aid clinicians in dealing with parents of adolescents presenting with behavioral problems:
- Support and nurture the parent
- Provide parents with an understanding of normal versus concerning behaviors given the adolescent's developmental phase
- Emphasize a parenting style that recognizes strengths of the child, uses positive reinforcement, actively ignores benign behaviors and provides effective limit-setting, and nonpunitive punishment (time out)
- Teach the power of positive parental attention
- Invite the parent to show you or tell you what they do and say
- Remind the parent of the importance of their behavior as a model for the child
- Provide or refer parenting programs accessible and convenient
- Share skills and techniques to help parents cope.

## Parent Child Interaction Therapy

An evidence-based treatment for children with severe disruptive behavior and their parents. It focuses on changing ineffective parent-child interaction patterns in two stages:
1. *Stage 1:* Focuses on child-directed interaction, strengthens the parent-child relationship, builds the child's self-esteem, and reinforces the child's prosocial behaviors.
2. *Stage 2:* Focuses on parent-directed interaction and introduces parent management training.

# TREATMENT OF OPPOSITIONAL DEFIANT DISORDER

## Family Intervention
In this, there is a direct training of the parent in child management skills and careful assessment of family interactions.

## Behavior Therapy
It emphasizes on teaching parents how to alter their behavior to discourage the child's oppositional behavior and encourage appropriate behavior. It also focuses on selectively reinforcing and praising appropriate behavior and ignoring undesired behavior.

## Individual Psychotherapy
The child is helped to learn new strategies to develop a mastery and success in social situations with peers and families. Effort is targeted in restoring child's self-esteem so that he indulges less in provocative behavior.

# TREATMENT OF CONDUCT DISORDER

The following models have been found useful: parent management training (PMT), problem solving skills training (PSST), and multisystemic therapy (MST).

## Parent Management Training
It aims to improve parenting skills. It addresses the parenting practices identified in research as contributing to conduct problems. It covers promoting play and positive relationship, praise and rewards for sociable behaviors, clear rules and clear commands, consistent and calm consequences for unwanted behaviors, and reorganizing the child's day to prevent trouble.

## Problem Solving Skills Training
It is a cognitive approach and includes anger management and modes to improve child's interpersonal skills, schemes for sorting difficulties at school, e.g., learning disabilities and other class room behaviors, deviant peer group reduction and placing youth with CD in groups with well-functioning youth, etc.

## Multisystemic Therapy
This differs from traditional family therapy in various regards. (1) Treatment is delivered in the situation where the patient lives, e.g., at home. (2) The therapist has a low case load (4–6 families) and the team is available round the clock. (3) The therapist is responsible for ensuring that appointments are kept and making change happen. (4) Regular written feedback on progress toward goal from multiple sources is gathered by the therapist and acted

upon. (5) There is a manual for therapeutic approach and adherence is checked weekly by the supervisor.

## Sociotherapy

It is reemerging as a treatment of DBD. It is a social science and form of social work that involves the study of groups of people, it's constituent individuals and their behaviors, using learned information in case and care management toward holistic life enrichment or improvement of social and life conditions. Sociotherapy has been used in the treatment and education of adolescents at Kanner Academy and Community Schools in Sarasota, Florida, USA. In these settings, the working definition of sociotherapy is the practice of promoting healthy growth and living by facilitating therapeutic communities, personal relationships, and positive peer culture. It is better known as the relationship therapy.

## Pharmacotherapy

Comorbidity in DBD should be looked for and should also be treated simultaneously. Some of the following drugs may be needed according to the indications.
- Antidepressants such as fluoxetine, paroxetine, fluvoxamine, and sertraline can be used for depression.
- For mania or mixed affective episode antiepileptics or lithium can be used.
- For hyperactivity/impulsivity stimulant drugs such as methylphenidate, dexamphetamine, and imipramine are given.

Situations requiring referral to psychiatrist or psychotherapists are listed in **Box 4**.

## ■ PROGNOSIS

Different set of circumstances play a role in how an individual shapes up. The study by Laub and Simpson on delinquent boys to age 70 showed how the individual can be steered away from antisocial path. The prognosis of CD is varied, usually due to learning problems; they drop out of school and hence have poor vocational qualification. They have low social economic status due to low income and in turn get more exposed to alcohol and drug abuse, with few friends and limited involvement with relatives. Episodes of deliberate self-harming behavior also occur commonly. Many of them develop into "antisocial personality disorder".

## ■ POINTS TO REMEMBER

- Occasional disruptive behaviors if repeated in a pattern that negatively affects others may then be a "DBD".

# CHAPTER 22: Disruptive Behavior Disorders in Adolescents: Management

- Early recognition and appropriate interventions are likely to help in effectively dealing with these behaviors and prevent their escalation into a disorder.
- Pediatricians can play a very important role by not avoiding the complaints of parents about such behaviors.
- Pediatricians can coordinate with various professionals such as psychiatrists, counselors, and social workers to extend appropriate care to these children and adolescents, and their families.

## SUGGESTED READING

1. Achenbach TH, Edelbrock CS. Manual for the child behavior checklist and revised child behavior profile. Burlington, VT: Queen City Printers; 1983.
2. American Psychiatric Association. Diagnostic and Statistical Manual of Mental Disorders, 5th edition. Washington, DC: American Psychiatric Association; 2022.
3. Benjamin JS, Virgenia AS, Pataki C. Disruptive behavior disorders. In: Benjamin JS, Virgenia AS (Eds). Kaplan and Sadock's Synopsis of Psychiatry: Behavioural Sciences/Clinical Psychiatry, 10th edition. Philadelphia: Lippincott Williams & Wilkins; 2007. pp. 1218-27.
4. Bloomquist ML, Schnell SV. Helping children with aggression and conduct problems: Best practices for intervention. New York: Guilford Press; 2002. pp. 114-74.
5. Conners CK, Wells KC, Parker JD, Sitarenios G, Diamond JM, Powell JW. A new self report scale for the assessment of adolescent psychopathology: factor structure, reliability, validity and diagnostic sensitivity. J Abnormal Child Psychol. 1997;25:487-97.
6. Friebous R-M. Sociotherapy in German social law. Indication, contents, and aspects of public health. Nervenarzt. 2003;74(7):596-600.
7. Kazdin AE. Child, parent and family dysfunction as predictors of outcome in cognitive-behavioural treatment of antisocial children. Behav Res Ther. 1995;33:271-81.
8. Kazdin AE. Treatment of antisocial behavior in children, current status and future directions. Psychol Bull. 1987;102:187-203.
9. Laub JH, Sampson RF. Understanding desistance from Crime. Crime Justice. 2001:28:1-69.
10. Lee RG, Kanner C. The Value of Connection: A Relational Approach to Ethics. United Kingdom: Gestalt Press; 2004.
11. Scott S. Classification of psychiatric disorders in childhood and adolescence, building castles in the sand? Adv Psychiatr Treat. 2002;8:205-13.
12. World Health Organization. The ICD-11 classification of mental and behavioural disorders: clinical descriptions and diagnostic guidelines. Geneva: World Health Organization; 2019.

# CHAPTER 23
# Management of Adolescent Suicidal Behavior in Office Practice

*Preeti M Galagali, Amitha Rao Aroor*

## ■ INTRODUCTION

Suicide among adolescents has emerged as a significant global health problem. As per the World Health Organization (WHO) global health estimates, suicide is the third leading cause of adolescent mortality in India and fifth leading cause globally. Due to the stigma attached to mental healthcare and existing shortage of mental healthcare professionals, pediatricians could be the first point of contact and hence play a crucial role in identifying and managing adolescents at risk of self-harm. Various terminologies related to self-harm are detailed in **Table 1**.

In India, one child dies of suicide every hour. Most adolescent suicides are impulsive. Adolescents commit suicide mainly by hanging, poisoning, drowning, and self-immolation. The important contributory causes are family problems, breakup in romantic relationships, physical and mental illness, failure in examinations, poverty, bereavement, hero worship, unemployment, and gender discrimination.

## ■ VULNERABILITY IN ADOLESCENCE

Adolescence is a period of heightened emotional reactivity that could result in suicidal behaviour. This is due to the early development of limbic system or emotional brain compared to the prefrontal cortex or reasoning brain (responsible for impulse control, decision making, and executive functions) that matures in young adulthood. Immature stress response and poor

**TABLE 1:** Terminologies related to self-harm.

| | |
|---|---|
| Suicidal ideation (SI) | Consideration of or desire to end one's own life. Can range from passive SI (wanting to be dead) to active SI (wanting to kill oneself) |
| Suicidal plans | Thoughts related to designing and engaging in the act of suicide |
| Suicide attempt | An action intended to deliberately end one's own life |
| Nonsuicidal self-injury (NSSI) | Deliberate destruction or alteration of body tissue without suicidal intent |

coping skills also contribute to impulsivity and vulnerability in adolescence. Adolescents are susceptible to suicide contagion, i.e., a process by which direct or indirect exposure to suicide of one or more persons influence others to attempt suicide. They may commit suicide in response to suicide reports in mass media, especially those that glorify suicide. Cyber bullying on social media, online availability of self-harm techniques, and online sexual solicitation also predispose to self-harm.

## ■ FACTORS ASSOCIATED WITH ADOLESCENT SUICIDE

Suicide is the end result of a complex interplay between genetic, psychiatric, and various other factors. Predisposing biological (serotonin imbalance), personality (perfectionism and impulsivity), and cognitive vulnerabilities (impaired problem solving) along with negative life events, lack of social support, and psychiatric disorders predispose adolescents to suicidal behavior **(Flowchart 1)**.

## ■ RISK AND PROTECTIVE FACTORS

There are multiple risk factors for adolescent suicide **(Table 2)**. All adolescents with suicidal ideation should be screened for underlying psychiatric illness. Previous self-harm or suicidal attempts increase the suicidal risk. These indicate that the person is capable of moving rapidly from suicidal thoughts to behavior. Protective factors promote resilience and reduce the potential for suicide.

## ■ CLINICAL ASSESSMENT OF SUICIDAL RISK

Pediatricians have a role **(Box 1)** in both management and prevention of suicide in adolescence. They need to maintain impeccable documentation

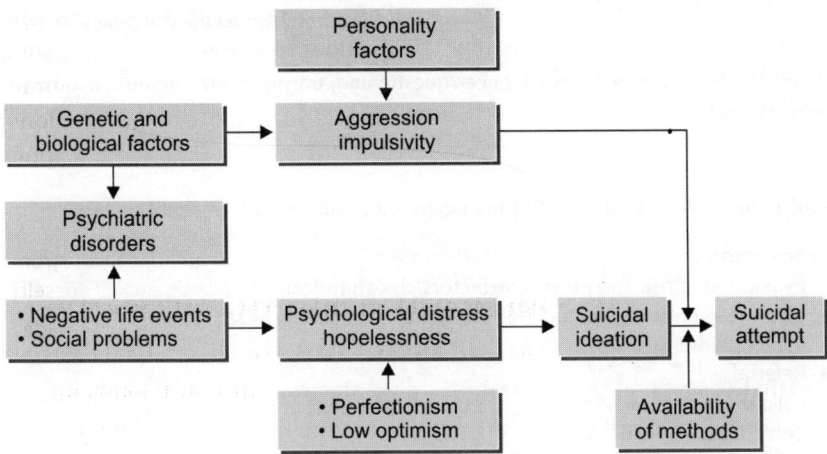

**Flowchart 1:** Biopsychosocial model of adolescent suicide.

**TABLE 2:** Risk and protective factors for adolescent suicide.

| Risk factors | Protective factors |
|---|---|
| *Individual* | |
| • Female sex<br>• School drop out<br>• Previous history of suicidal attempt<br>• Death wish/suicidal notes/online posts<br>• Child abuse/trafficking, bullying, cyberbullying<br>• Nonsuicidal self-injury<br>• Mental and physical illness<br>• Failed intimate relationship<br>• Substance use disorder<br>• Children in conflict with law and in need of care and protection<br>• Gender minority youth: LGBQTIA + marginalized youth | • Positive coping skills<br>• Emotional self-regulation skill<br>• High self-esteem<br>• Conflict resolution skill<br>• Involvement in hobbies and activities<br>• Employment<br>• Religious belief<br>• Good social skills<br>• Help seeking behavior |
| *School and peers* | |
| • Failure in exam<br>• Learning problems<br>• Violent peers<br>• Lack of school counseling services and social support | • Academic achievement<br>• Positive peer relationships<br>• Strong school connectedness<br>• Life skill education, suicide, and bullying prevention programs |
| *Family* | |
| • Family dysfunction and violence<br>• Child abuse and neglect<br>• Economic crisis, environmental disasters<br>• Family history of suicide, mental disorder, alcohol use disorder | • Family stability<br>• Authoritative parenting<br>• Strong family connectedness<br>• Positive discipline |
| *Community* | |
| • Access to means of suicide<br>• Unsafe media portrayal of suicide | • Access to adolescent friendly and mental health services<br>• Responsible media reporting<br>• Comprehensive national policy for suicide prevention |

(LGBQTIA: lesbian, gay, bisexual, queer/questioning, transgender/transsexual, intersex, and asexual)

**BOX 1:** Pediatrician's role in office management of suicidal adolescent.

- Screening
- Evaluation of risk and protective factors, risk stratification
- Brief intervention—immediate counseling with reassurance
- Safety planning
- Referral
- Follow-up
- Prevention

of case assessment and management. Adolescents usually do not reveal suicidal thoughts unless asked. Questions related to suicide should be asked during HEEADSSS screening. Establishing rapport, active listening, being nonjudgmental, and demonstrating empathy are important clinical skills to be used during the assessment. Research shows that asking youth about suicidal thoughts does not increase the risk of suicide; rather it makes them more comfortable to discuss it when they are distressed. The Indian Academy of Pediatrics (IAP) recommends routine screening of adolescents about suicidal ideation, thoughts and behaviors, and other risk factors associated with suicide. In addition to interviewing the adolescent alone, collateral information should be obtained from parents and other gatekeepers. Disclosure of suicidality entails breaking confidentiality and sharing this information with a trustworthy caregiver that the adolescent chooses to ensure safety and well-being.

Open-ended questions are asked to assess the risk of suicide **(Table 3)**. Normalizing the statements when introducing the topic facilitates disclosure. Suicidal ideation, intent, and plans have to be assessed. The presence of suicidal intent should be assessed in all those having ideation. Acts of self-harm might or might not be associated with true intent to commit suicide. They need to be specifically asked whether the self-harm behavior was intended to relieve psychological pain [nonsuicidal self-injury (NSSI)] or

**TABLE 3:** Screening for suicidal ideation, intent, and plan.

| Ideation | Intent | Plan |
|---|---|---|
| • Sometimes people think about hurting or killing themselves when they are upset. Have you anytime experienced such thoughts?<br>• How often do you get these thoughts and how long do they last?<br>• How difficult is it for you to distract yourself when you have such thoughts?<br>• What do you do when you have such thoughts? What coping strategies do you use?<br>• What is the worst that they have ever been? What did you do?<br>• Are there any triggering events?<br>• Do you have hope that things will get better? (significant hopelessness has increased suicidal risk) | • Have you ever thought of acting on your thoughts?<br>• How likely do you think you are to carry out your plan? | • Do you have a plan? If so, how are you planning to do it?<br>• Do you have the means that you would use?<br>• Is there something that would trigger the plan? |

whether there was an intention to commit suicide. Details of the plan, if present, should be asked.

If there is a history of a previous suicide attempt, the following details should be asked:
- The method used (unusual methods carry higher risk)
- Whether it was impulsive or planned
- The lethality of the method used
- The anticipated outcome
- Steps taken to decrease the likelihood of being discovered (signifies higher intent).

## ■ SCREENING TOOLS

Standardized screening instruments for suicidal ideation are available. They may complement but should never replace thorough clinical assessment. Ask Suicide-Screening Questionnaire (ASQ) is a validated four-item measure with good sensitivity and negative predictive value in identifying youth at risk for suicide. Others include the Columbia Suicide Screen, Suicidal Ideation Questionnaire, Beck Depression Inventory, and Patient Health Questionnaire-9-Adolescents.

## ■ EXAMINATION

Detailed clinical examination includes assessment of:
- General appearance (dressing, eye contact, grooming, facial expression) and vitals
- Injuries and hesitation cuts (self-inflicted superficial cuts made by those considering suicidal attempt)
- Attitude (cooperative/violent/avoidant)
- Activity (calm/restless)
- Mental status examination
- Features of child abuse and substance abuse
- Family interactions
- Evidence of systemic diseases.

## ■ WARNING SIGNS OF SUICIDE

A suicide warning sign indicates a heightened risk of suicide in the near-future (i.e., within minutes, hours, or days). Most adolescents with suicidal behavior do exhibit warning signs of suicide, if they are closely looked for. The American Association of Suicidology has developed the mnemonic "IS PATH WARM" to identify warning signs of suicide **(Table 4)**.

## ■ RISK STRATIFICATION

Assessing suicide risk level can be difficult because of multiple factors associated with the clinical presentation. Assessment needs evaluation of

**TABLE 4:** Warning signs of suicide (IS PATH WARM).

| | | |
|---|---|---|
| I | Ideation | Talking/writing about death, threatening to hurt or kill self, looking for ways to die, behaviors or statements indicating good-byes, including giving away prized possessions |
| S | Substance use | Increased substance use |
| P | Purposelessness | Having no reason to live; neglecting appearance and hygiene |
| A | Anxiety(worry/fear) | Anxiety, agitation, and unable to sleep |
| T | Trapped | Feeling like there is no way out of a bad situation, believing suicide is the only solution to one's problems |
| H | Hopelessness | Hopelessness about future |
| W | Withdrawal | From friends/family/society |
| A | Anger | Rage, uncontrolled anger, and seeking revenge |
| R | Recklessness | Engaging in risk activities, not caring for the consequences |
| M | Mood changes | Suddenly improving following a severe depression; dramatic mood changes |

suicidal thoughts, level of intent, existence of plan, access to means, stressors, family, and social support. All suicidal ideation and attempts must be taken seriously and require assessment by a mental health specialist.

Adolescents with suicidal thoughts are classified into three groups:
1. Low risk—suicidal ideation, thoughts of death only; no plan or behavior
2. Moderate risk—suicidal thoughts, limited suicidal intent, and no clear plan
3. High risk—suicide plan with preparatory behavior, past history of suicide attempt and/or NSSI, and multiple risk factors.

Passive ideation should not be ignored as it could progress to active ideation with plan. The management plan depends on the risk categorization **(Flowchart 2)**.

Urgency of mental health referral is according to risk categorization:
- Emergency mental health referral is needed if there is immediate threat to life, for patients assessed as moderate-to-high risk and with severe mental distress.
- Urgent mental health referral within 48–72 hours is needed for patients with low risk.

## RISK CATEGORIZATION IN PATIENTS WITH PREVIOUS SUICIDAL ATTEMPT/NONSUICIDAL SELF-INJURY

When determining the risk, it is essential to assess chronic and acute risk level. Chronic risk level is determined by history of suicidal/nonsuicidal

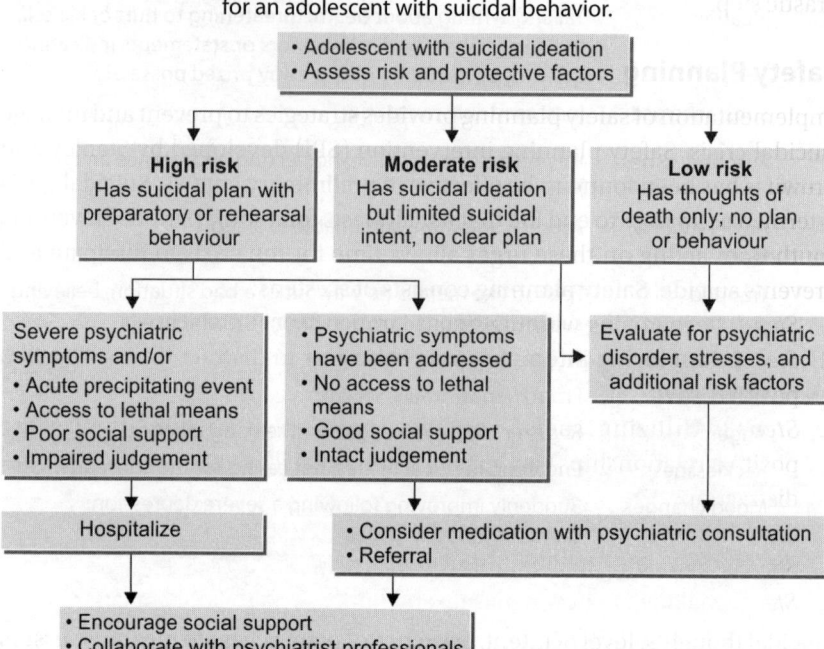

**Flowchart 2:** Risk categorization and management plan for an adolescent with suicidal behavior.

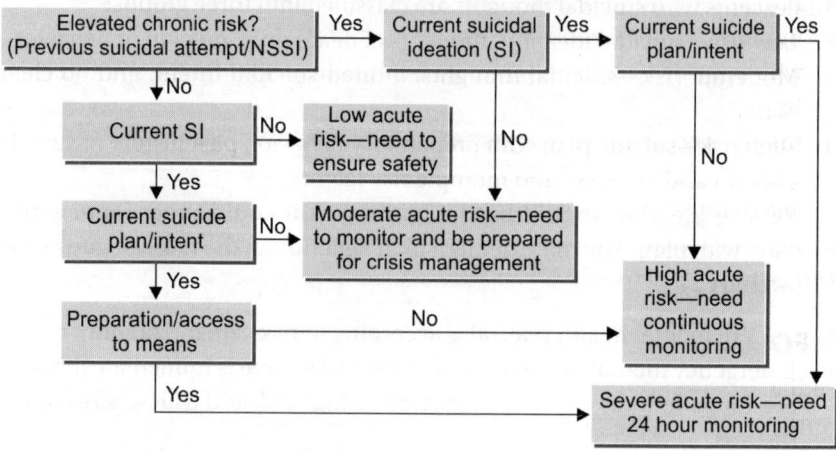

**Flowchart 3:** Risk stratification in patients with previous suicidal attempt/nonsuicidal self-injury (NSSI).

injury behaviors in the past. Risk stratification based on chronic and acute risk is shown in **Flowchart 3**.

## ■ MANAGEMENT

A simple method suggested to save lives from suicide is QPR. QPR refers to Question, Persuade, and Refer. Exploring suicidal thoughts, persuading to seek help, and making timely referral can prevent teens from taking the drastic step.

## Safety Planning

Implementation of safety planning provides strategies to prevent and manage suicidal crisis. Safety planning intervention (SPI) developed by Stanley and Brown is has been found to be effective in preliminary studies. Suicidal crisis is termed as an urge to end life that usually lasts for a short period. Preventing youth from acting on these urges allows time for the crisis to dissipate and prevents suicide. Safety planning consists of six steps:

1. *Step 1:* Recognizing warning signs of impending suicidal crisis.
2. *Step 2:* Employing internal coping strategies to distract themselves in a positive way.
3. *Step 3:* Utilizing social contacts (people with whom they share positive relationships) and social settings (mall, park, etc.) as means of distraction.
4. *Step 4:* Utilizing trusted adults to help resolve the crisis.
5. *Step 5:* Contacting health professionals/helpline.
6. *Step 6:* Making environment safe and limit access to lethal means.

Safety planning intervention forms the basis of the *cascade of care* recommended by the IAP for providing first responder emergency clinical care **(Fig. 1)** that includes:
- Providing emergency medical services, wound care, and appropriate immunization for those presenting with life-threatening conditions and with injuries.
- Imparting psychoeducation and counseling to foster hope and counter the feelings of hopelessness, helplessness, worthlessness, shame, and guilt. Counseling also reinforces protective factors and empowers to cope with stressors through life skills education.
- Activating psychosocial support and discussing lethal means counseling.
- Creating a safety plan with adolescent and the family **(Box 2)**.

## ■ FOLLOW-UP

Pediatricians should collaborate with psychiatrists, psychologists, social workers, educators, and counselors to formulate a follow-up plan. This includes life skills training, building resilience, and therapy for mental disorders along with training on positive parenting. Follow-ups are scheduled once a week for 2 months; later once a month in the first 1 year and twice in the second year.

According to a recent Cochrane review, there is uncertainty regarding effectiveness of various psychosocial interventions in preventing recurrence of self-harm although dialectical behavior therapy for adolescents (DBT-A)

## SECTION 3: Common Medical Problems

```
┌─────────────────────────┐
│ • Suicide risk          │
│ • Suicide attempt       │
│ • Self-harm             │
└─────────────────────────┘
             ↓
┌─────────────────────────────────────────┐
│ • Emergency treatment                   │
│ • Rule out medical disease              │
│ • Explain your role as coordinator of care │
│ • Assess degree of risk*                │
└─────────────────────────────────────────┘
             ↓
┌──────────────────────────────────────────────────────────┐
│ • Listen to the adolescent, develop rapport              │
│ • Reassure about help with difficulties**                │
│ • Instill HOPE                                           │
│ • Counsel caregivers on seriousness, discuss treatment plan, give support │
│   and impart lethal means counselling***                 │
│ • Make safety plan with parents/caregivers and patient** │
│ • Screen for mental health conditions (e.g., depression, psychosis, bullying, │
│   abuse, and substance use) and plan treatment           │
│ • Review risk assessment                                 │
└──────────────────────────────────────────────────────────┘
             ↓
┌─────────────────────────────────────────────┐
│ • Out-patient care                          │
│               or                            │
│ • In-patient care according to risk assessment │
└─────────────────────────────────────────────┘
             ↓
┌──────────────────────────────────────────────────────────┐
│ • Psychiatrist referral, urgency according to risk assessment │
│ • Motivation counseling to address worthlessness,        │
│   hopelessness, helplessness, shame, and guilt           │
│ • Treatment of underlying mental health conditions       │
│ • Resilience building with life skills with focus on coping and problem solving │
│ • Collaborative care with psychologist, educators, social workers, │
│   and nongovernmental organizations (NGOs)               │
└──────────────────────────────────────────────────────────┘
```

| First visit | | |
|---|---|---|
| *Risk assessment: clinical judgement | **Safety plan: supportive factors | ***Caregiver support and lethal means counselling |
| • Look for agitation, intoxication, triggering event, and lethality of means (e.g., poisoning and, hanging)<br>• Self-report on feelings: How do you feel about being alive? What can happen if you lose your life? After suicide attempt/self-harm, ask: Can you share why you attempted to kill/harm yourself? Do you regret what you did? Do you still feel that you want to end your life? If you face the same situation/ have same thoughts in future what will you do differently?<br>• Self-report on protective factors: What makes life worth living? How have you coped with stressors before? Which people have helped/supported you in the past? What change in your life/circumstances would make you change your mind against taking your life? What are your strengths? | • Psychoeducation to caregiver and adolescent: Suicidal behaviour indicates emotional distress. Psychosocial support can relieve distress. Suicides are preventable. Reassure about access to health care and counselling: share contact number and childline number 1098<br>• Appreciate strengths and build self-worth/self esteem<br>• Discuss coping with emotions, problem solving, and relaxation (e.g., deep breathing and, yoga) techniques<br>• Encourage a healthy lifestyle: regular exercise, 8–9 hours sleep, balanced diet, reduce media use, prayer, meditation<br>• Identify at least 2 two supportive adults and peers and encourage talking with them<br>• Emphasize the need for follow-up for 2 years<br>• Sign-up safety plan with adolescent and parents<br>*Sample provided as Box 2.* | Caregiver support: Validate feelings of distress, express empathy, counsel to be supportive, to avoid blaming and criticizing the adolescent. Discuss warning signs of suicide. Tell that asking for suicidal thoughts does not increase the risk of suicide. It makes the adolescent feel at ease to discuss feelings and seek help.<br>Impart lethal means counselling:<br>• Check the person and belongings for the means of suicide: weapon/blade/rope/poison/dupatta/saree<br>• Restrict access to the means of suicide<br>• Ensure 24 hours surveillance by supporting adults<br>• Ensure no lock on bathroom doors<br>• Ensure lock on window and doors and protective grill cover for balcony<br>• No access to alcohol and prescription medication |

**Fig. 1:** Cascade for emergency care of adolescent suicidal behavior.

**BOX 2:** Sample safety plan.

a. Warning signs like thoughts, images, persons, situations, events
   1.                      2.                      3.
b. What I can do to distract myself immediately even without involving other people (e.g., praying, relaxation, deep breathing, imagery, and reverse counting from 100 to 1)
   1.                      2.                      3.
c. Places and people who can help you to distract (e.g., grandparents, friends, playground, mall, neighbor, relative, music, and painting)
   1.                      2.                      3.
d. People whom I can ask for help
   1. Name:                         Phone no:
   2. Name:                         Phone no:
   3. Name:                         Phone no:
e. Doctors, clinic, hospital, and helpline that I can contact for help
   1. Child helpline                Phone no: 1098
   2. Name:                         Phone no:
   3. Name:                         Phone no:

*Reminder:* I am precious. My life is precious. The one thing that is very important for me and makes my life worth living for is ..................................................................................
........................................................................................................................................................

*Note:* Fill in the points as per your preference and choices. Think about what is practical and will work for you. Keep this safety plan handy for reference on your phone, pasted on your door, etc. So that you can remind yourself that you can keep yourself safe at all times.

Signature of adolescent    Signature of caretaker/s    Signature of pediatrician

and individualized cognitive behavior therapy have been found to be beneficial in a few research studies.

## ■ PREVENTION OF ADOLESCENT SUICIDE

Many of the teen suicides are preventable and it requires combined effort and education of the adolescent and the gate keepers. Suicide prevention can be primary prevention (to prevent the onset of suicidal thoughts) which include promoting resilience, promoting peer/family connectedness, helping teens overcome distress by using coping strategies, and secondary prevention to detect youth at risk of suicide and recognize those with warning signs. Some of the measures to reduce teen suicide are as follows:

- *Crisis care:* For those with suicidal ideation and/or with previous attempt.
- *Treatment of mental illness:* By psychotherapy (e.g., cognitive behavioral therapy) and pharmacotherapy. Those who are on selective serotonin reuptake inhibitor (SSRIs) need to be monitored for suicidal ideation during the initial weeks of therapy.

- *Training of pediatricians:* Pediatricians play an important role in suicide prevention by identifying behavioral and emotional problems, promoting positive parenting skills and by promoting resilience among youth and families.
- *Gatekeeper (adults who regularly interact with adolescents and who may recognize problems and help) training:* To identify at risk behavior and promote resilience.
- *School programs:* Focused on life skill education, knowledge about warning signs, and promote help seeking.
- *Community programs:* To promote mental health and reduce the stigma associated with mental illness.
- *Role of media:* Responsible reporting of suicide by media, detecting youth with suicide risk with their social media posts, running youth awareness campaigns on social media, and disseminating information regarding suicide helplines and online consultations.
- *Means restriction:* Restricting the access to common means of suicide, e.g., restricting the sale of organophosphorus insecticides and firearms.
- *Comprehensive national suicide prevention program and maintaining a suicide registry:* These are currently under consideration by the Government of India.

Pediatricians have a major role to play in prevention of adolescent suicide. Timely intervention, along with counseling and safety planning in cases presenting with suicidal behavior can save lives.

## POINTS TO REMEMBER
- Suicide is one of the top causes of adolescent mortality in India and is the result of interplay of genetic and multiple environmental factors.
- Adolescents do not reveal suicidal thoughts unless asked and hence screening is essential.
- Management depends on risk stratification.
- Pediatricians should discuss safety planning interventions with adolescents and caregivers and impart counseling to counter hopelessness and build hope before referring them to a mental health specialist.
- Adolescent suicides can be prevented with adequate training of "gate keepers".

## ACKNOWLEDGMENT

**Table 2**, **Figure 1**, and **Box 2** were originally published in the article Galagali PM, Dinakar C, Bala P, Shah D, Gupta P, Rao C, et al. Indian Academy of Pediatrics Consensus Guidelines on Prevention and Management of Suicidal Behavior in Adolescents. Indian Pediatr. 2022;59:553-62. The material is reproduced by authors after taking permission from Indian Pediatrics.

## SUGGESTED READING

1. Benton TD, Muhrer E, Jones JD, Lewis J. Dysregulation and suicide in children and adolescents. Child Adolesc Psychiatr Clin N Am. 2021;30:389-99.
2. Cha CB, Franz PJ, Guzmán ME, Glenn CR, Kleiman EM, Nock MK. Annual Research Review: Suicide among youth—epidemiology, (potential) etiology, and treatment. J Child Psychol Psychiatry. 2018;59:460-82.
3. Demaso DR, Walter HJ, Wharff EA. Suicide and attempted suicide. In: Kleigman RM, Geme JS (Eds). Nelson Textbook of Paediatrics 21st edition. Amsterdam, Netherlands: Elsevier; 2019. pp. 159-62.
4. Dilillo D, Mauri S, Mantegazza C, Fabiano V, Mameli C, Zuccotti GV. Suicide in pediatrics: epidemiology, risk factors, warning signs and the role of the pediatrician in detecting them. Ital J Pediatr. 2015;41:1-8.
5. Galagali PM, Dinakar C, Bala P, Shah D, Gupta P, Rao C, et al. Indian Academy of Pediatrics Consensus Guidelines on Prevention and Management of Suicidal Behavior in Adolescents. Indian Pediatr. 2022;59:553-62.
6. Garg K, Kumar CN, Chandra PS. Number of psychiatrists in India: Baby steps forward, but a long way to go. Indian J Psychiatry. 2019;61:104-5.
7. Horowitz L, Tipton MV, Pao M. Primary and secondary prevention of youth suicide. Pediatrics. 2020;145:S195-203.
8. Klein DA, Goldenring JM, Adelman WP. HEEADSSS 3.0: The psychosocial interview for adolescents updated for a new century fueled by media. Contemp Paediatr. 2014;31:16-28.
9. Kommu JVS, Jacob P. Specialty training in child and adolescent psychiatry in India. Eur Child Adolesc Psychiatry. 2020;29:89-93.
10. Korczak DJ; Canadian Pediatric Society, Mental Health and Developmental Disabilities Committee. Suicidal ideation and behavior. Paediatr Child Health. 2015;20:257-60.
11. National Crime Records Bureau. (2020). Accidental Deaths and Suicide in India 2020. [online] Available from https://ncrb.gov.in/sites/default/files/ADSI_2020_FULL_REPORT.pdf. [Last accessed January, 2023].
12. Pettit JW, Buitron V, Green KL. Assessment and Management of Suicide Risk in Children and Adolescents. Cogn Behav Pract. 2018;25:460-72.
13. Shain B; Committee on Adolescence. Suicide and Suicide Attempts in Adolescents. Pediatrics. 2016;138: e20161420.
14. Taliaferro LA, Oberstar JV, Borowsky IW. Prevention of youth suicide: The role of the primary care physician. J Clin Outcomes Manag. 2012;19:270-85.
15. Vijayakumar L, Chandra PS, Kumar MS, Pathare S, Banerjee D, Goswami T, et al. The national suicide prevention strategy in India: context and considerations for urgent action. Lancet Psych. 2022;9:160-8.
16. Witt KG, Hetrick SE, Rajaram G, Hazell P, Taylor Salisbury TL, Townsend E, et al. Interventions for self-harm in children and adolescents. Cochrane Database Syst Rev. 2021;3:CD013667.
17. World Health Organization. India Adolescent Mortality Rates. [online] Available from https://www.who.int/data/maternal-newborn-child-adolescent-ageing/indicator-explorer-new/mca/adolescent-mortality-ranking—top-5-causes-(country). [Last accessed January, 2023].

# 24. Anemia in Adolescents

*Piyali Bhattacharya*

## INTRODUCTION

Anemia is defined as reduction in the oxygen carrying capacity of blood due to reduced hemoglobin (Hb) concentration and red cell mass (hematocrit) leading to tissue hypoxia.

Optimal Hb concentration required to meet physiologic needs also varies as per age, sex, smoking habits, pregnancy status, or the altitude of residence.

The World Health Organization (WHO) defines adolescent age as the period between the age of 10 years and 19 years. The recently released The National Family Health Survey-5 (NFHS-5) data (2019–21) reveal that the prevalence of anemia has increased among children, women of all age groups including pregnant women, and men in almost all the states. According to the WHO, anemia affects 24.8% of the global population. 27% of adolescent females in poor countries and 6% of adolescent females in affluent nations are affected.

Anemia was found to be related to poor living conditions exacerbated by substandard housing and sanitary services, number of siblings, high prevalence of parasitic diseases along with undernutrition. With the increase in number of household members, the opportunity of receiving nutritious food decreases, and appropriate childcare is also absent.

As adolescence includes formative developmental years, anemia during this phase has long-term implications on physical growth, immunity, cognitive function, menstrual cycle, and subsequent poor pregnancy effects in girls. Higher prevalence of anemia has been linked to some medical conditions such as essential hypertension, hypothyroidism, congestive heart

**TABLE 1:** The World Health Organization (WHO) definition of anemia.

| Age | 5–11 years | 12–14 years | 15–19 years |
|---|---|---|---|
| Hemoglobin (g/dL) | <11.5 | <12 | Girls: <12<br>Boys: <13 |

failure, coronary artery disease, and rheumatoid arthritis. However, if treated early, most anemia-related consequences can be avoided.

*Factors contributing to development of anemia in the adolescent include:*
- Adolescent growth spurt with hormonal changes and mismatched diet (e.g., testosterone peaks during adolescence and affects erythropoiesis).
- In adolescent boys, rapidly increasing muscle mass requires high amount of iron.
- In adolescent girls, menstrual losses, increased demand for iron due to growth spurt, and teenage pregnancy (50% of our adolescent girls are married) are responsible for iron deficiency anemia (IDA).
- Changing lifestyle, newly acquired freedom, irregular meal timings, peer pressure regarding food choices, and consumption of junk foods.
- Gender bias with reduced availability of nutritious food to the adolescent girl child.
- *Body image issues:* Fear and anxiety of weight gain leading to decrease in proper diet in adolescents. Adolescent girls want a zero-waist figure and all boys want six pack abs.
- Minimal visits to doctors and poor compliance to treatment (in both sexes).
- *Food habits:* Predominantly vegetarian food poor in heme iron, inadequate intake of fruits and vegetable, and consuming tea/coffee along with meals (interferes with iron absorption). Phytates present in cereals and legumes also reduce absorption of iron.

By far, the most common cause of anemia in adolescents is nutritional deficiency, particularly the deficiency of iron (IDA) which occurs due to accelerated growth and hormonal changes often compounded by malnutrition. Deficiency of folate, vitamin A, and vitamin B12 are also important causes. Other causes such as infectious diseases (e.g., malaria, tuberculosis, etc.) and parasitic infections may also be significantly responsible for anemia in adolescents.

Adolescent girls face a greater challenge because of onset of menarche and ensuing menstrual blood losses. This is additive to the increased demand of iron caused by abrupt increase in lean body mass and total blood volume. More frequent and heavy bleeding were found responsible for low Hb concentrations in girls. Individual factors associated with anemia were short-cycle length of mensuration period (16–20 and 21–25 days).

Compared to 54.1% in NFHS-4, anemia in females aged 15–19 years was found to be 59.1% in NFHS-5 **(Fig. 1)**. The numbers were more in rural India (58.7%) as compared to urban India (54.1%).

West Bengal and Gujarat had the highest prevalence of anemia among adolescent girls **(Fig. 2)**.

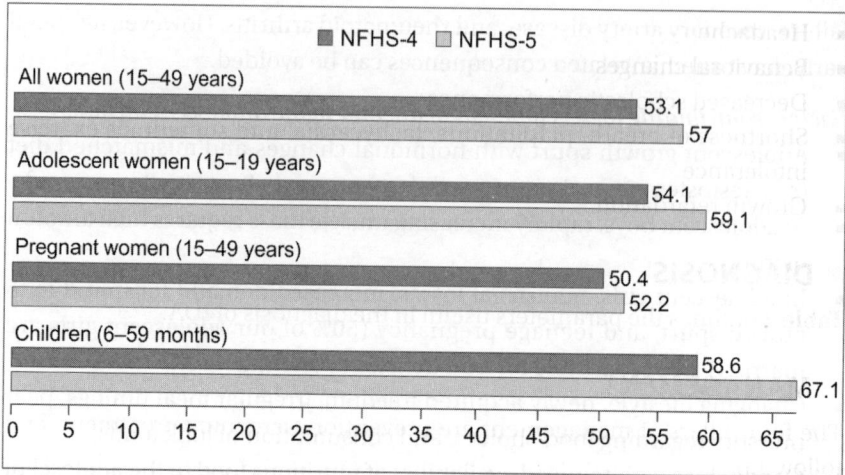

**Fig. 1:** Prevalence of anemia among women and children in India (NFHS-4 vs. NFHS-5).
*Source:* The National Family Health Survey (NFHS).

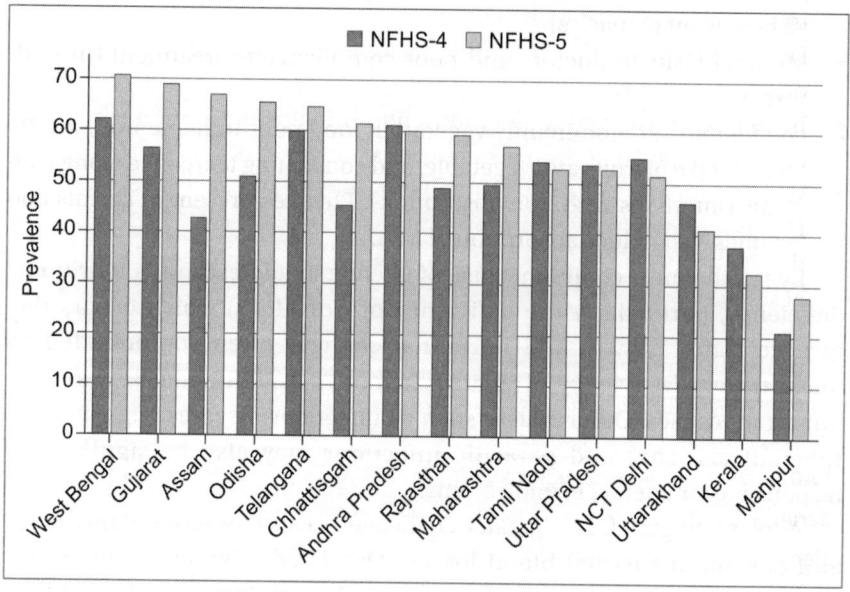

**Fig. 2:** Prevalence of anemia among adolescent women (15–19 years) (NFHS-4 vs. NFHS-5).
*Source:* The National Family Health Survey-5 (NFHS-5).

## SIGNS AND SYMPTOMS

- Pallor
- Irritability
- Fatigue, dizziness, and fainting
- Jaundice may occur

- Headache
- Behavioral changes
- Decreased scholastic performance
- Shortness of breath, palpitations, tachycardia, and sometimes exercise intolerance
- Growth retardation.

## DIAGNOSIS

Table 2 outlines the parameters useful in the diagnosis of IDA.

## MANAGEMENT

The four pillars of management are prevention, screening, treatment, and follow-up.

### Screening and Prevention

- Screening of adolescents by Hb estimation (clinical examination may miss mild/moderate anemia).
- Deworming of all adolescents twice a year can contribute to a significant decrease in anemia.
- Increased consumption of food rich in iron, fortification of commonly consumed food (e.g., iron fortified flour).
- Weekly iron and folate supplementation.
- Dietary interventions, e.g., community awareness programs on healthy dietary habits and reduced consumption of junk food for adolescents and at schools.
- Prevention of adolescent pregnancies by delaying age of marriage and providing family planning strategies are important for improving the state of anemia in young women.

**TABLE 2:** Diagnostic parameters for iron deficiency anemia.

| Serum markers | Iron deficiency anemia (IDA) |
| --- | --- |
| Hemoglobin (Hb) | <130 g/L males<br><129 g/L females<br><110 g/L in pregnancy |
| Serum iron | Decreased |
| Ferritin | <30 µg/L<br>(<100 µg/L in inflammation) |
| Total iron binding capacity (TIBC) | Increased |
| Transferrin | Increased |
| Mean corpuscular volume (MCV) | Decreased |
| Transferrin saturation | <20% |

## Treatment

It consists of iron replenishment which can be done via three routes depending on severity and tolerance to medication:
1. Oral iron supplementation
2. Parenteral iron
3. Transfusion of packed red cells.

### Oral Iron

First-line therapy for iron replenishment is oral iron preparation. It is cheap, available in multiple preparations, has good bioavailability, and has been shown to correct anemia and replenish iron stores effectively. Gastrointestinal (GI) side effects of constipation or nausea and diarrhea may result in decrease of patient adherence leading to cessation and thus, inadequate treatment. Milk or dairy products should be avoided for 1 hour before and 2 hours after each dose to avoid interference with iron absorption.

The Government of India has been addressing the problem through programs like "Anemia Mukt Bharat" designed on the technical and operational evidence from National Iron Plus Initiative (NIPI) and Weekly Iron and Folic Acid Supplementation (WIFS) programs. This program was launched under National Health Mission as part of Intensified National Iron plus Initiative (I-NIPI) in 2018 **(Table 3)**. The action plan is to provide micronutrients such as iron-folic acid (IFA), calcium, and vitamin A along with albendazole to children. Few states like Haryana launched the Anemia Mukt Haryana program under the name "Atal Abhiyaan" (Assuring Total Anemia Limit Abhiyaan) to reduce anemia in all age group across Haryana in 2019.

*Weekly iron and folic acid supplementation:* Key features of the WIFS are as follows:
- Weekly iron (100 mg) and folic acid (500 μg) to adolescent boys and girls 52 weeks a year.
- Administered in schools, every monday; out of school adolescents also need to be supplemented.
- Biannual deworming (albendazole 400 mg), 6 months apart, for control of worm infestation.
- Information and counseling for improving dietary intake and for taking actions for prevention of intestinal worm infestation.

**TABLE 3:** The Intensified-National Iron Plus Initiative (I-NIPI).

| Age | Iron-folic acid | Frequency | Albendazole |
|---|---|---|---|
| 10–19 years | 100 mg elemental iron + 500 μg folic acid | Once a week | One tablet to be chewed at bedtime |

## Parenteral Iron

Parenteral iron is used in selected cases only when oral iron is not well tolerated or rapid increase in Hb is desired, e.g., in adolescent pregnancy with anemia. The primary advantage of intravenous iron is that it bypasses the GI tract absorption avoiding any mucosal inflammation and producing fewer side effects.

Older approved intravenous iron therapies such as low-molecular-weight iron dextran, iron sucrose, ferric gluconate, and ferric derisomaltose require multiple infusions or injections given over a period of weeks/months. These preparations bind iron less tightly, and therefore can only be given in small doses of <250 mg at a time, over periods of weeks. Parenteral iron therapy needs calculation of total iron requirement of the patient.

$$\text{Iron requirement (mg)} = 4.4 \times \text{body weight (kg)} \times \text{Hb deficit g/dL}$$

Newer parenteral preparations, ferric carboxymaltose and ferumoxytol overcome limitations of older preparations and are recommended for total treatment courses of two doses (dose loads up to 1,500 mg (ferric carboxymaltose) and 1,020 mg (ferumoxytol)). These newer preparations have carbohydrate shells that bind elemental iron more tightly and have a distinct advantage over the adverse event profile. They also enable to complete iron replacement doses in 1 hour or less over a two-dose course of treatment.

## Red Blood Cell Transfusion

*Indication:*
- Hb ≤4 g/dL
- Adolescents with Hb 4–6 g/dL who are hemodynamically unstable and/or have associated comorbid conditions, e.g., dehydration, shock, impaired consciousness, heart failure, deep and labored breathing, or very high malarial parasitemia [>10% of red blood cell (RBC)].

Packed cells 10 mL/kg over 3–4 hours are preferred. If packed cells are not available, whole blood 20 mL/kg over 3–4 hours with diuretics may be used with close monitoring for volume overload.

## Follow-up

All adolescents who have successfully completed treatment with recovery of Hb levels should be followed up for the next 3 months.

## ◼ NEED TO RE-LOOK

Questions remain over the cutoffs and resultant overdiagnosis, the WHO Hb cutoffs to define anemia are five decades old and based predominantly on five studies on white adult populations. Considering this fact, a re-look of the existing cutoffs in the context of a healthy population of Indian adolescents becomes mandatory. A group of researchers from multiple institutions across India say that there is a possibility that anemia is being overdiagnosed in India due to a wrong (higher than appropriate) Hb diagnostic cutoff.

The Comprehensive National Nutrition Survey (CNNS), a large, nationally representative, survey of children and adolescents aged 0–19 years, was launched in 2019 in India. The CNNS survey collected blood samples from 49,486 participants between 24th February 2016 and 26th October 2018. Anemia prevalence with the study cutoffs was 19.2% points lower than with WHO cutoffs in the entire CNNS sample. These findings support the reexamination of the WHO Hb cutoffs to define anemia in the Indian perspective.

## ■ RECOMMENDATIONS

Anemia among adolescents is a major public health concern and must be addressed through effective public health policies. There is a felt need to disseminate information about anemia-related programs, such as NIPI, through mass media. Health measures such as awareness programs on improved dietary choices and nutrition and IFA supplementation in schools are effective ways of combating anemia. Iron supplementation is a lifecycle approach starting in infancy and continuing to the end of adolescence for boys and into adulthood for girls. All pediatricians and physicians must examine and prescribe iron supplements to adolescent children during their visit to the clinic.

## ■ SUGGESTED READING

1. Auerbach M, Deloughery T. Single-dose intravenous iron for iron deficiency: a new paradigm. Hematology Am Soc Hematol Educ Program. 2016;2016:57-66.
2. Bathla S, Arora S. Prevalence and approaches to manage iron deficiency anemia (IDA). Crit Rev Food Sci Nutr. 2021;7:1-14.
3. Fernández-Gaxiola AC, De-Regil LM. Intermittent iron supplementation for reducing anaemia and its associated impairments in adolescent and adult menstruating women. Cochrane Database Syst Rev. 2019;1:CD009218.
4. Kapil U, Bhadoria AS. National Iron-plus initiative guidelines for control of iron deficiency anaemia in India, 2013. Natl Med J India. 2014;27:27-9.
5. Lee TW, Kolber MR, Fedorak RN, van Zanten SV. Iron replacement therapy in inflammatory bowel disease patients with iron deficiency anemia: a systematic review and meta-analysis. J Crohns Colitis. 2012;6:267-75.
6. Ministry of Health and Family Welfare. National Family Health Survey (NFHS-5) 2019–21. Compendium of fact sheets. Key indicators. New Delhi: Ministry of Health and Family Welfare, Government of India; 2022.
7. Ramzi M, Haghpanah S, Malekmakan L, Cohan N, Baseri A, Alamdari A, et al. Anemia and iron deficiency in adolescent school girls in Kavar urban area, southern Iran. Iran Red Crescent Med J. 2011;13:128-33.
8. Sachdev HS, Porwal A, Acharya R, Ashraf S, Ramesh S, Khan N, et al. Haemoglobin thresholds to define anaemia in a national sample of healthy children and

adolescents aged 1–19 years in India: a population-based study. Lancet Glob Health. 2021;9:e822-31.
9. Sarna A, Porwal A, Ramesh S, Agrawal PK, Acharya R, Johnston R, et al. Characterisation of the types of anaemia prevalent among children and adolescents aged 1–19 years in India: a population-based study. Lancet Child Adolesc Health. 2020;4:515-25.
10. Sedlander E, Long MW, Mohanty S, Munjral A, Bingenheimer JB, Yilma H, et al. Moving beyond individual barriers and identifying multi-level strategies to reduce anemia in Odisha India. BMC Public Health. 2020;20:457-72.
11. Snook J, Bhala N, Beales ILP, Cannings D, Kightley C, Logan RP, et al. British Society of gastroenterology guidelines for the management of iron deficiency anemia in adults. Gut. 2021;70:2030-51.

# CHAPTER 25

# Menstrual Disorders in Adolescence

*J Shyamala, Chitra Dinakar, Shilpa Chandrashekhar*

## ■ NORMAL MENSTRUAL CYCLE

Menstruation is the cyclic, orderly sloughing of the uterine lining, in response to a complex feedback system involving the hypothalamus, pituitary, and ovaries (HPO axis). During normal menstrual cycles, the sequence of events involves release of gonadotropin-releasing hormone (GnRH) from the hypothalamus, which, acting on the anterior pituitary, releases the follicle-stimulating hormone (FSH). This acts on the ovary to recruit and mature an ovarian follicle. The ovarian follicle secretes estradiol during the first half of the cycle, which causes endometrial hyperplasia. Following a mid-cycle surge of luteinizing hormone (LH), ovulation occurs and the follicle is converted to the corpus luteum. The corpus luteum secretes progesterone that helps in stabilizing the endometrium in anticipation of pregnancy. In case the ovum is not fertilized, hormonal levels rapidly decline by 2 weeks post ovulation, which results in endometrial regression and shedding, heralding the beginning of the next menstrual cycle.

## ■ MENSTRUAL CYCLES IN ADOLESCENT GIRLS

Menarche, or the first menstrual cycle, usually occurs within 2–3 years after breast budding/thelarche. It usually occurs at Tanner stage IV of breast development and is generally rare before Tanner stage III, the median age being 12–13 years. The length of a menstrual cycle is the number of days between the first day of menstrual bleeding of one cycle to the onset of menses of the next cycle. Menstrual cycles are often irregular in adolescence, particularly the initial few cycles, and first 2 years. This is due to the immaturity of the HPO axis during the early years after menarche and the fact that these cycles are anovulatory. Bleeding may last 2–7 days during the first menses. 90% of cycles will last 21–45 days, although cycles of <20 days or >45 days may occur. Majority of them follow the adult pattern by the end of the 2–3 years post menarche. **Box 1** summarizes the characteristics of normal menstrual cycles in adolescent girls.

**BOX 1:** Normal menstrual cycles in adolescent girls.

- Menarche (median age): 12.43 years
- Mean cycle interval: 32.2 days in first gynecologic year
- Menstrual cycle interval: Typically 21–45 days
- Menstrual flow length: 7 days or less
- Menstrual product use: Three to six pads or tampons per day

Problems associated with menstruation are seen in nearly 75% of girls at some time in adolescence. These will be discussed under four main headings—amenorrhea, abnormal uterine bleeding (AUB), dysmenorrhea, premenstrual disorders (premenstrual syndrome and premenstrual dysphoric disorder).

## Amenorrhea

Amenorrhea is marked by the complete absence or cessation of menses. It is divided into primary and secondary types. Primary amenorrhea may be defined as the absence of menses at age of 15 years. Secondary amenorrhea is defined as absence of menstrual flow for least 3 months in those with previously regular menses, or for over 6 months in those who previously had irregular menses. There may be various causes: anatomical or functional anomalies of the genital tract, hormonal disorders, or multifactorial.

Based on regulatory processes occurring at the HPO axis and outflow tract, primary or secondary amenorrhea may follow when there is any disturbance of the normal signaling within the axis. At the level of the hypothalamus, the GnRH is responsible for the hormonal surge required for onset of puberty. Thelarche is the first sign of puberty which signals that the HPO axis has been activated. Delayed breast development compared to peers is seen in females with constitutional delay of puberty. GnRH from the hypothalamus promotes release of FSH and LH from the pituitary. At the pituitary level, variations in prolactin level either due to central or peripheral causes lead to amenorrhea. In any female with amenorrhea, headaches and vision changes, space occupying lesions and tumors of the pituitary should be excluded. At the ovarian level, low reserve before or after puberty results in amenorrhea as in Turner syndrome.

Polycystic ovarian syndrome (PCOS) is the most common endocrine disorder in either primary or secondary amenorrhea and affects 3.6–15% of reproductive age women. Adolescent females who have attained full height and pubertal potential, but not attained menarche, may have PCOS. Menstrual irregularities such as amenorrhea or oligomenorrhea may occur along with severe acne and hirsutism. Amenorrhea in PCOS occurs due to the effects of hyperandrogenism on GnRH secretion with resultant elevated LH. Other neurotransmitters such as neurokinin B and dynorphins may also affect LH activity. PCOS in this age group (where anovulatory cycles are

**TABLE 1:** Etiologies of primary and secondary amenorrhea.

| Primary amenorrhea | Secondary amenorrhea |
|---|---|
| • Genetic abnormalities:<br>  – Turner syndrome<br>  – Gonadal dysgenesis<br>• Kallman syndrome<br>• Anatomic<br>  – Imperforate hymen<br>  – Transverse vaginal septum<br>  – Mayer–Rokitansky–Küster–Hauser syndrome<br>• Hypothalamic/pituitary<br>  – Functional hypothalamic amenorrhea<br>  – Idiopathic hypogonadotropic hypogonadism<br>  – Delayed adrenarche and gonadarche<br>  – Constitutional delay<br>• Ovarian<br>  – Primary ovarian insufficiency<br>  – Autoimmune oophoritis<br>  – Polycystic ovary syndrome<br>• Systemic diseases<br>  – Craniopharyngioma<br>  – Germinoma<br>  – Langerhans cell histiocytosis<br>• Sellar masses<br>• Deficiencies<br>  – Androgen insensitivity syndrome<br>  – 5-alpha reductase deficiency<br>  – 17-alpha hydroxylase deficiency | • Pregnancy<br>• Breastfeeding<br>• Hypothalamic<br>  – Functional hypothalamic amenorrhea<br>  – Tumors of the hypothalamus<br>• Pituitary<br>  – Hyperprolactinemia<br>  – Sheehan syndrome<br>  – Radiation<br>  – Pituitary gland lesions<br>• Uterine<br>  – Asherman syndrome<br>• Ovarian<br>  – Premature ovarian failure<br>  – Polycystic ovary syndrome<br>• Systemic<br>  – Chronic diseases<br>  – Type 1 diabetes mellitus<br>  – Celiac disease<br>• Thyroid<br>  – Hypothyroidism (more common)<br>  – Hyperthyroidism<br>• Adrenal disease<br>• Tumors<br>• Medications<br>  – Psychotropics<br>  – Contraceptives |

typical in the early postmenarchal years) needs to be diagnosed with caution. Some increase in facial hair growth and androgens during normal puberty can further confuse the picture.

Eliciting a proper medical history and performing a thorough clinical examination of the adolescent is essential in deciphering the cause of amenorrhea

**Table 1** shows the different causes of amenorrhea with some degree of overlap.

## Abnormal Uterine Bleeding

Abnormal uterine bleeding is defined as bleeding from uterus that is abnormal in duration, volume, frequency and/or regularity, common in adolescents because of immaturity of the HPO axis.

Heavy menstrual bleeding (HMB) is the most common form of AUB and is defined as excessive menstrual blood loss interfering with a woman's physical, social, emotional, or quality of life. Other signs of HMB include need for pad or tampon change more often than every 1–2 hours, use of double-hygiene protection, frequent soiling of clothes or bed sheets and blood clots more than one inch (2.5 cm) in diameter. Average blood loss in a normal cycle may range from 5 to 80 mL, while >80 mL maybe termed heavy. The FIGO Working Group on Menstrual Disorders in 2011 classified HMB using the mnemonic *"PALM-COEIN"*-*P*olyp, *A*denomyosis, *L*eiomyoma, *M*alignancy–*C*oagulopathy, *O*vulatory dysfunction, *E*ndometrial, *I*atrogenic and *N*ot yet classified. "PALM" encompasses structural causes (rarely seen in adolescents) and hyperplasia and COEIN includes non-structural causes.

Abnormal uterine bleeding may also be classified as acute or chronic. An episode of heavy bleeding severe enough quantitatively to require urgent intervention so as to prevent further blood loss is referred to as acute AUB. Chronic AUB may be defined as abnormalities in quantity, regularity and/or timing of the bleed in the last 6 months. Chronic menstrual bleeding exceeding 80 mL will usually result in anemia. Causes of abnormal uterine bleeding in adolescents are listed in **Table 2**.

**TABLE 2:** Causes of abnormal uterine bleeding in adolescents.

| | |
|---|---|
| Endocrine | • Anovulatory bleeding<br>• PCOS<br>• Thyroid disorders<br>• Hyperprolactinemia |
| Bleeding disorders | • Von Willebrand disease<br>• Platelet dysfunction<br>• Thrombocytopenia<br>• Clotting factor deficiency |
| Pregnancy | • Abortion<br>• Ectopic pregnancy<br>• First trimester bleeding<br>• Gestational trophoblastic disease |
| Infections | • Cervicitis<br>• Endometritis<br>• Sexually transmitted disease |
| Uterine pathology | • Polyp<br>• Leiomyoma<br>• Adenomyosis<br>• Malignancy |
| Medications | • Anticoagulants<br>• Depot medroxyprogesterone implants<br>• Intrauterine devices |
| Trauma | Foreign bodies |

(PCOS: polycystic ovarian syndrome)

## Dysmenorrhea

Dysmenorrhea, or menstrual pain, considered the most common menstrual symptom among adolescent girls, is categorized as primary and secondary. *Primary dysmenorrhea* being more common is characterized by painful menstruation in the absence of pelvic pathology. It typically begins when ovulatory cycles occur, usually within 6-12 months of menarche. Pain starts just before menses and is limited to 1-2 days of menses. Prostaglandins and leukotrienes, both mediators of inflammation, contribute to the pathophysiology. Patients with severe dysmenorrhea may complain of headaches, nausea, vomiting, diarrhea, muscle cramps and poor sleep quality which may lead to school absenteeism. In a study of Japanese high school students, the rates of prevalence of premenstrual syndrome and premenstrual dysphoric disorder increased with the severity of dysmenorrhea.

Secondary dysmenorrhea is characterized by painful menses due to pelvic pathology or a recognized medical condition, the most common cause being endometriosis. Adenomyosis, infection, myomas, Müllerian anomalies, obstructive reproductive tract anomalies, or ovarian cysts are other possible causes of secondary dysmenorrhea.

## Premenstrual Syndrome and Premenstrual Dysphoric Disorder

Premenstrual syndrome (PMS) and premenstrual dysphoric disorder (PMDD) are the two disorders marked by both physical and psychological symptoms which occur during the luteal phase of the menstrual cycle, before the onset of menses. Being more common of the two, PMS affects 20-40% of menstruating women and manifests with symptoms of low mood, fatigability, abdominal bloating, breast tenderness, acne, and changes in appetite and food cravings. PMDD affects a smaller percentage of women and is marked by more severe symptoms, mostly psychiatric. It is listed as a depressive disorder in the Diagnostic and Statistical Manual of Mental Disorders, Fifth Edition (DSM-5) and leads to periodic interference with day-to-day activities and interpersonal relationships. Pathophysiology of these disorders remains unclear. Many factors are believed to play a role such as hormonal fluctuations, abnormal serotonergic activity, irregularity in progesterone and the neurotransmitter gamma aminobutyric acid (GABA), etc.

## APPROACH AND EVALUATION OF AN ADOLESCENT WITH MENSTRUAL DISORDERS

### History and Physical Examination

A thorough knowledge of menstrual patterns of adolescent girls, the ability to distinguish between normal and abnormal menstruation, and the skill and expertise to evaluate adolescent girls will aid general pediatricians and primary healthcare physicians in counseling them and facilitating their smooth transition to adulthood.

Menstrual cycle may be considered as an additional vital sign and identifying abnormal menstrual patterns in adolescence may be as important as measuring blood pressure, heart rate, or respiratory rate in early identification of potential health concerns in an adult.

Age of onset of menarche is in itself a milestone and should always be asked for along with pubertal development—thelarche, adrenarche, and menarche. Aiding the differential diagnosis of amenorrhea is to make a distinction between primary and secondary amenorrhea, along with noting the presence, or absence of secondary sexual characteristics. Genetic and familial disorders, menstrual histories of female family members should be elicited. A complete review of systems—weight changes, headaches, vision problems, appetite, exercise, galactorrhea, drug intake and stress—should be asked for. An accurate history of patient's cycles including cycle length, variability over time, and the amount of menstrual bleeding is important for diagnosis.

After building a good rapport, sexual history should be elicited. Pregnancy and its related complications should also be part of the initial investigation in girls presenting with AUB. In majority of adolescents, abnormal bleeding may be attributable to anovulatory cycles, yet severe bleeding cannot be neglected and may be the first sign of an underlying pathological condition. Excessive bleeding during menarche may also be attributable to an underlying bleeding disorder. Up to 36% of adolescents with AUB may have an underlying coagulopathy. The most common bleeding disorders in adolescent girls with HMB are Von Willebrand disease, platelet function defects, thrombocytopenia, and clotting factor deficiencies. PCOS, another cause of anovulatory cycles, is a common underlying etiology in AUB and can easily be missed in this age group. AUB is a diagnosis of exclusion.

Menstrual abnormalities that suggest the need for further evaluation are listed in **Box 2**.

Distinguishing features of primary versus secondary dysmenorrhea are indicated in **Table 3**. When there is no reduction in dysmenorrhea within 3-6 months of therapy, treatment adherence should be checked while also working up for possible secondary causes. Secondary dysmenorrhea should also be suspected in patients in whom there is lack of response to medical measures, those with progressively worsening dysmenorrhea, heavy and irregular bleeding, pain during or after the cycles or acyclic pain, family history of endometriosis, a renal anomaly, and other congenital anomalies (spine, cardiac, or gastrointestinal).

Diagnosis of PMS and PMDD is a challenge as there is no objective diagnostic test. It depends on accurately recording symptoms over two cycles

**BOX 2:** Menstrual abnormalities that may require evaluation.

Menstrual periods that
- Have not started within 3 years of thelarche
- Have not started by 14 years of age with signs of hirsutism
- Have not started by 14 years of age with a history or examination suggestive of excessive exercise or eating disorder
- Have not started by 15 years of age
- Occur more frequently than every 21 days or less frequently than every 45 days
- Occur 90 days apart even for one cycle
- Last more than 7 days
- Require frequent pad or tampon changes (soaking more than one every 1–2 hours)
- Are heavy and are associated with a history of excessive bruising or bleeding or a family history of a bleeding disorder

**TABLE 3:** Primary vs. secondary dysmenorrhoea

| Differentiating Features | Primary dysmenorrhoea | Secondary dysmenorrhoea |
| --- | --- | --- |
| Onset | Within 2 years of menarche, marked during adolescence | Around 4th to 5th decade, rarely during adolescence |
| Definition | Recurrent lower abdominal cramps and pain that occurs during menses in the absence of underlying pathology | Recurrent lower abdominal pain that can occur before or during menses in presence of a demonstrable pelvic pathology |
| Other associated symptomatology | Nausea, vomiting, diarrhoea, headache, fatigue | Dyspareunia, infertility, menstrual irregularities |
| Pelvic findings | Normal | Congestion and variable findings depending upon the cause |
| Management | • Reassurance<br>• Analgesics-NSAIDS<br>• OC pills | Treat the underlying cause |
| Prognosis | Improves with age | Will subside only on treating the cause |

and the timing of symptoms during the luteal phase of the menstrual cycle. Symptoms disappear by the end of menstruation and do not recur before ovulation, giving the patient a symptom-free interval of at least 1 week. PMS is cyclical and occurs in most menstrual cycles. Substantial impairment of daily activities at work or school, social activities and hobbies and interpersonal relationships is a key feature.

On physical examination of an adolescent with amenorrhea, growth parameters should be plotted on appropriate charts. Short stature is invariably found in females with Turner syndrome. Further causes of amenorrhea can be possibly diagnosed by assessing the sexual maturity rating. Dermatological findings such as acne and hirsutism in the setting of amenorrhea can suggest hyperandrogenism seen in PCOS, so also acanthosis suggestive of hyperinsulinism. Bodily habitus, lack of subcutaneous fat, dysmorphism, fundoscopic examination, sense of smell, and neurocutaneous findings are noted. The genitourinary examination includes inspection of the genital area and a detailed internal examination if indicated.

## Laboratory Evaluation

*Amenorrhea:* Laboratory evaluation of an adolescent with primary and secondary amenorrhea are presented in **Flowcharts 1 and 2**.

In constitutional growth delay, the adolescent is otherwise healthy but hormonal evaluation will reveal a low-to-low normal gonadotropin levels. Bone age is delayed compared to the chronological age. In Turner syndrome, significantly high FSH levels are detected with low or almost absent estradiol levels. For diagnosis of PCOS to be made in adolescents, use of Rotterdam criteria (clinical or biochemical evidence of hyperandrogenism, anovulation or oligomenorrhea and ultrasound findings of polycystic ovarian appearance) is not appropriate, since research shows that polycystic ovarian morphology may be seen in many healthy adolescents in the early postmenarchal years. As per the international consensus diagnostic criteria, PCOS should be considered in adolescents who have a combination of the

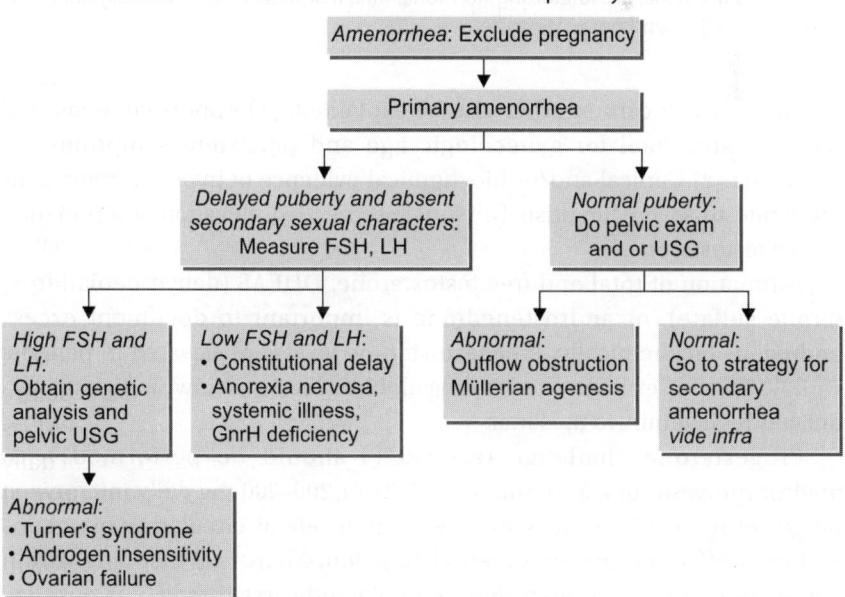

**Flowchart 1:** Evaluation of an adolescent with primary amenorrhea.

(GnRH: gonadotropin-releasing hormone, FSH: follicle-stimulating hormone; LH: luteinizing hormone; USG: ultrasonography)

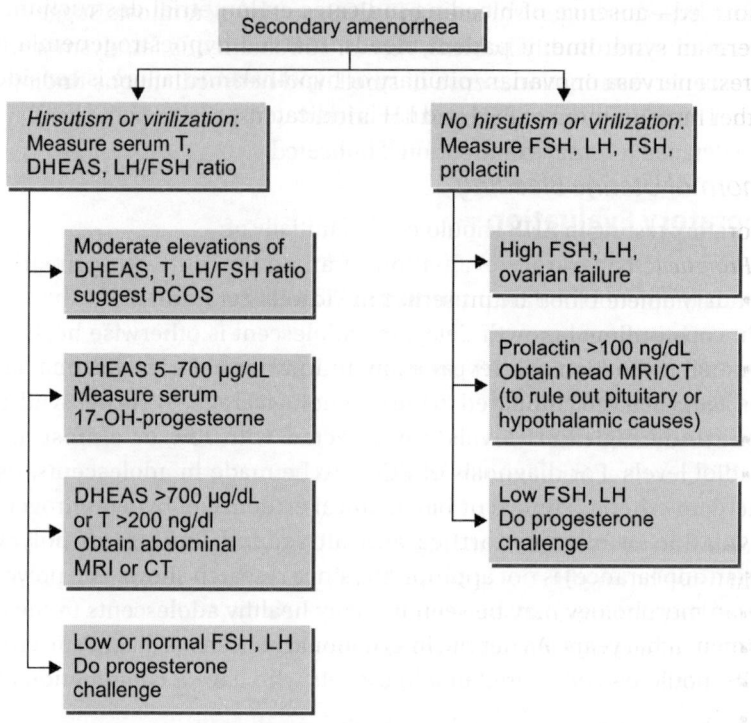

**Flowchart 2:** Evaluation of an adolescent with secondary amenorrhea.

(CT: computed tomography; DHEAS: dehydroepiandrosterone sulfate; FSH: follicle-stimulating hormone; LH: luteinizing hormone; MRI: magnetic resonance imaging; PCOS: polycystic ovarian syndrome; T: testosterone,

following which cannot otherwise be explained: (1) Abnormal menstrual pattern (abnormal for gynecologic age and persistent symptoms for 1-2 years; (2) Clinical and/or biochemical evidence of hyperandrogenism-moderate-to-severe hirsutism (hirsutism score >15), elevation of serum total or free testosterone.

Estimation of total and free testosterone, DHEAS (dehydroepiandrosterone sulfate), or androstenedione is important to document excess androgens biochemically. Free testosterone levels are elevated in patients with PCOS and sex hormone-binding globulin levels are low since testosterone has high affinity to the latter.

Progesterone challenge test (PCT) should be performed with medroxyprogesterone 5-10 mg once daily or 200-300 mg daily micronized progesterone for 7-10 days to assess the levels of circulating estrogens and their effect on the endometrial function. Menstrual bleeding within 1 week of cessation of progesterone intake indicates that PCT is positive, signifying that estrogen production by the ovaries is sufficient to stimulate endometrial proliferation and that anovulation is the cause for amenorrhea.

If PCT is negative, challenge with sequential estrogen–progestin regimen is performed—absence of bleeding indicates endometrial destruction, e.g., Asherman syndrome; if patient bleeds, marked hypoestrogenemia as in anorexia nervosa or ovarian/pituitary or hypothalamic failure is considered. Further measurement of FSH and LH is indicated.

## Abnormal Uterine Bleeding

Laboratory testing in AUB should consist initially of:
- *Routine tests:*
  - Complete blood count including platelet count to assess the severity of bleeding
  - Prothrombin time (PT), activated partial thromboplastin time (aPTT), and bleeding time
  - Pregnancy test
  - Screening for sexually transmitted infections–cervical cultures for chlamydia and gonorrhea
- *Secondary laboratory studies:* Done in those not responding to therapy or in those having findings suggestive of a systemic disorder:
  - Thyroid-stimulating hormone (TSH) test
  - Fasting blood glucose, liver and renal function tests
  - Prolactin
  - LH, FSH, and androgen levels (DHEAS and free testosterone)
  - Adrenal function tests [e.g., cortisol, 17-alpha hydroxyprogesterone (17-OHP)]
- *Imaging studies:* Done for adolescents who do not respond to routine treatment.
  - Pelvic ultrasound is useful for demonstrating structural abnormalities of the uterus, endometrial thickness and adnexal areas, to rule out PCOS, and early fibroid.
  - Magnetic resonance imaging (MRI)/computed tomography (CT) scanning—only rarely superior to ultrasonography.

## Dysmenorrhea

Laboratory testing or imaging is not routinely required to make a diagnosis of primary dysmenorrhea. Specific investigations may be ordered when:
- Secondary dysmenorrhea is suspected, to confirm the clinical diagnosis and find out the extent of the underlying disease.
- For girls who suffer from dysmenorrhea refractory to first-line therapy.

Pelvic ultrasound may show a mass or an obstructing Müllerian malformation but cannot detect subtle signs of organic diseases such as uterosacral ligament tenderness or nodules and cervical motion tenderness. In such cases, MRI is a useful option.

## ■ MANAGEMENT OF MENSTRUAL DISORDERS
## Amenorrhea
Counseling and reassurance are important to alleviate anxiety of adolescent patients and caretakers. Therapy is directed at treating the underlying cause of amenorrhea.

### In Girls with No Pubertal Development
Due to hypoestrogenism either due to ovarian failure, hypopituitarism or hypothalamic disorders, estrogen therapy is given in three phases:
1. *Phase 1:* For induction of breast development, lower doses of estradiol 25 µg as patches and conjugated estrogens 0.3 mg for 6–12 months. Oral contraceptives are not recommended for initial therapy as they contain higher levels of estrogen, and progestin throughout the cycle which is not physiological.
2. *Phase 2:* Establishment of normal menses, completion of breast development and acquisition of normal bone mass: Estradiol 50 µg patches, 0.625 mg of conjugated estrogens, or 20 µg ethinyl estradiol. A short course of progestin 5 or 10 mg medroxyprogesterone may be added within 2–3 months of phase 2 for 5 days in a month. This dose of progestin is given only until breast development is completed in 6–12 months and then the progestin dose is increased to 10 days and ultimately 12–14 days.
3. *Phase 3:* Long-term maintenance of a normal estrogen state—both estrogen and progestin are continued until the expected age of menopause. Estrogen as 50–100 µg estradiol patches, 0.62–1.25 mg conjugated estrogens or 20 µg ethinyl estradiol daily plus progestin for 12–14 days each month or oral contraceptive pills (OCPs) are given. Most adolescents prefer monthly menses and hence can be prescribed daily estrogen, cycled every 60–90 days with progestin for 14 days. If the girl is well estrogenized with anovulation as the cause of amenorrhea, menstrual cycles can be induced with cyclic progestins every 1–3 months

### Polycystic Ovary Syndrome
Dietary modifications and weight loss, treatment of hyperandrogenism, and relief of hirsutism may help in the resumption of menses and fertility. The drug of choice to induce ovulation is clomiphene citrate. In case there is no hirsutism, an intermittent progestin (e.g., medroxyprogesterone acetate 5–10 mg/day po for 10–14 days) or oral contraceptives are used.

### Endocrine Disorders
Hypothyroidism is treated with levothyroxine. Surgery is required for tumors of the pituitary, hypothalamus, ovary, and adrenal glands, as also

for some genital tract malformations. e.g., hematocolpos. Pulsatile GnRH is used for treatment of hypothalamic amenorrhea. Gonadotropins are used in management of amenorrhea secondary to pituitary disease (excluding prolactinomas). In case of documented adrenal hyperfunction or enzyme defects in the steroidogenic pathway, glucocorticoids are indicated. Hyperprolactinemia is managed with dopamine receptor agonists such as bromocriptine and cabergoline.

Calcium and vitamin D supplementation daily should be advised. Lifestyle changes and exercise to promote bone formation and cardiovascular fitness. Cognitive behavioral therapy, psychological and nutritional rehabilitation are the cornerstones in management of anorexia nervosa.

## Surgical Therapy

In case of ovarian cysts or uterine problems such as intrauterine adhesions/transverse vaginal septum—hysteroscopic lysis of adhesions, surgical excision of the septum, etc. can be performed. For vaginal agenesis, manual dilators maybe used to create a functional vagina/surgical creation of neovagina (vaginoplasty) to accord the girl an opportunity to have a normal sexual life. Surgery in patients with testicular feminization should be performed after attainment of puberty, to allow for breast development and attainment of the maximum expected adult stature. Estrogen replacement therapy should be given after gonadectomy.

## Abnormal Uterine Bleeding

The goals of management of AUB include establishment and or maintenance of hemodynamic stability, correction of acute or chronic anemia, return to a pattern of normal menstrual cycles, prevention of recurrence and of long-term consequences of anovulation. The preferred treatment of abnormal uterine bleeding in adolescence is medical. Management of AUB based on severity of bleeding is summarized in **Table 4**.

## Dysmenorrhea

### Primary Dysmenorrhea

Aggressive and evidence-based treatment is warranted to prevent school absence and loss of productivity. Pharmacological measures—use of nonsteroidal anti-inflammatory drugs (NSAIDs) such as mefenamic acid, ibuprofen, and naproxen are considered the first-line therapy **(Table 5)**. NSAIDs should be started at the beginning of menses and continued for the first 1–2 days of menstrual cycle or for the usual duration of crampy pain. In case of severe symptoms, NSAIDs should be started 1–2 days prior to onset of menses. If NSAIDs do not control symptoms after two to three

**TABLE 4:** Management of AUB based on severity of bleeding.

|  | Mild bleeding | Moderate bleeding | Severe bleeding with moderate anemia | Severe bleeding with severe anemia |
|---|---|---|---|---|
| Hb | >11 g/dL | 10–11 g/dL | 8–10 g/dL | <7 g/dL |
| Anemia correction | Oral iron | Oral iron | Oral iron | Blood transfusion |
| Treatment | Reassurance | Progestin/OCPs | Progestin/OCPs | OCPs/conjugated estrogen |
| OCPs dosage | 1 pill daily for 21 days | 1 pill BD till bleeding stops and then 1 pill OD for 21 days | 1 pill qid for 2–4 days and then 1 TDS for 3 days then 1 BD for 2 weeks till Hb normal | 1 pill 4–6 hourly till bleeding slows then 1 qid for 2–4 days, 1 tds for 3 days, 1 BD for 2 weeks till Hb is normal |
| D and C | Never done | Not done | Not required | Required for recurrence or treatment failure |
| Follow-up | Monthly | Weekly then monthly | Weekly then monthly | Daily then monthly |

(AUB: abnormal uterine bleeding; Hb: hemoglobin; OCP: oral contraceptive pill)

**TABLE 5:** Medications to treat dysmenorrhea.

| | |
|---|---|
| *Propionic acid group:* | |
| • Ibuprofen | 400–600 mg Q4–6H |
| • Naproxen sodium | 550 mg load then 275 mg Q6H |
| • Naproxen | 500 mg load then 250 mg Q 6–8H |
| *Fenamate group:* Mefenamic acid | 500 mg loading dose then 250 mg Q6H |

cycles, a trial of OCPs may be indicated. Antiemetics are prescribed in case of nausea or vomiting. Rest, adequate sleep, hot fomentation, yoga, aerobic exercise, and other nonpharmacological measures may be helpful in some women.

### *Secondary Dysmenorrhea*

Treatment of the underlying cause is important. The primary management is medical with prostaglandin synthetase inhibitors, oral contraceptives (monophasic OCP such as norgestrel 0.3 mg/ethinyl estradiol 30 µg, levonorgestrel 0.15 mg/ethinyl estradiol 30 µg), danazol and progestins. A narrow cervical os may be dilated to give temporary relief for about 3–6 months (simultaneous diagnostic curettage may be done if needed).

Other surgical measures such as myomectomy, polypectomy, laparoscopy for endometriosis, presacral neurectomy, and division of the sacrouterine ligaments are not usually required in adolescent girls.

For all patients, it is recommended to maintain a menstrual calendar noting duration and extent of blood loss. General measures to improve the health status—proper balanced diet, adequate rest during menses, and oral iron supplementation to replenish iron stores—may be tried.

## PMS and PMDD

It is important to distinguish PMS and PMDD from mental health disorders such as anxiety and depression. Validated tools including DSM-V criteria exist to diagnose these disorders.

Treatment is required if PMS symptoms are affecting patients' day-to-day activities. Lifestyle changes including dietary modifications (e.g., low fats, high protein, complex carbohydrates, reducing salty foods, avoiding caffeine and alcohol), adequate rest, and sleep are advised. In severe cases, medications may be required in addition. Management based on severity is summarized in **Table 6**.

## ■ ANTICIPATORY GUIDANCE

Primary care clinicians should include pubertal development in their anticipatory guidance to female children (and their parents) as early as

**TABLE 6:** Treatment of PMS according to severity.

| Mild cases | Severe cases |
| --- | --- |
| • Patient education about relationship of symptoms to menstrual cycle<br>• Stress management and psychological counseling<br>• Exercise, aerobic activity, brisk walking, cycling, swimming can help improve overall health and alleviate symptoms such as fatigue and a depressed mood<br>• Deep breathing exercises to help reduce headaches, anxiety, or insomnia<br>• Calcium, magnesium, vitamin B-6, vitamin E are also known to be effective in soothing the symptoms of PMS | • Common medications for PMS include nonsteroidal anti-inflammatory drugs (NSAIDs)<br>• Selective serotonin reuptake inhibitors e.g., Fluoxitine 10–20 mg daily continuously or intermittently beginning at ovulation when symptoms begin and ending when symptoms resolve<br>• Hormonal therapy is effective in some patients. Oral contraceptives; progesterone for 10–12 days premenstrually; a long-acting progestin (e.g., medroxyprogesterone acetate 200 mg IM every 2–3 monthly); or a gonadotropin-releasing hormone agonist with low-dose estrogen-progestin "add-back" therapy to eliminate cyclic changes can be used |

(PMS: premenstrual syndrome)

8–10 years, when they start developing secondary sexual characteristics. It is important to educate them about the usual progression of puberty. This includes information about breast growth (may initially be unilateral, slightly tender, some asymmetry is normal; females will likely begin to menstruate approximately 2–2.5 years after breast development begins), development of pubic hair (increase in amount over time and become thicker and curlier), and about menarche.

### Menstrual Calendar (Either App Based or Physical)

Adolescents should be encouraged to chart their menstrual bleeding from the time of menarche, with dates and number of days of the cycle and menstrual flow. This helps clinicians to differentiate normal from abnormal enabling early identification of potential health concerns. This is also a valuable tool to assess response to therapy, especially related to irregularity and heavy flow, when treatment details are juxtaposed with flow details in the same calendar.

### Menstrual Hygiene

Poor menstrual hygiene is linked to urinary tract infections, sexually transmitted infections, and cervical cancer. Studies on Indian adolescent girls from an urban slum reveal that about 76–84% are unaware of the anatomy and physiology of menstruation. 30% of Indian adolescents from a slum were found to have poor menstrual hygiene practices. Given the NFHS-5 report of median marriageable age for girls being 19.2 years, there is a window of opportunity for pediatricians to create awareness of menstrual health and hygiene along with reproductive health issues (covering areas of fertility period [9th–16th day of a 28 day cycle], contraceptive options, and planned pregnancy).

Menstrual hygiene encompasses use of hygienic methods to collect flow, adequate options for privacy to wash and dry private parts, reusable pads as frequently as needed and safe and sustainable disposal of used products. There is a menstrual hygiene scheme under the national health mission which is scaling up to support these needs. Menstrual cups, now available in small sizes for adolescents/women yet to be sexually active should be promoted as a cheap, safe, and sustainable method. Pediatricians should enquire, guide, and advocate on hygiene practices at every opportunity and bust myths associated with menses that can interfere with hygiene.

### Myths Associated with Menses

There are rampant myths associated with menses, primarily related to restrictions, in 80% adolescents (religious activities, kitchen access, and social isolation). In a study on urban Indian adolescents, 67% had dysmenorrhea,

50% had tiredness, and 27% had backache. Menses being both a physical and psychological experience, there is a need to treat and counsel about these common issues to minimize disruptions to school, work, and also promote mental well-being.

Empowering adolescent girls with knowledge of reproductive physiology and menstrual disorders is a powerful tool that helps them feel comfortable about handling their growing bodies, opens channels for reliable communication and lays a good foundation for their sexual and reproductive health. Such empowerment has intergenerational effects for positive outcomes not only for women but also their children and families as a whole.

## ■ POINTS TO REMEMBER

- Menstrual disorders are common and maybe seen in up to 75% of adolescent girls.
- Irregularity in menstrual cycles is well known in adolescence due to immaturity of the hypothalamus, pituitary, and ovaries (HPO) axis and due to anovulatory cycles.
- Amenorrhea, either complete absence or cessation of menses, may be primary or secondary. Causes include anatomical or functional anomalies of the genital tract, hormonal disorders, and sometimes multifactorial.
- Heavy menstrual bleeding (HMB) is the most common form of abnormal uterine bleeding. Nonstructural causes such as coagulopathy, ovulatory dysfunction, pregnancy complication, endometrial disease and "not yet classified" are more common. Structural causes including fibroids are rare.
- Dysmenorrhea is one of the most common menstrual symptoms among adolescent girls and can be primary (no pelvic pathology) or secondary (pelvic pathology or a recognized medical condition exists).
- Premenstrual syndrome (PMS) and premenstrual dysphoric disorder (PMDD) occur due to the hormonal fluctuations during the luteal phase of the cycle and increased sensitivity to the same. It is important to distinguish them from mental health disorders like anxiety and depression. Diagnosis is a challenge as there is no objective diagnostic test.
- Accurate menstrual history, complete review of systems, and physical examination should precede hormonal investigations and imaging.
- Appropriate management and counseling can be offered only after accurate diagnosis of the underlying disorder.
- All adolescents will need "adolescent-friendly approach and counseling".

## ■ CONCLUSION

A thorough understanding of menstrual patterns of adolescent girls and skills in evaluation will help them weather a stormy phase in their development.

Anticipatory guidance of parents and their daughters as soon as they develop secondary sexual characteristics helps allay anxieties, opens channels for reliable communication and lays a good foundation for sexual and reproductive health of adolescents.

## ■ SUGGESTED READING

1. Akgül S, Kanbur N. Premenstrual disorder and the adolescent: clinical case report, literature review, and diagnostic and therapeutic challenges. Int J Adolesc Med Health. 2015;27(4):363-8.
2. American College of Obstetricians and Gynecologists. ACOG Committee Opinion No. 557: Management of acute abnormal uterine bleeding in nonpregnant reproductive-aged women. Obstet Gynecol. 2013;121:891-6.
3. American College of Obstetricians and Gynecologists. Menstruation in girls and adolescents: using the menstrual cycle as a vital sign. Committee Opinion No. 651. Obstet Gynecol. 2015;126:e143-6.
4. Benjamins LJ. Practice guideline: evaluation and management of vaginal bleeding in adolescents. J Pediatr Health Care. 2009;23:189-93.
5. Biro FM, Huang B, Crawford PB, Lucky AW, Striegel-Moore R, Barton BA, et al. Pubertal correlates in black and white girls. J Pediatr. 2006;148:234-40.
6. Dabadghao P. Polycystic ovary syndrome in adolescents. Best Pract Res Clin Endocrinol Metab. 2019;33(3):101272.
7. Dangal G. Menstrual disorders in Adolescents: J Nepal Med Assoc. 2004;35:76-8.
8. Data from NFHS (National Family Health Survey)-5-2019-21 report. India. P 208, 115, 116.
9. Deligeoroglu E, Karountzos V. Abnormal Uterine Bleeding including coagulopathies and other menstrual disorders. Best Pract Res Clin Obstet Gynaecol. 2018;48:51-61.
10. Deshpande TN, Patil SS, Gharai SB, Patil SR, Durgawale PM. Menstrual hygiene among adolescent girls–A study from urban slum area. J Family Med Prim Care. 2018;7(6):1439.
11. Dysmenorrhea and endometriosis in the adolescent. ACOG Committee Opinion No. 760. American College of Obstetricians and Gynecologists. Obstet Gynecol. 2018;132:e249-58.
12. Finer LB, Philbin JM. Trends in ages at key reproductive transitions in the United States, 1951-2010. Womens Health Issues. 2014;24:271-9.
13. Fraser IS, Critchley HO, Broder M. The FIGO recommendations on terminologies and definitions for normal and abnormal uterine bleeding. Semin Reprod Med. 2011;29:383-90.
14. Gray SH, Emans SJ. Abnormal vaginal bleeding in adolescents. Pediatr Rev. 2007;28:175-82.
15. Gray SH. Menstrual disorders. Pediatr Rev. 2013;34(1):6-18.
16. Greydanus D, Omar H, Tsitsika A, Patel DR. Menstrual disorders in adolescent females. In: Omar H, Greydanus D, Tsitsika A, Patel DR, Merrick J (Eds). Pediatric and adolescent sexuality and gynecology. New York: Nova Science Publishers Inc, 2010. pp. 315-411.
17. Gupta P, Menon PSN, Ramji S, Lodha R. Adolescent Health. In: Gupta P, (Eds). Postgraduate textbook of Pediatrics, 2nd edition, NewDelhi: Jaypee Brothers Medical Publishers (P) Ltd.; 2017. pp.1183-92.

18. Haamid F, Sass AE, Dietrich JE. Heavy menstrual bleeding in adolescents. J PediatrAdolesc Gynecol. 2017;30:335-40.
19. Hickey M, Balen A. Menstrual disorders in adolescence: Investigation and management. Hum Reprod Update. 2003;9:493-504.
20. Itriyeva K. Premenstrual syndrome and premenstrual dysphoric disorder in adolescents. Curr Probl Pediatr Adolesc. 2022;52(5):101187.
21. Kitamura M, Takeda T, Koga S, Nagase S, Yaegashi N. Relationship between premenstrual symptoms and dysmenorrhea in Japanese high school students. Arch Womens Ment Health. 2012;15:131-3.
22. Kumar S, Padubidri VG, Daftary SN. Common disorders of menstruation. In: Shaw's textbook of Gynaecology, 17th edition. NewDelhi: Jaypee Brothers Medical Publishers (P) Ltd.; 2019. pp. 122-27.
23. Laufer MR, Goitein L, Bush M, Cramer DW, Emans SJ. Prevalence of endometriosis in adolescent girls with chronic pelvic pain not responding to conventional therapy. J Pediatr Adolesc Gynecol. 1997;10:199-202.
24. Munro MG, Critchley HO, Broder MS, Fraser IS; FIGO Working Group on Menstrual Disorders. FIGO classification system (PALM-COEIN) for causes of abnormal uterine bleeding in nongravid women of reproductive age. Int J Gynaecol Obstet. 2011;113:3-13.
25. Newbery G, Neelakantan M, Cabral MD, Omar H. Amenorrhea in adolescents: a narrative review. Pediatr Med. 2019;2.
26. (NICE guideline) National Institute for Health Institute for Health and Care Excellence. Heavy menstrual bleeding: assessment and management.
27. Omidvar S, Amiri FN, Bakhtiari A, Begum K. A study on menstruation of Indian adolescent girls in an urban area of South India. J Family Med Prim Care. 2018;7(4):698.
28. Reid RL, Yen SS. Premenstrual syndrome. Am J Obstet Gynecol. 1981;139(1):85-104.
29. Rosenfield RL. Perspectives on International Recommendations for the diagnosis and Treatment of polycystic ovarian syndrome in adolescence. J Pediatr Adolesc Gynecol. 2022:S1083.
30. Slap GB. Menstrual disorders in adolescence. Best Pract Res Clin Obstet Gynaecol. 2003;17:75-92.
31. Vijayakumar M, Upadhyay Z, Sakamuri K. Menstrual irregularities. IAP Standard Treatment Guidelines. Mumbai: Indian Academy of Pediatrics; 2022. pp. 1-8.
32. World Health Organization Task Force on Adolescent Reproductive Health. World Health Organization multicenter study on menstrual and ovulatory patterns in adolescent girls. II. Longitudinal study of menstrual patterns in the early post menarchal period, duration of bleeding episodes and menstrual cycles. J Adolesc Health Care. 1986;7:236-44.
33. Yaşa C, Uğurlucan FG. Approach to Abnormal Uterine Bleeding in Adolescents. J Clin Res Pediatr Endocrinol. 2020;12(Suppl 1):1-6.

# CHAPTER 26

# Relationship Counseling

*MKC Nair, Shyamal Kumar, Riya Lukose*

## ■ INTRODUCTION

"Human relations" are quite intriguing and even so delicate. It is a complicated one to explain in simple words. For psychologists, "human relation" includes an overview of basic psychological and cultural concepts related to human behavior interactions and dealing with principles of communication, listening, and conflict resolution, with an emphasis on skill development to improve relationships. The notion of "human relations" is one of the important theoretical movements of the 1960's and RE Miles was responsible for much of the work on crystalizing the notion of "human relations". For communication scholars, the human relations perspective sees communication as a tool that can be used by management to "buy" cooperation from subordinates.

Relationship counseling includes any form of psychotherapy which is focused on improving the relationship between individuals and thus helping them resolve interpersonal/intrapersonal issues and modify maladaptive patterns of interactions, thereby fostering the healthy psychosocial growth of all individuals. It is thus a broader term encompassing components as family therapy and couple therapy. This was first described by US social worker Jessie Taft (1882–1960) and child psychiatrist Frederick H Allen (1890–1964).

## ■ HUMAN RELATIONS COUNSELING MODEL

Carl Roger described counseling relationship in the context of developing a nonhostile environment which is necessary for an individual to integrate experiences into their self-structure. The human relations counseling model emphasizes on a client-centered approach in helping relationship along with mutual identification of objectives, goals, and intervention strategies that can ultimately be evaluated from the point of view of the client's observable behavioral change. These approaches use a variety of techniques and strategies, but the major vehicle for change is the development and maintenance of a warm and empathic relationship with the client through

the six necessary and sufficient conditions for constructive personality change very aptly proposed by Roger.
1. The two concerned persons should be in psychosocial contact.
2. The person seeking counseling (the client), is in a state of incongruence, being vulnerable or anxious.
3. The "the counselor", is *congruent* or integrated in the relationship.
4. The counselor has complete *unconditional positive regard* for the client.
5. The counselor experiences an *empathic understanding* of the client's internal frame of reference and endeavors to communicate this experience to the client.
6. The counselor should achieve "empathic understanding" and "unconditional positive regard" for client's current mental status.
   - *Congruence:* As per Roger's the definition of congruence state stands as a close matching between the counselor's real experience, what is present in the counselor's awareness, and what is expressed to the client. It includes the therapist's openness and attunement to the moment-by-moment experience and the counselor's genuine expression of empathy and unconditional positive regard toward the client.
   - *Unconditional positive regard:* It is the warm acceptance of every aspect of the client's experience. This reflects the counselor's fundamental belief in the self-actualizing tendency of the client.
   - *Empathic understanding:* It is a process of "entering the personal perceptual world of the client and becoming thoroughly at home at it while being sensitive, and sensible, to the changing feelings which flow in this other person, and also communicating your sensing's of his/her world".

The counselor must learn how and when to use a battery of techniques and strategies with the client in order to deal as fully as possible with the client's affective, cognitive, and behavioral domains. The imperative goal of the whole counseling process is to help the client become emotionally and cognitively aware of his/her responsibility and choices and translate this awareness into action. This evolving relationship is the foundation of the helping process and as long as there is an effective helping relationship that communicates the helper's strength, understanding and ability to give permission and protection to the client, flexibility to use, select, and even fail with different strategies is possible. The ultimate strengths of a counselor in this counseling model are the abilities to hear verbal messages, interpret nonverbal signs/signals, and respond to these messages verbally and nonverbally.

## ASSUMPTIONS OF HUMAN RELATIONS COUNSELING MODEL

Many people believe that one should only seek relationship counseling when separation or divorce is looming. But that is often too little, too late.

Relationship therapy should begin as soon as the problems get in the way of one's daily life. Here are some high points in a "human relationship counseling model":
- Almost all the problems occur from unfinished issues from the past and it shapes who you are and the effects of which come years later, especially in reference to childhood issues.
- Problems often also originate from what one faces when he/she is an integral part of the system or society.
- The immediate environment has a lot to do with everything a person goes through and some, especially with mental illness may not be capable of making their own sound decisions.
- Young people are capable of learning new behaviors, eliminate the old ones, and are able to reinforce themselves.
- Young people are capable of making their own decisions within their environmental factors.
- Young people are striving to meet their needs and their behaviors are purposeful and goal oriented.
- Young people want to feel good about themselves but they often need confirmation from others.

## ■ BOY/GIRL RELATIONSHIP

A boy/girl relationship usually starts, when a boy and a girl meet and they develop an attraction or a feeling of liking toward each other and in many such cases, the relationship in a school may not lead to courtship. The laws of boy-girl relationships include:
- *The law of attraction:* We as humans are easily attracted to that which is hard to get, and belittle things which are easily obtained. This is a factual nature of humans.
- *The law of difference:* There is difference in the way boys and girls think about love and affection and this difference lies not only in the obvious, outward differences, but in their thinking process as well. For example, the boy thinks of love in terms of physical intimacy; a girl thinks of love in terms of romance.
- *The law of self-image:* We all are controlled by the way we see ourselves inwardly. If we regard ourself as not being worth much, we are definitely going to act that very same way. We all manage to remember all the "put downs" we have experienced.

### How to have a Healthy Boy-girl Relationship (Tips for Adolescents)

In order to develop a good boy-girl relationship one has to love oneself, accept oneself as you are, become good friend of yourself, be respectful to others, socialize and meet more friends, be cheerful always, and be socially pleasant.

- Being compassionate in understanding the feeling of the other family members, respecting the elders and caring younger ones, and in the process developing their trust and confidence.
- Honesty builds trust as trust is an integral part of a happy relationship.
- Maintain an even balance between your relationship and other aspects in life.
- In a healthy relationship, you need to talk openly to other members.
- It is important to accept and be comfortable with what you have and who you are engaged to in a relationship.
- Respect means you value the beliefs, opinions, and ideas of your colleague and other members.

The things that are essential for any relationships are:
- Trust—the most important ingredients of a happy and healthy relationship
- Respect—respecting the individuality of your partner
- Caring—love, attention, and effective communication.

## TYPES OF RELATIONSHIPS

The most common relationship types are:
- Monogamous relationships
- Polyamorous relationships
- Open relationships
- Long-distance relationships
- Casual sex relationships
- "Friends with benefits" relationships
- Asexual relationships
- True caring love relationships.

## DIFFERENT TYPES OF LOVE RELATIONSHIPS

Seven types of love include:
1. Liking (intimacy)
2. Infatuation (passion)
3. Empty love (commitment)
4. Romantic love (passion + intimacy)
5. Fatuous love (commitment + passion)
6. Companionate love (intimacy + commitment)
7. Consummate love (passion + intimacy + commitment).

## TYPES OF BOY-GIRL RELATIONSHIPS

Types of boy/girl relationship include:
- Compatible relationship
- Codependent relationship

- Complicated relationship
- Distracted relationship—invisible to each other
- Friends with benefits—no commitments
- May-December relationships—one of the partner is at least 10–15 years older or younger
- Emotional relationship
- Sacrificial relationship—unconditional love in its worst form
- Imperfect relationship
- Held-by-loss relationship—often a rebound relationship
- Long-distance relationship—minimal physical intimacy
- Love-hate relationship
- Negotiation relationship
- Open relationship
- *Toxic relationships:* Looks pleasant only from outside
- *Insecure relationship:* One may assume cheating
- Time pass fling
- Asexual relationship—traditional Indian view
- Sexual affair—no emotional connect
- Trophy relationship—just to impress others
- Unhappy relationship
- Controlling relationship
- Abusive relationship
- Spiritual love relationship—lot of caring

Top 10 teenage relationship problems include:
1. Serious love or just a date
2. How to tell your parents about your feelings
3. Limited money
4. Jealousy and trust issues
5. Lack of maturity
6. Parents
7. Peer pressure
8. Fear of losing first love
9. Social media
10. Breakup

Eight ways physical relationship before marriage affect relationship are:
1. Could be giving away all you have
2. Could get pregnant
3. Feeling trapped
4. Focus on other responsibilities after marriage, e.g., family, income, and children

5. A healthy relationship is equally controlled by both the partners; however, a physical relationship before marriage may end up with one of the partner with lot of disbelief and self-doubt.
6. Might not go any further in a relationship
7. Relationship could end up being just about sex
8. Sex makes the relationship stronger.

Although, it is true, that the vast majority of those who had physical relationship before marriage are capable of safeguarding themselves emotionally, at least some of them may be troubled by distrust, guilt, low self-esteem, paranoia, scepticism, self-doubt, sexual dysfunction, shame, and most importantly unsatisfactory sex.

## ■ INTERVENTION STRATEGIES

The feasible intervention strategies include family life education at high school level, adolescent guidance and counseling, premarital and newlywed counseling, and partner-relationship counseling (couple counseling) using Partner-relationship Assessment Scale Trivandrum (PAST—abridged–13 item and full version–26 items).

The goal of couple counseling is to build an existential base to their lives; identify and communicate their sense of purpose, priorities, and values; what they hold to be sacred; missions, ethics, and morality; philosophy of life and religion; legacy from their families; and culture and meaning of how to move through time together.

## ■ POINTS TO REMEMBER

- The human relationship counseling model follows Roger's client-centered approach, where the client forms the core part of therapy process.
- A boy-girl relationship follows certain laws—"laws of attraction, difference, and self-image".
- The boy-girl relationship can be of multiple types, and these have their own set of relationship issues.
- A healthy boy-girl relationship is formed on the grounds of honesty, compassion, finding right balance, talking openly, and having mutual respect.
- Physical relationship before marriage can affect postmarriage relationship.

*There will be lot of boys/girls to "love" you, but very few to take lifelong responsibility; multicolor fantasy of youth will become black and white reality later on.*

## SUGGESTED READING

1. Miles RE. Human relations or human resources? Harv Bus Rev. 1965;43(4):148-57.
2. Mini G, Kumari A, Nair MKC. Development of a tool on partner relationship and estimation of prevalence of marital disharmony among married people (Ph.D Thesis) Submitted to University of Kerala; 2020.
3. Nair MKC, George B, Indira MS, Sumaraj L. Adolescent Counselling, 1st edition. New Delhi: Jaypee Brothers Medical Publishers (P) Ltd; 2016. pp. 73-87.
4. Nair MKC, Russell P, George B, Sumaraj L. Adolescent Pediatrics, 1st edition. New Delhi: Noble Vision Medical Book Publishers; 2017. pp. 202-13; 225-32.
5. Okun BF. (1981). Effective Helping-The Human Relations Counseling Model' (From Correctional Counseling and Treatment, P 213-222, 1981, by Peter C Kratcoski See NCJ-74557). [online] Available from https://www.ojp.gov/ncjrs/virtual-library/abstracts/effective-helping-human-relations-counseling-model-correctional. [Last accessed January, 2023].
6. Pejaver RK, Nair MKC. Adolescence and Family Life Education, 1st edition. Karnataka: Prism Books Private Limited; 2001. pp. 97-146.
7. Rogers C. The necessary and sufficient conditions of therapeutic personality change. J Consult Psychol. 1957;21(2):95-103.
8. Thompson HP, Fedewa AL. Counseling and Psychotherapy with Children and Adolescents, 5th edition. Hoboken, New Jersey: John Wiley & Sons, Inc.; 2015. pp. 95-7.

# CHAPTER 27

# Office Management of Substance Abuse

*Jayashree K, Preeti M Galagali*

## ■ INTRODUCTION

Adolescence is a period of exploration and experimentation. Many risky behaviors like substance abuse have their onset in adolescence. These habits usually track into adulthood. Substance use before the age of 18 years is associated with an eightfold greater likelihood of developing substance dependence in adulthood. Even the first use of a psychoactive substance may result in tragic consequences of injury, victimization, or even fatality. Substance use disorder (SUD) is associated with problems in all spheres of an adolescent's life namely individual, family, school, and society. Substance abuse can cause a fall in academic performance, juvenile delinquency, rape, promiscuous sexual behavior, human immunodeficiency virus (HIV), hepatitis, family conflict, runaway behavior, depression, or suicide attempts. Drug-crime correlation has been noted with the consumption of substances, e.g., cannabis intake is linked with murder, inhalants with rape, and opioids with snatching-related crimes.

## ■ SITUATIONAL ANALYSIS

In the US, 21% of teens between 12 and 17 years have tried a tobacco product, including use of traditional cigarettes (13%), electronic cigarettes (11%), cigars (8%), hookahs (7%), and smokeless tobacco (4%). In India as per the National Survey on Extent and Pattern of Substance Use 2019, the prevalence of various substance uses in children between 10 and 17 years were alcohol (1.3%), cannabis (0.9%), opioid (1.8%), and sedatives (1.7%).

Despite the problems associated with substance abuse in adolescents still, it has not been researched well in India. The Ministry of Social Justice and Empowerment, Government of India through the National Drug Dependence Treatment Center (NDDTC), All India Institute of Medical Sciences (AIIMS), New Delhi 2018, conducted a national survey on the extent and pattern of substance use in India by the reported prevalence of substance use separately for adolescent subpopulation as shown in **Table 1**. Prevalence of inhalants use was noted to be higher among adolescents than in adults.

**TABLE 1:** Magnitude of substance use in the population and adolescent group.

| Drug | Prevalence in the population | Prevalence in adolescents |
|---|---|---|
| Alcohol | 14.6% | 1.3% |
| Cannabis | 2.8% | 0.9% |
| Opioids | 2.1% | 1.8% |
| Inhalants | 0.7% | 1.17% |

A major source of information about these products is available online, especially on the widely accessed YouTube video platform. 55% and 88% of adolescents in treatment for SUD meet criteria for a psychiatric disorder, namely conduct disorder, attention deficit hyperactivity disorder (ADHD), depression, and anxiety.

Based on effects on the central nervous system, drugs are classified as depressants, hallucinogens, and stimulants.
- *Depressants:* These drugs include alcohol, OxyContin, opioids, marijuana, tranquillizers, barbiturates, solvents and inhalants including petrol, glue, paint thinners, and lighter fluid.
- *Hallucinogens:* This group of substances contains psychoactive drugs that distort reality by triggering hallucinations, delusional thinking, and/or skewed experiences of time and space. These substances include d-lysergic acid diethylamide (LSD), peyote, mescaline, mushrooms (psilocybin), and dimethyltryptamine (DMT).
- *Stimulants:* These include methylphenidate, cocaine, narcotics like Fortwin, buprenorphine, morphine, pethidine, Spasmo Proxyvon, codeine containing cough syrups, cocaine, amphetamine, club drugs, anabolic steroids, electronic cigarettes, and hookahs are commonly being used by adolescents.

*Electronic nicotine delivery systems (ENDS) or e-cigarettes* are battery powered devices used to smoke or vape which contains nicotine and other harmful chemicals as flavoring agents. In 2019, among high school students the estimated prevalence of e-cigarette use (27.5%), middle school students (10.5%), and the estimated prevalence of smoking cigarettes was 5.8% and 2.3%, respectively.

Nicotine exposure in adolescents can result in nicotine addiction, nicotine toxicity, and harmful long-term effects to the developing brain, including negative effects on cognition. Potential harms of e-cigarette use also include lung injury known as e-cigarette or vaping product use-associated lung injury (EVALI) and death, depending on the ingredients included in e-cigarette fluids. Use of ENDS can open a gateway for new tobacco addiction which is a potential threat to the country's tobacco control laws and on-going tobacco control programs. As per Indian council of Medical Research there is complete prohibition (including procuring, production, marketing, promotion, and sale) on ENDS or e-cigarettes. As per US Preventive Services Task Force (USPSTF), behavioral interventions may reduce the likelihood of smoking initiation in nonsmoking children and adolescents.

Adolescents who abuse drugs, particularly those involved in the juvenile justice system, should be screened for other psychiatric disorders. Neurodevelopmental vulnerability of adolescents to drug use in adolescence, there is a general "imbalance" in functional development across brain regions, with earlier development occurring in posterior regions (reward center) and anterior regions (prefrontal cortex) progressing later, which leads to underdeveloped connections between midbrain cortico-limbic (reward) and frontal (inhibitory) region circuits. This "imbalance" enables heightened risk-taking behavior, particularly when the behavior results in immediate rewards. Adolescents with high alcohol consumption, on long-term drug abuse noted to have structural changes in the brain associated with cognitive impairment and anxiety-like behavior. The risk factors and protective factors for substance abuse are given in **Table 2**.

Having a family member who uses substances; enjoyment and curiosity are cited as major influences in decisions by adolescents to use substances.

Drug-specific clues for substance use are provided in **Table 3**.

The Diagnostic and Statistical Manual of Mental Disorders, Fifth edition (DSM-5) has 11 criteria for diagnosis of SUDs as given in **Box 1**.

## ROLE OF PEDIATRICIAN

### Screening for Substance Use Disorder

The primary care setting provides a unique opportunity to screen adolescents for SUD. The *HEEADSSS* interview focuses on assessment of the **H**ome environment, **E**ducation and employment, **E**ating, peer-related **A**ctivities, **D**rugs, **S**exuality, **S**uicide/depression, and **S**afety from injury and violence. During HEADSSS screening of an adolescent, anticipatory guidance reinforcing avoidance of drug use should be given to abstinent adolescents. The goal of motivational interviewing is to assess the patient's readiness to make a change, help him/her to identify reasons for change, and support his/her autonomy to do so. The desired change may be discontinuation of substance use or may focus on risk reduction, depending upon the patient's level and risks of use.

### Therapeutic Intervention

Pediatricians should have a high index of suspicion for substance abuse. Such an adolescent can present in an outpatient, inpatient, or emergency setting. USPSTF recommended that primary care clinicians provide interventions, including education or brief counseling, to prevent initiation

**TABLE 2:** Risk factors and protective factors for substance abuse.

| Risk factors | | Protective factors |
|---|---|---|
| • Externalizing and internalizing disorders<br>• High impulsivity and sensation seeking<br>• Rebelliousness and alexithymia<br>• Low intellectual development<br>• Lack of perception of harm from substances<br>• Family history of substance use disorder (SUD)<br>• Adverse childhood experience<br>• Poor academic performance | Individual factors | • Higher self-efficacy<br>• Average intelligence<br>• Good social skills<br>• Spirituality/religiosity<br>• Good coping skills and problem-solving |
| • Parental SUD<br>• Parenting style<br>• Parental psychopathology<br>• Single parent<br>• Parental separation<br>• Parental neglect/authoritarian style<br>• Low parental education<br>• Family mental illness<br>• Poverty<br>• Overcrowding | Family factors | • Authoritative parenting style<br>• Fewer siblings<br>• Parental presence<br>• Family cohesion<br>• Parental value toward schooling and risk behaviors |
| • Deviant peer group<br>• Social isolation from peers<br>• Neighborhood<br>• Cultural factors<br>• Exposure to violence<br>• Easy access to substances | Community factors | • Peers with prosocial norms<br>• School with drug policies<br>• Access to role models<br>• Access to healthcare and education<br>• Employment opportunities for adults<br>• Clear expectation of behaviors |

of tobacco use among school-aged children and adolescents. In 2016, the American Academy of Pediatrics endorsed the simple to use and implement Screening, Brief Intervention, and Referral to Treatment (SBIRT) model to manage substance use in adolescence.

## History of Comorbid High-risk Behavior

- Look for co-occurring mental disorders.
- Specific drug history including type of the drug/s used, extent of use, setting of use and degree of social, educational and vocational disruption.
- Look for flag signs as mentioned in **Table 3**.
- Use the Screening to Brief Intervention Tool (S2BI Tool) is as follows:

## CHAPTER 27: Office Management of Substance Abuse

| Screening | Brief intervention | Referral to treatment |
|---|---|---|
| Quickly assess the severity of substance use and identify the appropriate level of treatment. | Increase insight and awareness of substance abuse, motivation toward behavioral change. | Provide those identified as needing more extensive treatment with access to specialty care. |

The S2BI tool (**Flowchart 1**) uses a stem question and forced-response options (none, once or twice, monthly, and weekly or more) in a sequence to reveal the frequency of past-year use of tobacco, alcohol, and marijuana.

**TABLE 3:** Drug-specific clues.

| Drug used | Physical symptoms | Look for |
|---|---|---|
| Alcohol | Black outs, gastritis, slurred speech, relaxed inhibitions, and impaired coordination | Smell of alcohol on clothes or breath, intoxicated behavior, hangover, and glazed eyes |
| Marijuana | Flu-like symptoms, red conjunctiva, abnormal pupils, increased appetite for sweets, gynecomastia, small testes, and irregular periods | Rolling papers, pipes, dried plant material, odor of burnt hemp rope, and roach clip |
| Cocaine | Brief intense euphoria, raised blood pressure and tachycardia, restlessness, and excitement | Glass vials, glass pipes, razor blades, white crystalline powder, syringes, and needle marks |
| Hallucinogens (lysergic acid diethylamide, psilocybin, and MDMA) | Altered mood and perceptions, focus on detail, anxiety, panic, nausea, synesthesia (e.g., smell colors, and see sounds) | Capsules, tablets, microdots, and blotter squares |
| Narcotics (opium, heroin, and codeine) | Euphoria, drowsiness, insensitivity to pain, pinpoint pupil, cold moist skin, and runny nose | Needle marks on arms, needles, syringes, and spoons |
| Stimulants (amphetamines, nicotine, and caffeine) | Alertness, talkativeness, wakefulness, increased blood pressure, chest pain, tachycardia, loss of sleep and appetite, and hyperactivity | Pills and capsules |
| Date rape drugs, e.g., flunitrazepam, ketamine, and barbiturates | Amnesia | Tablets, ampules, and syringes |

**BOX 1:** The Diagnostic and Statistical Manual of Mental Disorders, Fifth edition (DSM-5) has following criteria for diagnosing substance abuse disorders.

- Substance is often taken in larger amounts and/or over a longer period than the patient intended
- Persistent attempts or one or more unsuccessful efforts made to cut down or control substance use
- A great deal of time is spent in activities necessary to obtain the substance, use the substance, or recover from effects
- Craving or a strong desire or urge to use the substance
- Recurrent substance use resulting in a failure to fulfil major role obligations at work, school, or home
- Continued substance use despite having persistent or recurrent social or interpersonal problem caused or exacerbated by the effects of the substance
- Important social, occupational, or recreational activities given up or reduced because of substance use
- Recurrent substance use in situations in which it is physically hazardous
- Substance use is continued despite knowledge of having a persistent or recurrent physical or psychological problem that is likely to have been caused or exacerbated by the substance
- Tolerance, as defined by either of the following:
  - Markedly increased amounts of the substance in order to achieve intoxication or desired effect
  - Markedly diminished effect with continued use of the same amount
- Withdrawal, as manifested by either of the following:
  - The characteristic withdrawal syndrome for the substance
  - The same (or a closely related) substance is taken to relieve or avoid withdrawal symptoms

*Mild:* 2–3 symptoms present
*Moderate:* 4–5 symptoms present
*Severe:* 6+ symptoms present

Management according to the severity of drug use is as follows:
- *No substance use:* Pediatricians should give positive reinforcement, encourage being "drug free" and discuss the risks of drug use and skills to withstand negative peer pressure. Talk to teens about life skills, self-awareness, self-esteem, and problem-solving.
- *Mild-to-moderate SUD:* Pediatrician should give brief intervention by creating insight regarding the consequences of drug use. Discuss and deal with "stressors" that trigger drug usage and reduce other risky behavior. Advice on stress management as shown in **Figure 1**.
- *Severe SUD:* Here the pediatrician should give motivational intervention. This is based on the principles of expressing empathy, developing discrepancy between life goals and the need to use drugs which could be stumbling blocks toward reaching the goals, enhancing self-efficacy to

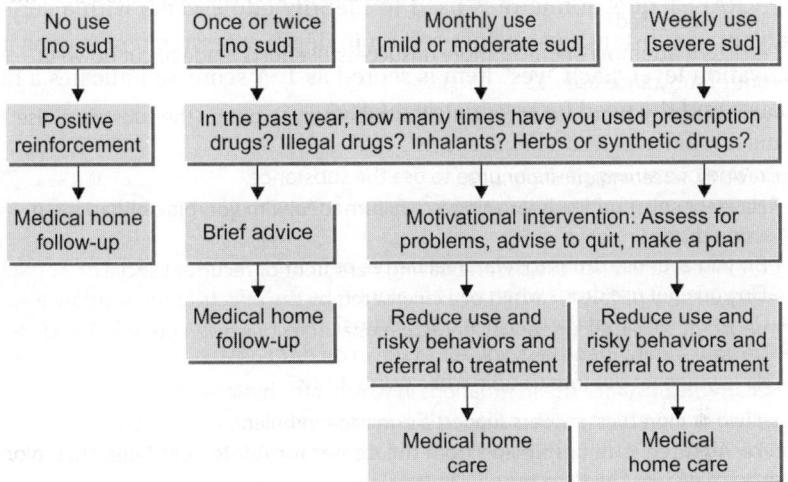

**Flowchart 1:** The S2BI-based approach to clinical SBIRT.

(S2BI: Screening to Brief Intervention; SBIRT: Screening, Brief Intervention, and Referral to Treatment; SUD: substance use disorder)
*Source:* Levy S, Shrier L. Boston, MA: Boston Children's Hospital. Copyright 2014, Boston Children's Hospital.

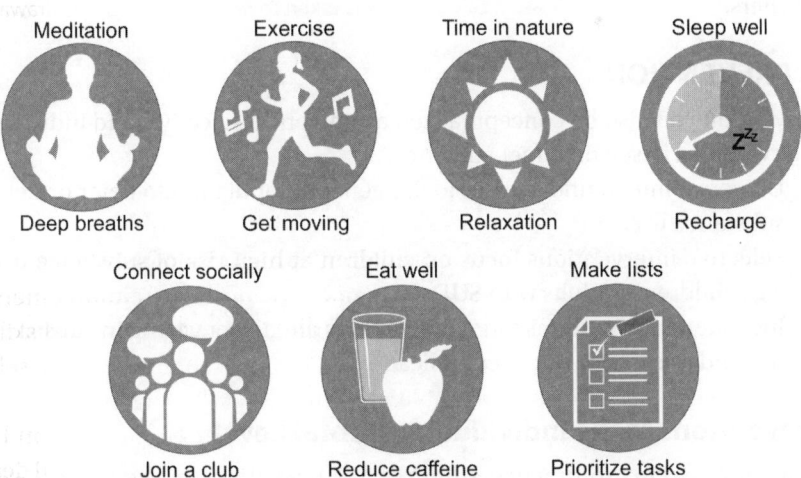

**Fig. 1:** Stress management.

resist drug use and rolling with resistance, if the adolescent refuses to get motivated to decrease/stop drug use. Few other therapies in the form of cognitive behavior therapy (CBT), pharmacotherapy, and family therapy also needed.

# THE CRAFFT QUESTIONNAIRE: A BRIEF SCREENING TEST FOR ADOLESCENT SUBSTANCE ABUSE

The CRAFFT questionnaire is used to identify adolescents with a serious problem of substance use, who need an in depth assessment of staging and motivation level. Each "yes" item is scored as 1. A score >2 indicates a high risk use and the need for psychiatric referral.

> *The CRAFFT screening questionnaire:*
> C—Have you ever ridden in a car driven by someone who was high or had been using drugs?
> R—Do you ever use drugs to relax, feel better, or fit in?
> A—Do you ever use drugs when you are alone?
> F—Do you ever forget things while using drugs?
> F—Do your family/friends ask you to cut down on drug use?
> T—Have you ever got into trouble while using drugs?
>
> *Note:* Two or more "yes" answers suggest a significant problem.
> *Source:* Adapted with permission from the Center for Adolescent Substance Abuse Research, CeASAR, Children's Hospital Boston.

*Severe SUD:* Pediatrician should refer such cases to an adolescent friendly psychiatrist for cognitive behavior therapy, motivational intervention, family therapy in the form parental support, love, better communication, reduced blame, and encouragement for the change. School support from peers and teachers.

## ■ PREVENTION

Prevention can also be conceptualized as universal, selective, and indicated interventions based on target audience.
- Universal interventions cater to the general population to deter or delay substance use;
- Selective interventions focus on children at high risk of substance use, e.g., children of adults with SUD;
- Indicated interventions target individuals already engaging in substance use and are at high risk of complications.

### Prevention: At the Individual–parental Level

Coaching parents to practice authoritative parenting and be a good role model for their teens. Teach adolescents life skills and to be goal oriented.

### Prevention: At Community Level
- School-based drug prevention programs
- Teaching life skills and resilience coaching at schools and school bonding

- Good role models in school and society
- Community cohesion by helping adolescents to overcome substance abuse.

## LAWS RELATED TO ALCOHOL, TOBACCO, AND PSYCHOTROPIC DRUGS

- Various states have age limit 18–25 years. Dry states: Bihar, Gujarat, Tripura, Lakshadweep, Mizoram, and Nagaland. Dry days: August 15, January 26, October 2, and others. Alcohol level for drink and driving: blood alcohol content (BAC) 0.03% per 100 mL (60 mL whiskey, 200 mL wine, and 660 mL beer for 65 kg person).
- *Tobacco laws in India:* Cigarette and Other Tobacco Products Act (COTPA): The age limit for using tobacco is >18 years. Advertising through most forms of media is prohibited. Health warning on packet covering 85% of both sides with picture and text. No sale within 100 yards of the educational institute. Law prohibits E-cigarettes in any form.
- Narcotic Drugs and Psychotropic Substances Act 1985 (NDPS Act): Prohibit production, manufacturing, cultivation, possession, sale, purchase, transport, storage, and consumption of a narcotic drug. Punishment: Imprisonment for 1 year, fine of 10,000 for small quantities. Imprisonment for 10 years and a fine of up to 1 lakh rupees for commercial quantity.
- Nasha Mukt Bharat Abhiyaan (NMBA) is for 272 districts across 32 state/union territories identified as the most vulnerable in terms of the usage of drugs in the country based on finding of Comprehensive National Survey and the inputs provided by the Narcotics Control Bureau (NCB).
- *mCessation programme:* Quit tobacco out of life: Ministry of Health and Family Welfare in partnership with the World Health Organization and the International Telecommunications Union has started an initiative utilizing mobile technology for tobacco cessation via registering for the session by giving a missed call to 011-22901701.

## CONCLUSION

Substance abuse is a medico-social-economic problem that can start during adolescence and into adulthood. Pediatricians should partner with parents, schools, and community in prevention strategies. More adolescent awareness programs and life skills training should be conducted. Pediatricians can play a vital role in early recognition and treatment/referral. Treatment requires a multidisciplinary approach along with parental and peer support. Well-equipped deaddiction centers must be made available in every district to cater to adolescents and youth with substance abuse.

## POINTS TO REMEMBER

- In adolescents' substance use begins as a part of curiosity or peer pressure.
- Creating awareness among adolescents, parents, and teachers is the need of the hour.
- Pediatrician should screen every adolescent for substance use.
- Behavioral interventions help in prevention of substance use.

## SUGGESTED READING

1. Ambekar A, Agrawal A, Rao R, Mishra AK, Khandelwal S, Chadda RK. Magnitude of substance use in India. New Delhi: Ministry of Social Justice and Empowerment, Government of India; 2019.
2. Ambrose BK, Day HR, Rostron B, Conway KP, Borek N, Hyland A, et al. Flavored tobacco product use among US youth aged 12-17 years, 2013-2014. JAMA. 2015;314(17):1871-3.
3. American Psychiatric Association. Diagnostic and Statistical Manual of Mental Disorders, Fifth edition. Arlington, VA: American Psychiatric Publishing; 2013.
4. Botvin KW. Preventing substance use among children and adolescents. In: Miller S (Ed). The ASAM Principles of Addiction Medicine, 6th edition. Philadelphia: Wolters Kluwer; 2019. pp. 3730-43.
5. Chakma JK, Dhaliwal RS, Mehrotra R. Indian Council of Medical Research. White Paper on Electronic Nicotine Delivery System. Indian J Med Res. 2019;149(5):574-83.
6. Defoe IN, Dubas JS, Figner B, van Aken MA. A meta-analysis on age differences in risky decision-making adolescents versus children and adults. Psychol Bull. 2015;141:48-84.
7. Department of Social Justice and Empowerment. Annual Report 2018-19. [online] Available from: http://socialjustice.gov.in/writereaddata/UploadFile/Social_Justice_AR_2018-19_English.pdf. [Last accessed February, 2023].
8. Galagali PM, Somashekar AR. Substance use in adolescence. In: Galagali PM (Ed). Mission Kishore Uday 2018–2019. Mumbai, India: Indian Academy of Pediatrics; 2019. pp. 48-52.
9. Grella CE, Hser Y, Joshi V, Rounds-Bryant J. Drug treatment outcomes for adolescents with comorbid mental and substance use disorders. J Nerv Ment Dis. 2001;189(6):384-92.
10. Hingson RW, Zha W. Age of drinking onset, alcohol use disorders, frequent heavy drinking, and unintentionally injuring oneself and others after drinking. Pediatrics. 2009;123(6):1477-84.
11. Levy S, Weiss R, Sherritt L, Ziemnik R, Spalding A, Hook SV, et al. An electronic screen for triaging adolescent substance use by risk levels. JAMA Pediatr. 2014;168(9):822-8.
12. Mason MJ, Aplasca A, Morales-Theodore R, Zaharakis N, Linker J. Psychiatric comorbidity, and complications. Child Adolesc Psychiatr Clin N Am. 2016;25(3):521-32.
13. Nackers KA, Kokotailo P, Levy SJ. Substance Abuse, General Principles. Pediatr Rev. 2015;36(12):535-44.

14. Selph S, Patnode C, Bailey SR, Stoner R, Chou R. Primary Care-Relevant Prevention and Cessation in Children and Adolescents Updated Evidence Report and Systematic Review for the US Preventive Services Task Force. JAMA. 2020;323(16):1599-608.
15. Shuja QS, Goel RK, Jagjeet S, Ahluwalia SK, Pathak R, Bashir H. Prevalence and pattern of substance abuse among school children in Northern India: a rapid assessment study. Int J Med Sci Public Health. 2013;2:273-82.
16. Spear LP. Consequences of adolescent use of alcohol and other drugs: studies using rodent models. Neurosci Biobehav Rev. 2016;70:228-43.
17. Tims FM, Dennis ML, Hamilton N, Buchan BJ, Diamond G, Funk R, et al. Characteristics and problems of 600 adolescent cannabis abusers in outpatient treatment. Addiction. 2002;97(Suppl 1):46-57.
18. Tsering D, Pal R, Dasgupta A. Licit and illicit substance use by adolescent students in eastern India: prevalence and associated risk factors. J Neurosci Rural Pract. 2010;1:76-81.
19. van Duijvenvoorde AC, Jansen BR, Visser I, Huizenga HM. Affective and cognitive decision-making in adolescents. Dev Neuropsychol. 2010;35:539-54.

# SECTION 4
# Chronic Diseases in Adolescents

28. **Tuberculosis in Adolescents**
    *Utkarsh Bansal, Gowrishankar NC, Dhakshayani RV*
29. **Asthma in Adolescents**
    *S Lakshmi Velmurugan, Utkarsh Sharma, S Kalpana*
30. **Pneumonia in Adolescents**
    *V Poovazhagi, Kamal Kumar Singhal*
31. **Psychotic Disorders in Adolescents**
    *Megha Mahajan, Vinayak Koparde*

# CHAPTER 28

# Tuberculosis in Adolescents

*Utkarsh Bansal, Gowrishankar NC, Dhakshayani RV*

## ■ INTRODUCTION

Tuberculosis (TB) is one of the most ancient diseases known to mankind and remains a major public health challenge in the world, particularly in developing countries. In 2020, globally about 10 million people were diagnosed with TB, including 5.6 million men, 3.3 million women, and 1.1 million children. The National Tuberculosis Elimination Programme (NTEP) of India has screened >80 million people for TB, treated 15 million patients, and saved millions of lives. Still, India contributes the largest number of TB patients (26%), and TB-related deaths in the world [38% of global TB deaths among human immunodeficiency virus (HIV)-negative people and 34% of the combined total number of TB deaths in HIV-negative and HIV-positive people]. In high-incidence settings, children and adolescents experience a huge burden of TB. Young children suffer more from severe and disseminated disease associated with risk of death or long-term disability, while adolescents commonly develop adult-type pulmonary TB (ATpTB), and are highly infectious, contributing significantly to community transmission.

## ■ ETIOLOGY

*Mycobacterium tuberculosis (M. tb)* bacilli are pleomorphic, weakly gram positive, nonspore-forming, nonmotile, obligate aerobic, and 2–4 µm long curved rods. *M. tb* cell wall has a high lipid content (60%) which contains mycolic acid, making it impervious to Gram staining. Acid-fast stains such as Ziehl–Neelsen, or fluorescent stains such as auramine stain *M. tb*. It grows more slowly in egg-based solid media such as Lowenstein–Jensen (LJ), and solid agar-based such as Middlebrook 7H11 or 7H10, and slightly faster in liquid media such as Middlebrook 7H9 or 7H12. Currently, *Mycobacterium* Growth Indicator Tube™ (MGIT) culture is used and is a WHO-recommended automated liquid culture for quicker results.

## EPIDEMIOLOGY

Tuberculosis bacterium is ubiquitous and is estimated that one-fourth of the world's population is infected by it. But, active TB diseases occur in about 5–15% of these people. The remaining with latent TB infection are noninfectious to others. The risk of developing TB disease is higher in infants and immunocompromised, especially HIV-positive individuals. In 2020, the estimated incidence of all forms of TB in India was 188 per 100,000 population (129–257 per 100,000 population). TB has an estimated incidence of 333,000 cases annually among Indian children in the 0–14 years age group (28% of global childhood TB burden), with boys being more commonly infected. Though children have a higher proportion of extrapulmonary TB (EPTB) when compared to adults, still pulmonary TB (PTB) is the most common type to be encountered. Children up to 14 years of age constitute about 25.4% of the Indian population and are expected to be 13% of the cases but only account for 6% of the cases reported to the NTEP. In 2021, India was the home of 373 million children up to 14 years and 242 million adolescents aged 10–19 years. In 2019, a gap of 55% in notification was established as the NTEP reported 150,000 cases in children up to 14 years. Globally, adolescents account for an estimated 800,000 incident TB cases annually, while 1 million young adults (20–24 years of age) develop TB disease every year. Adolescents and young adults (AYAs, ages 10–24 years) are hugely affected by TB and this essential phase of life is critical for laying the foundation for a healthy and productive adulthood, thus underlining the importance to prevent and control TB in this period.

Transmission of *M. tb* is from person to person, airborne through a symptomatic pulmonary case, with higher infectivity in those who are acid-fast sputum smear positive.

Children with primary PTB disease are usually noninfectious due to paucibacillary disease and poor ability to cough. Adolescents tend to be more infectious due to higher bacillary load and the development of cavitary PTB. Their ability to cough and have a large social circle are very important reasons for the dissemination of bacilli. The most heartening aspect of this disease is that most infectious patients become noninfectious within 2 weeks of starting effective treatment.

## CLINICAL MANIFESTATIONS

Tuberculosis infection (TBI) describes the asymptomatic stage of infection with *M. tb*. The immunological tests are positive, but the chest radiograph is normal or shows healed infection (calcification). TB disease indicates the presence of clinical signs and symptoms and/or an abnormal chest radiograph or other extrapulmonary manifestations. The interval between TBI and the onset of the disease may be several weeks in children or many decades in adults.

**Flowchart 1:** Pathophysiology of tuberculosis infection.

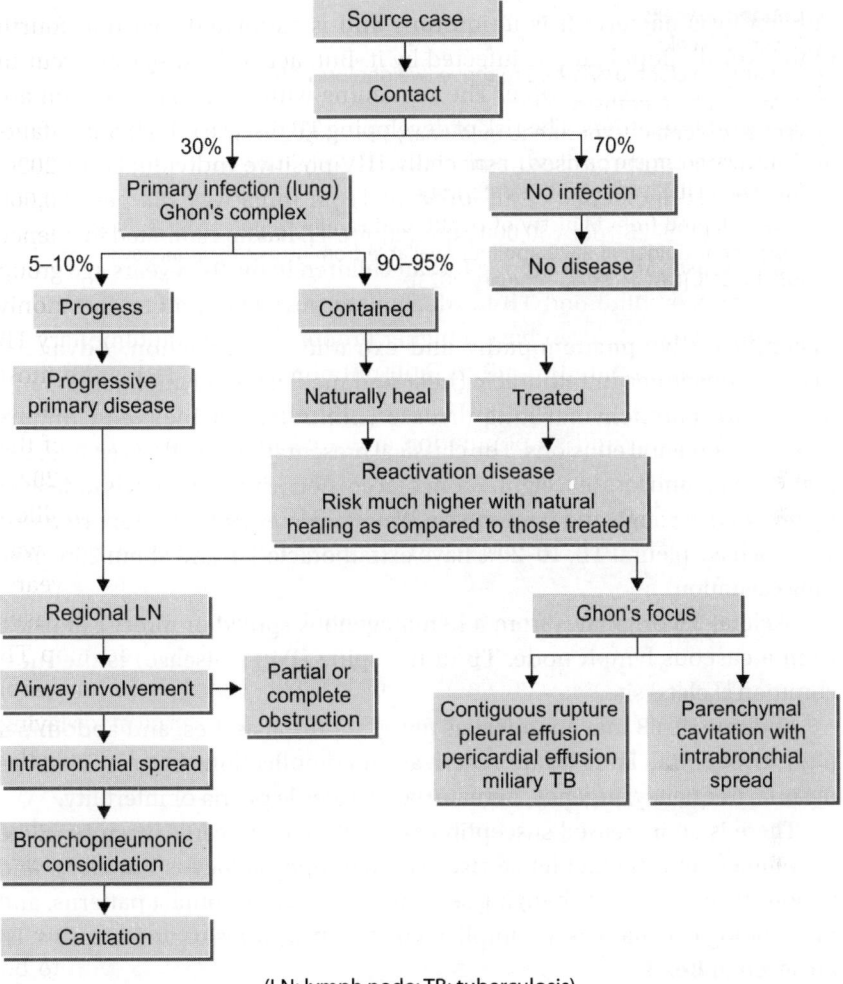

(LN: lymph node; TB: tuberculosis)

*Source:* Adapted from Ministry of Health and Family Welfare. (2019). RNTCP Updated Paediatric TB Guidelines 2019. [online] Available from: https://www.scribd.com/document/426087947/Updated-Pediatric-TB-Guidelines-2019-Guidance-Document#. [Last accessed February, 2023].

Children usually have an asymptomatic primary TB infection. Progressive primary disease is primary pneumonia that develops shortly after the initial infection. It may sometimes progress in infants to disseminated miliary disease or central nervous system (CNS) infection. Pulmonary cavitation is rare in children while it is typical with reactivation PTB in adolescents and adults **(Flowchart 1)**.

Reactivation PTB most commonly involves the apical segments of the upper lobes or superior segments of the lower lobes. There is usually

> **BOX 1:** Symptoms of presumptive TB.
>
> - Cough >2 weeks
> - Fever >2 weeks
> - Definitive weight loss/failure to thrive (weight loss of 5% in 3 months or no weight gain in past 3 months)
> - History of contact/exposure to pulmonary TB in past 2 years
> - Gradually enlarging painless lymph node, especially in the neck
> - Swelling in the back—gibbus deformity
>
> *Source:* Adapted from Ministry of Health and Family Welfare. (2022). Paediatric TB Management Guideline 2022. [online] Available from https://tbcindia.gov.in/showfile.php?lid=3668. [Last accessed February, 2023].

insignificant lymphadenopathy and extrathoracic infection. Advanced disease constitutes intrathoracic (hilar and mediastinal) lymphadenopathy along with parenchymal lung disease (infiltrates, cavities, and miliary disease), or pleural effusions. The classical presentation is with fever, malaise, night sweats, and loss in weight. Bronchial erosion with cavitation is indicated by productive cough and hemoptysis. Among adolescents, it is reported that 10–20% have pleural TB, 10–20% have extrathoracic TB, and about 25% have lung cavitation.

Skeletal TB originates from a hematogenous spread or direct extension from a caseous lymph node. TB of the spine (Pott's disease) is the most common skeletal site.

Abdominal TB may manifest as fever, anorexia, ascites, and abdominal pain. Urogenital TB is a late reactivation complication that manifests as dysuria, frequency, urgency, hematuria, and sterile pyuria or infertility.

There is an increased susceptibility to TB in adolescents when both the prevalence and the incidence rise. The pathophysiology is not clear, and various factors such as changing sex hormones, social contact patterns, and immunological changes are implicated. The symptoms of presumptive TB are given in **Box 1**.

## ■ DIAGNOSIS

The conventional gold standard for the diagnosis of TB is the demonstration of acid-fast bacilli (AFB) on smear or isolation of *M. tb* by the culture of an appropriate specimen.

Chest X-ray should be done for presumptive TB cases. Highly suggestive chest X-ray refers to miliary shadows, lymphadenopathy (hilar or mediastinal), or chronic fibrocavitary shadows.

### Skin Test for Tuberculosis

Tuberculin skin test (TST), an immunological test to elicit delayed type IV hypersensitivity, is done by injecting 2TU RT23 PPD intradermally. Test positivity is a marker of present or past infection with *M. tb*, but does not discriminate between active and latent TBI. Thus, TST is an ancillary test, used in conjunction with a contact history, screening of children exposed to TB or at increased risk of TB infection, and HIV-infected children.

## Rapid Diagnostic Tests

Cartridge-based nucleic acid amplification test (CBNAAT) and line probe assay (LPA) are preferred over smear microscopy. Truenat™ MTB-RIF Dx™, Xpert Rif™, and Xpert Rif UltraTM are the available CBNAAT tests. LPA is used in drug-resistant TB (DR-TB) cases. The first-line LPA (FL-LPA) is used to detect resistance to R and H—MTB DRplus™ and the second-line LPA (SL-LPA) is used to detect resistance to class FQ and class SLI—MTBDRsl™.

Adolescents usually expectorate sputum samples for investigations, but those who are unable to do so may require gastric aspirate (GA) or induced sputum (IS) to obtain adequate samples. Nebulized hypertonic saline-induced coughing increases the culture yields compared to conventional sputum samples.

Currently, liquid cultures like MGIT cultures are used and recommended as they give results relatively earlier than the traditional solid culture like LJ medium.

## Interferon γ Release Assays

This is an immune reaction test against *M. tb* specific antigens such as ESAT-6, CFP-10, and Tb7.7. It cannot distinguish between infection and disease. Interferon γ release assay (IGRA) is expensive and more resource demanding.

For presumptive PTB and EPTB cases, microbiological confirmation should be attempted **(Flowchart 2)**. Appropriate specimens from the presumed sites of involvement must be obtained for CBNAAT/smear microscopy/culture and drug sensitivity testing (DST) for *M. tb*/histopathological examination.

## ■ TREATMENT

Conventionally antitubercular treatment (ATT) is biphasic:
- *Intensive phase (IP):* initially the bacterial load is higher and also the chances of naturally occurring mutants. Thus, more drugs are given in the initial stage of the disease. They swiftly kill *M. tb*, reducing infectivity and worsening of disease, and preventing death.
- *Continuation phase (CP):* Lesser drugs are needed to eliminate the residual bacilli. It reduces failures and relapses.

There is a paradigm shift in TB treatment with the understanding that rifampicin-resistant strains when treated with first-line ATT lead to treatment failure and a paradoxical rise in acquired resistance to other drugs too. Thus

**Flowchart 2:** Diagnostic algorithm for pulmonary TB.

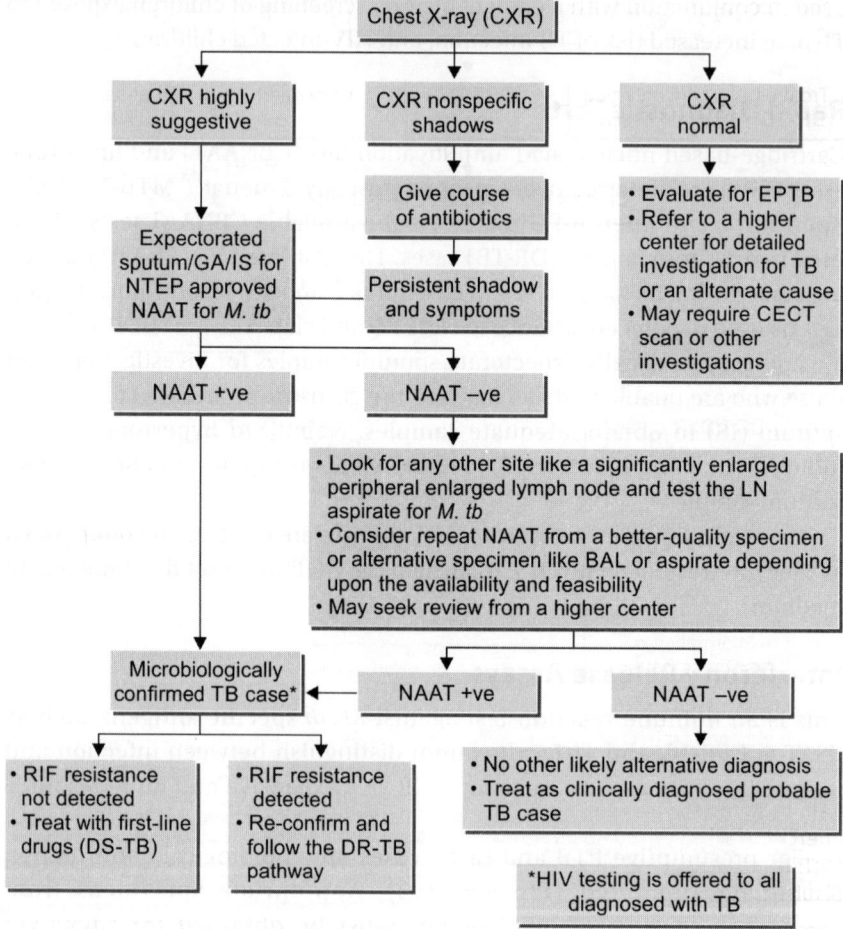

(BAL: bronchoalveolar lavage; CECT: contrast-enhanced computed tomography; DR-TB: drug-resistant tuberculosis; DS-TB: drug-sensitive tuberculosis; EPTB: extrapulmonary tuberculosis; GA: gastric aspirate; HIV: human immunodeficiency virus; IS: induced sputum; LN: lymph node; *M. tb*: *Mycobacterium tuberculosis*; NAAT: nucleic acid amplification test; NTEP: National Tuberculosis Elimination Programme; RIF: rifampicin; TB: tuberculosis)

*Source:* Adapted from Ministry of Health and Family Welfare. (2022). Paediatric TB Management Guideline 2022. [online] Available from https://tbcindia.gov.in/showfile.php?lid=3668. [Last accessed February, 2023].

universal drug sensitivity testing (UDST) upfront is recommended in all cases before initiation of the first-line ATT **(Flowchart 3)**. Case definitions are given in **Box 2**.

Patients are thus labeled rifampicin resistance detected (RR-TB) or rifampicin resistance not detected (RS-TB). The RS-TB cases are given first-line ATT even in relapse or default cases. The RR-TB cases need to be tested for other

**Flowchart 3:** Algorithm to approach of treatment of tuberculosis.

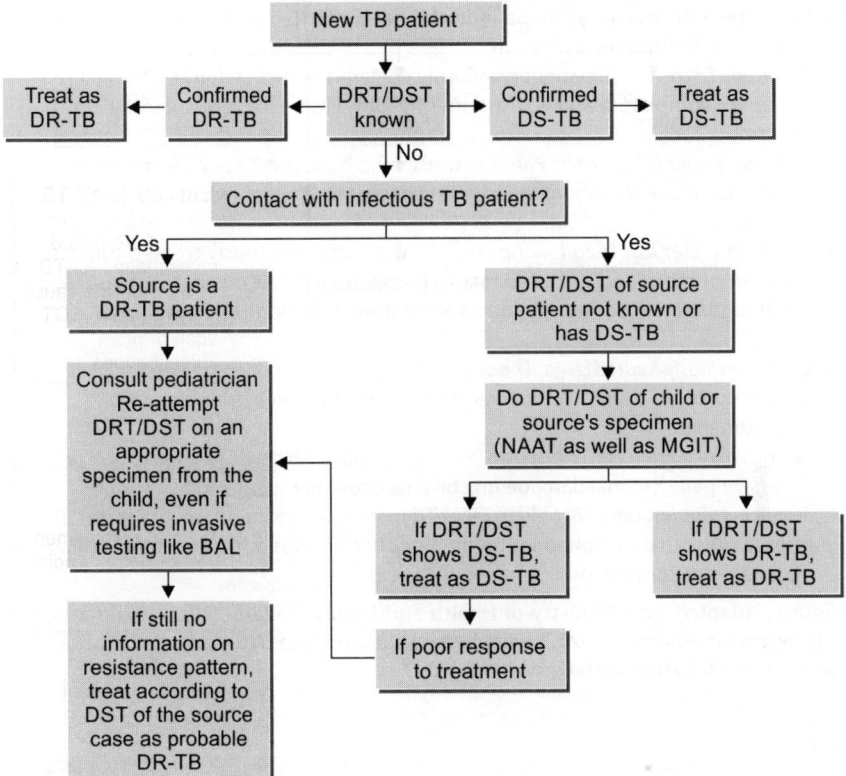

(BAL: bronchoalveolar lavage; DRT: drug-resistant testing; DR-TB: drug-resistant tuberculosis; DST: drug susceptibility testing; DS-TB: drug-sensitive tuberculosis; MGIT: *Mycobacterium* Growth Indicator Tube™; NAAT: nucleic acid amplification test; TB: tuberculosis)

*Source:* Adapted from Ministry of Health and Family Welfare. (2022). Paediatric TB Management Guideline 2022. [online] Available from https://tbcindia.gov.in/showfile.php?lid=3668. [Last accessed February, 2023].

drugs including isoniazid (INH) (mono or poly) and are treated with a DR-TB regimen. Furthermore, in cases of poor or nonresponse patient needs testing for DR-TB instead of a routine extension of IP. Now daily treatment has replaced alternate-day therapy using fixed drug combination (FDC) tablets (pediatric and adult) for better patient compliance **(Tables 1 to 3)**. The ideal weight should be employed to compute the dose in obese adolescents.

## DRUG-RESISTANT TUBERCULOSIS INCLUDING MULTIDRUG-RESISTANT TUBERCULOSIS

It is speculated that the prevalence of multidrug-resistant TB (MDR-TB) is about 2.8% among new cases and 14% among previously treated cases **(Flowchart 4)**. The DR-TB in comparison to drug-susceptible TB (DS-TB)

**BOX 2:** Case definitions.

- *New case:* A tuberculosis (TB) patient who has never had treatment for TB or has taken anti-TB drugs for <1 month
- *Recurrent TB case:* A TB patient previously declared as successfully treated (cured/treatment completed) and is subsequently found to be microbiologically confirmed TB case
- *Treatment after failure case:* Patients those who have previously been treated for TB and whose treatment failed at the end of their most recent course of treatment
- *Treatment after lost to follow-up case:* A TB patient previously treated for TB for 1 month or more and declared lost to follow-up in their most recent course of treatment and subsequently found to be a microbiologically confirmed TB case
- *Other previously treated cases:* Those who have previously been treated for TB, but the outcome after their most recent course of treatment is unknown or undocumented
- *Extensive (or advanced) TB disease:* Presence of bilateral cavitary disease or extensive parenchymal damage on chest radiography
- *Severe extrapulmonary TB:* Miliary TB or TB meningitis, extrapulmonary forms of disease other than lymphadenopathy (peripheral nodes or isolated mediastinal mass without compression)

*Source:* Adapted from Ministry of Health and Family Welfare. (2022). Paediatric TB Management Guideline 2022. [online] Available from https://tbcindia.gov.in/showfile.php?lid=3668. [Last accessed February, 2023].

**TABLE 1:** Regimen for rifampicin sensitive tuberculosis (RS-TB) case.

| Type of patient[a] | Regimens |
|---|---|
| - New microbiologically confirmed RS pulmonary TB<br>- New clinically diagnosed pulmonary TB (probable RS-TB)<br>- New microbiologically confirmed RS extrapulmonary TB<br>- New clinically diagnosed extrapulmonary TB (probable RS-TB)<br>- Drug sensitive previously treated TB[c] (recurrent, treatment after loss to follow-up, treatment after failure) | 2HRZE + 4HRE[b] |

[a]Molecular testing shall be done in all new cases in children with suspected TB at diagnosis and RS-TB (rifampicin resistance not detected) cases included in this regimen.
[b]In the case of neuro and spinal TB, the continuation phase is extended to 10 months.
[c]All these categories of children shall be evaluated as DR-TB suspects and assessed as per the DR-TB algorithm. Drug sensitivity testing (DST)-based treatment shall be followed. If they are found to be rifampicin [and isoniazid (INH)] sensitive, they shall be restarted on the regimen as for a new case. This group was earlier treated with category II regimen, which is now withdrawn from the National Tuberculosis Elimination Programme (NTEP).
*Source:* Adapted from Ministry of Health and Family Welfare. (2022). Paediatric TB Management Guideline 2022. [online] Available from https://tbcindia.gov.in/showfile.php?lid=3668. [Last accessed February, 2023].

**TABLE 2:** Dosing of first-line antitubercular drugs.

|  |  | Range (mg/kg/day) | Average (mg/kg/day) | Maximum dose (mg) |
|---|---|---|---|---|
| Rifampicin | R | 10–20 | 15 | 600 |
| Isoniazid | H | 7–15 | 10 | 300 |
| Pyrazinamide | Z | 30–40 | 35 | 2,000 |
| Ethambutol | E | 15–25 | 20 | 1,500 |
| Streptomycin | S | 15–20 | 20 | 1,000 |

*Source:* Adapted from Ministry of Health and Family Welfare. (2022). Paediatric TB Management Guideline 2022. [online] Available from https://tbcindia.gov.in/showfile.php?lid=3668. [Last accessed February, 2023].

**TABLE 3:** Drug dosage for DS-TB in FDCs according to weight.

*Drug dosage for pediatric DS-TB*

|  | Number of tablets (FDCs) | | | |
|---|---|---|---|---|
|  | Intensive phase | | Continuation phase | |
|  | HRZ | E | HR | E |
| Weight band (kg) | 50/75/150 | 100 | 50/75 | 100 |
| 4–7 | 1 | 1 | 1 | 1 |
| 8–11 | 2 | 2 | 2 | 2 |
| 12–15 | 3 | 3 | 3 | 3 |
| 16–24 | 4 | 4 | 4 | 4 |
| 25–29 | 3 + 1 A | 3 | 3 + 1 A | 3 |
| 30–39 | 2 + 2 A | 2 | 2 + 2 A | 2 |

*Drug dosage for adult DS-TB*

|  | HRZE | HRE |
|---|---|---|
| Weight band (kg) | 75/150/400/275 | 75/150/275 |
| 25–34 | 2 | 2 |
| 35–49 | 3 | 3 |
| 50–64 | 4 | 4 |
| 65–75 | 5 | 5 |
| >75 | 6 | 6 |

(DS-TB: drug-susceptible tuberculosis; FDCs: fixed drug combinations)
*Source:* Adapted from Ministry of Health and Family Welfare. (2022). Paediatric TB Management Guideline 2022. [online] Available from https://tbcindia.gov.in/showfile.php?lid=3668. [Last accessed February, 2023].

**Flowchart 4:** Algorithm to approach of treatment of drug-resistant tuberculosis.

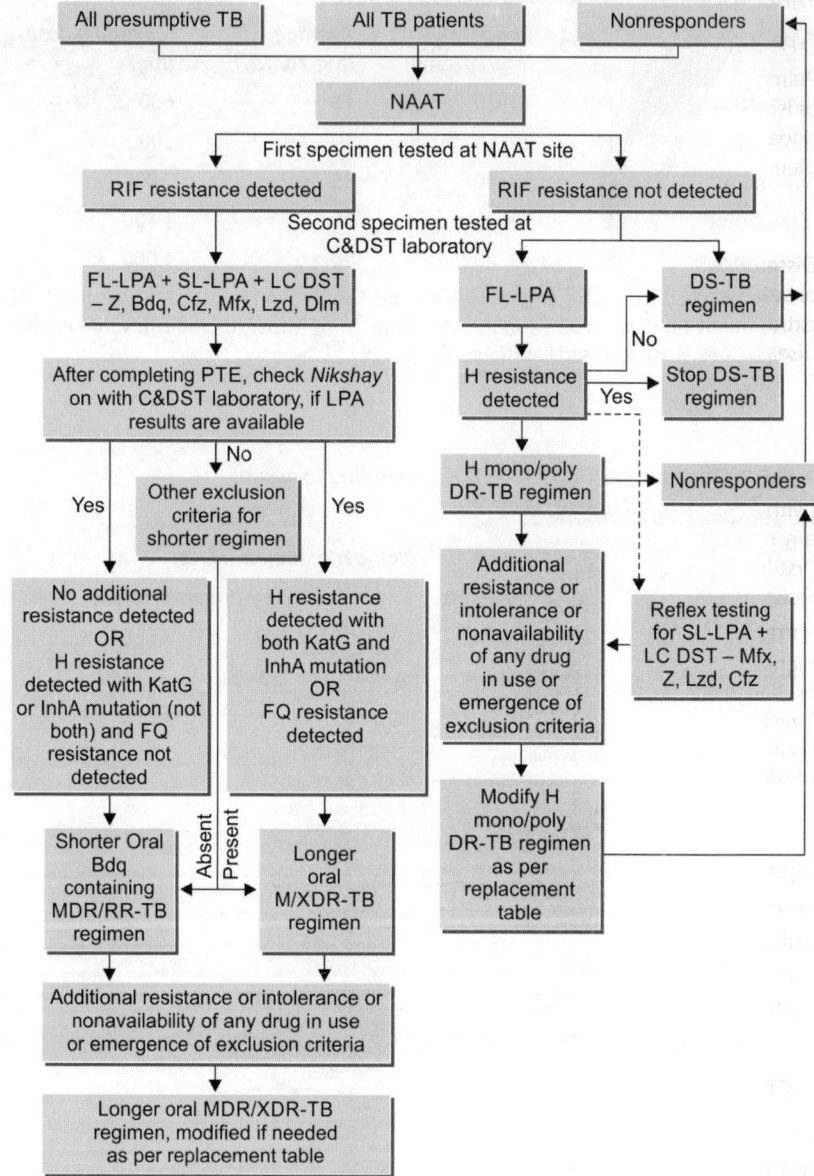

(C&DST: culture and drug susceptibility test; DST: drug susceptibility testing; DS-TB: drug-sensitive tuberculosis; DR-TB: drug-resistant tuberculosis; FL-LPA: first-line-line probe assay; FQ: fluoroquinolone; H: isoniazid; LC: liquid culture; MDR-TB: multidrug-resistant tuberculosis; NAAT: nucleic acid amplification test; PTE: pretreatment evaluation; RIF: rifampicin; SL-LPA: second-line-line probe assay; TB: tuberculosis; XDR-TB: extensively drug-resistant tuberculosis)

*Source:* Adapted from Ministry of Health and Family Welfare. (2022). Paediatric TB Management Guideline 2022. [online] Available from https://tbcindia.gov.in/showfile.php?lid=3668. [Last accessed February, 2023].

**TABLE 4:** Regimens for drug-resistant TB (DR-TB) case.

| Type of TB case | Treatment regimen | Special considerations |
|---|---|---|
| Pulmonary cases or isolated lymph node disease or pleural effusion | *Intensive phase* (4–6) Lfx, Cfz, Z, E, H[h], Eto (6) Bdq *Continuation phase* (5) Lfx, Cfz, Z, E | • Not for EPTB other than isolated lymph node disease or pleural effusion<br>• Not for children under 6 years<br>• Lf to be replaced by Mfx[h] if FQ class resistance |
| Disseminated or severe extrapulmonary disease | (18–20) Lfx, Lzd, Cfz, Cs (6) Bdq (6 m or longer) | • Modification shall be needed if additional FQ resistance<br>• Bdq can be replaced by Dlm if needed<br>• Individualized regime with drug replacement based on resistance pattern and tolerability as per PMDT guidelines |
| Resistance to INH (with or without any non-rifampicin first-line drug resistance) | (6) Lfx R E Z *Uniphasic regime* | • Can be extended to 9–12 months in:<br>• Extensive pulmonary disease<br>• Extrapulmonary disease like bone or intracranial |

(EPTB: extrapulmonary tuberculosis; FQ: fluoroquinolone; H[h]: high-dose isoniazid; Mfx[h]: high-dose moxifloxacin; PMDT: programmatic management of drug-resistant tuberculosis; SLI: second-line injectable)
*Source:* Adapted from Ministry of Health and Family Welfare. (2022). Paediatric TB Management Guideline 2022. [online] Available from https://tbcindia.gov.in/showfile.php?lid=3668. [Last accessed February, 2023].

requires a lengthy course, more drugs, and adverse effects. Thus treatment adherence is lower and the outcome is poor, including death **(Tables 4 and 5)**. Children below 10 years had a higher proportion of successful treatment outcomes (94% versus 60%) compared to adolescents. The MDR-TB case definitions are given in **Box 3**.

# ■ CONSIDERATIONS FOR ADOLESCENTS

Adolescence is a critical phase of development that is accompanied by rapid physical and mental growth. This phase is characterized by autonomy and impulsivity. The short-term social benefits outweigh the potential long-term health benefits, making adherence to the long-term treatment required for TB difficult. Before the commencement of therapy, adolescents need to be counseled on several aspects, which include medication compliance and assuring regular follow-up, the detrimental effect of unhealthy behaviors (including substance use), repercussions of isolation (social and medical), interference with work or schooling, and stigma associated with the disease.

**TABLE 5:** Grouping of drugs recommended for use in MDR-TB regimen.

| Groups and steps | Medicine | Abbreviation |
|---|---|---|
| Group A: Include all three medicines | • Levofloxacin OR Moxifloxacin<br>• Bedaquiline<br>• Linezolid | Lfx<br>Mfx<br>Bdq<br>Lzd |
| Group B: Add one or both medicines | • Clofazimine<br>• Cycloserine OR Terizidone | Cfz<br>Cs<br>Trd |
| Group C: Add to complete the regimen and when medicines from Group A and B cannot be used | • Ethambutol<br>• Delamanid<br>• Pyrazinamide<br>• Imipenem-cilastatin OR Meropenem<br>• Amikacin OR Streptomycin<br>• Ethionamide OR Prothionamide<br>• p-aminosalicylic acid | E<br>Dlm<br>Z<br>Ipm-Cln<br>Mpm<br>Am<br>S<br>Eto<br>Pto<br>PAS |

*Source:* Adapted from Ministry of Health and Family Welfare. (2022). Paediatric TB Management Guideline 2022. [online] Available from https://tbcindia.gov.in/showfile.php?lid=3668. [Last accessed February, 2023].

**BOX 3:** Multidrug-resistant tuberculosis (MDR-TB) case definitions.

- *Mono-resistance TB (MR-TB):* Resistant to one first-line anti-TB drug only.
- *Isoniazid-resistant TB (Hr-TB):* Resistant to isoniazid and susceptibility to rifampicin has been confirmed.
- *Poly-drug resistance TB (PDR-TB):* Resistant to more than one first-line anti-TB drugs, other than both H and R.
- *Rifampicin resistance (RR):* Resistant to R, with or without resistance to other anti-TB drugs. It includes any resistance to R, in the form of mono-resistance, poly-resistance, MDR or XDR.
- *Multidrug resistance TB (MDR-TB):* Resistant to both H and R with or without resistance to other first-line anti-TB drugs. MDR-TB patients may also have additional resistance to any/all fluoroquinolone (FQ) or any/all second-line injectable (SLI) anti-TB drugs.
- *Pre-extensively drug-resistant TB (Pre-XDR-TB):* An MDR/RR-TB patient additionally resistant to any FQ.
- *Extensive drug resistance (XDR):* An MDR-TB patient additionally resistant to at least a FQ (Ofx, Lfx, and Mfx) and SLI anti-TB drugs (Km, Am, and Cm).

*Source:* Adapted from Ministry of Health and Family Welfare. (2022). Paediatric TB Management Guideline 2022. [online] Available from https://tbcindia.gov.in/showfile.php?lid=3668. [Last accessed February, 2023].

Adolescents with TB and comorbidities such as HIV, diabetes, or DR-TB are the most challenging patients, as their treatment compliance and adherence to appointments is an essential aspect of successful treatment. But, due to the plethora of side effects and the prolonged duration of therapy, good compliance is seldom achieved. Psychosocial assistance is of paramount importance in cases of DR-TB, as they face social exclusion, depression, stigmatization, and poor morale.

Isolation is required in the early phase of PTB treatment to prevent transmission, which may lead to the absence of the adolescent from education or employment. This short-term default may have long-term socioeconomic outcomes. But exclusion from work or school in purely EPTB is unnecessary and should be avoided. There should be a provision of educational support for adolescents who cannot attend school due to the disease.

A comprehensive history of other comorbidities, medications, and behaviors (like substance abuse) is essential for the success of TB treatment, as they may decrease the effectiveness or increase the adverse effects of the treatment. Adolescents addicted to substance abuse should be specifically dealt with care and should be educated that alcohol use can increase hepatotoxicity. They should be guided to avoid sharing cigarettes while smoking to prevent the spread of infection to peers.

In sexually active adolescent girls, it is prudent to do pregnancy testing before treatment initiation and to counsel them to use nonhormonal contraception options, as hormonal contraception may be adversely affected by rifamycin, and cannot be depended on. During HIV testing, adolescents can be offered testing and counseling for other sexually-transmitted infections. An adolescent-friendly approach that upholds confidentiality should be incorporated into TB treatment to allow the adolescents to reveal their mental health issues, sexual activity, and substance use which may be unreported in the presence of caregivers.

## ■ SEQUELAE POST-TUBERCULOSIS

The long-term ramifications of TB on the health of adolescents are unexplored. The effect of school or work absence due to the disease has not been studied, nor has the evaluation of post-TB lung health in adolescents for long-term effects. Post-TB meningitis sequelae have been reported in 54–66% of patients ≤18 years. The DR-TB injectable agents induced irreversible hearing loss are reported.

The psychosocial impact of TB is again an uncharted sea in adolescence. There are detrimental effects on education, occupation, and relationships. Adolescents are very sensitive to social isolation. The stigma and discrimination can lead to extreme and enduring impacts on their life. Adolescents have a hard time accepting the diagnosis and during hospitalization, they face anxiety and sadness. Apprehension of the future, shame, and negative self-esteem sprout in them. But positive relationships with physicians, caregivers, and peers negate the impacts of TB diagnosis and hospitalization on adolescents' mental well-being.

The Adolescent Friendly Health Clinics (AFHCs) under the Rashtriya Kishor Swasthya Karyakram (RKSK) are perfect platforms to support the adolescents suffering from TB with the help of peer educators (PEs) or *Saathiya* who not only can promote early health seeking behavior but also acceptance and resilience toward the disease process.

## ■ INTERNATIONAL AND NATIONAL EFFORTS

Sustainable Development Goal (SDG) Target 3.3 includes ending the TB epidemic by 2030. The end TB strategy defines milestones (for 2020 and 2025) and targets (for 2030 and 2035) for reductions in TB cases and deaths. "The targets for 2030 are a 90% reduction in the number of TB deaths and an 80% reduction in the TB incidence rate (new cases per 100,000 population per year), compared with levels in 2015. The milestones for 2020 are a 35% reduction in the number of TB deaths and a 20% reduction in the TB incidence rate. The strategy also includes a 2020 milestone that no TB patients and their households face catastrophic costs as a result of TB disease."

The political declaration of the UN high-level meeting included four new global targets:

- Treat 40 million people for TB disease in the 5-year period 2018–2022 (including 3.5 million children and 1.5 million people with DR-TB, including 115,000 children)
- Reach at least 30 million people with TB preventive treatment for a latent TB infection in the 5-year period, 2018–2022 (including 6 million people living with HIV, 4 million children aged under 5 years, and 20 million people in other age groups, who are household contacts of people affected by TB)
- Mobilize at least US $13 billion annually for universal access to TB diagnosis, treatment, and care by 2022
- Mobilize at least US $2 billion annually for TB research.

The optimal management of pediatric TB requires a collaboration of multiple health agencies and utilization of the existing primary child health programs, as proposed by the National Strategic Plan 2017–2025.

## ■ INTEGRATED HEALTH SERVICES DELIVERY FRAMEWORK

The idea is to utilize and orchestrate activities of the existing health programs of the country such as NTEP, Rashtriya Bal Swasthya Karyakram (RBSK), and RKSK with the purpose to provide comprehensive services aiding elimination of TB.

**Flowchart 5:** Algorithm for an approach toward an adolescent with presumptive tuberculosis.

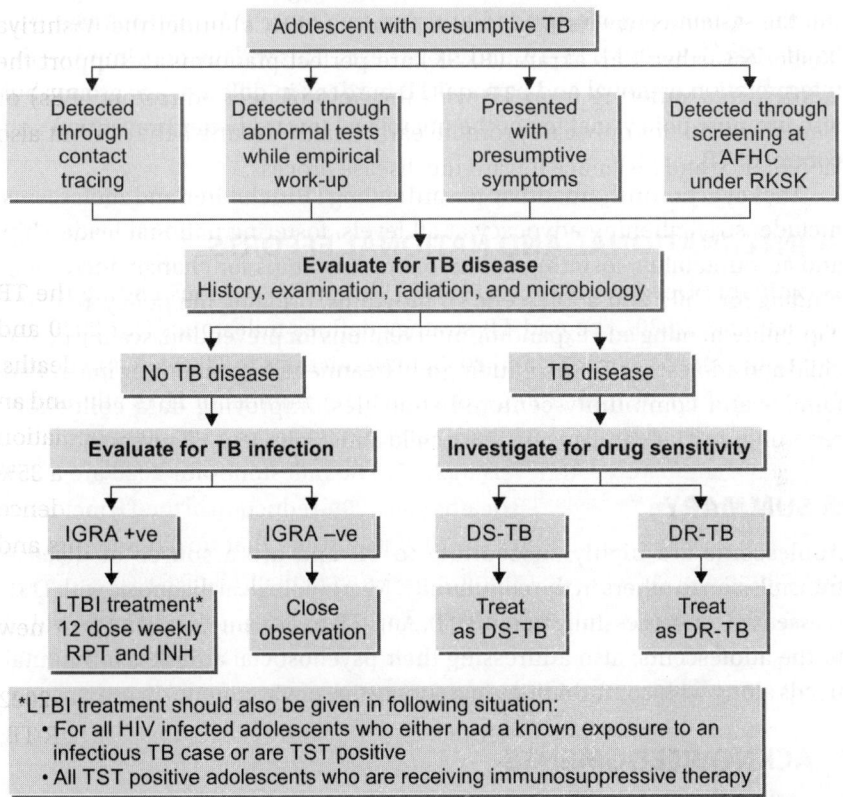

(AFHC: adolescent friendly health clinics; DR-TB: drug-resistant tuberculosis; DS-TB: drug-sensitive tuberculosis; HIV: human immunodeficiency virus; IGRA: interferon γ release assay; INH: isoniazid; LTBI: latent tuberculosis infection; RKSK: Rashtriya Kishor Swasthya Karyakram; RPT: rifapentine; TB: tuberculosis; TST: tuberculin skin test)

## Goal

To reduce TB-associated morbidity and mortality in children and adolescents through prevention, early detection, and prompt and complete management of TB.

## Approaches

- Enhancing community awareness of TB in children and adolescent population
- Generating demand and promoting disease prevention and early health-seeking behavior
- Increasing the early detection of children and adolescents with TB symptoms and further tracking for timely TB diagnosis and treatment initiation **(Flowchart 5)**.

Traditionally, the case notification data for TB was reported within three age bands: 0–4, 5–14, and 15–24 years for children and young adults. But the system is now upgraded to report in a more informative 5-year age bands: 0–4, 5–9, 10–14, 15–19, and 20–24 years. This will not only improve the interpretation of global and national TB burdens in different age groups but also promote policy-making at the microlevel toward better prevention and control of TB.

The key action in the roadmap toward ending TB in children and adolescents include: strengthening advocacy at all levels, fostering national leadership and accountability, fostering functional partnerships for change, increasing funding for child and adolescent TB programs, bridging the policy–practice gap, implementing and expanding interventions for prevention, scaling up the child and adolescent TB case-finding and treatment, implementing integrated family- and community-centered strategies, improving data collection, reporting, and use, and encouraging child and adolescent TB research.

## SUMMARY

Adolescents are highly susceptible to TB and are a source of disease transmission to others in the community. Microbiological diagnosis with DST is essential for successfully treating TB. Anti-TB treatment should be provided to the adolescents, also addressing their psychosocial and developmental needs along with comorbidities in a supportive environment.

## ACKNOWLEDGMENTS

We acknowledge the Pediatric TB Management Guideline 2022 and the NTEP workshop organized by the Indian Academy of Pediatrics in collaboration with NTEP, Ministry of Health and Family Welfare, Government of India, which have been quite helpful in completing this chapter.

## POINTS TO REMEMBER

- There is an increased susceptibility to TB in adolescence.
- Adolescents can be a major source of transmission of diseases due to their large social connections and hence contact tracing should be done keeping it in mind.
- Every effort should be made to make a microbiological diagnosis of TB along with DST upfront.
- Adolescents should be provided psychosocial, educational, and economic support while on treatment to ensure medication compliance and adherence to follow-up.
- A history of comorbidities such as HIV, diabetes, substance abuse, and sexually transmitted diseases is essential as they may alter the effectiveness of drugs or increase the side effects.

## SUGGESTED READING

1. Chiang SS, Khan FA, Milstein MB, Tolman AW, Benedetti A, Starke JR, et al. Treatment outcomes of childhood tuberculous meningitis: a systematic review and meta-analysis. Lancet Infect Dis. 2014;14(10):947-57.
2. Detjen AK, DiNardo AR, Leyden J, Steingart KR, Menzies D, Schiller I, et al. Xpert MTB/RIF assay for the diagnosis of pulmonary tuberculosis in children: a systematic review and meta-analysis. Lancet Respir Med. 2015;3(6):451-61.
3. Dhakulkar S, Das M, Sutar N, Oswal V, Shah D, Ravi S, et al. Treatment outcomes of children and adolescents receiving drug-resistant TB treatment in a routine TB programme, Mumbai, India. PLoS One. 2021;16(2):e0246639.
4. Ford CA, Millstein SG, Halpern-Felsher BL, Irwin CE. Influence of Physician Confidentiality Assurances on Adolescents' Willingness to Disclose Information and Seek Future Health Care: A Randomized Controlled Trial. JAMA. 1997;278(12):1029-34.
5. Franck C, Seddon JA, Hesseling AC, Schaaf HS, Skinner D, Reynolds L. Assessing the impact of multidrug-resistant tuberculosis in children: an exploratory qualitative study. BMC Infect Dis. 2014;14(1):1-10.
6. Graham SM, Marais BJ, Amanullah F. Tuberculosis in Children and Adolescents: Progress and Perseverance. Pathogens. 2022;11(4):392.
7. Isaakidis P, Paryani R, Khan S, Mansoor H, Manglani M, Valiyakath A, et al. Poor Outcomes in a Cohort of HIV-Infected Adolescents Undergoing Treatment for Multidrug-Resistant Tuberculosis in Mumbai, India. PLoS One. 2013; 8(7):e68869.
8. Kronman MP, Crowell CS, Vora SB. Tuberculosis. In: Marcdante K, Schuh A, Kliegman RM (Eds). Nelson Essentials of Pediatrics, 9th edition. Philadelphia: Elsevier; 2023. pp. 473-8.
9. Ministry of Health and Family Welfare,. (2021). Collaborative Framework to Address the Burden of Tuberculosis among Children and Adolescents. [online] Available from https://tbcindia.gov.in/WriteReadData/l892s/522270886Collaborative%20Framework%20to%20Address%20the%20Burden%20of%20Tuberculosis%20among%20Children%20and%20Adolescents.pdf. [Last accessed February, 2023].
10. Ministry of Health and Family Welfare. (2017). National Strategic Plan for Tuberculosis Elimination 2017–2025. [online] Available from: https://tbcindia.gov.in/WriteReadData/NSP%20Draft%2020.02.2017%201.pdf. [Last accessed February, 2023].
11. Ministry of Health and Family Welfare. (2020). National Strategic Plan to End TB in India 2020-25. [online] Available from https://tbcindia.gov.in/showfile.php?lid=3577. [Last accessed February, 2023].
12. Ministry of Health and Family Welfare. (2022). National TB Prevalence Survey India (2019-2021). [online] Available from https://tbcindia.gov.in/showfile.php?lid=3659. [Last accessed February, 2023].
13. Ministry of Health and Family Welfare. (2022). Paediatric TB Management Guideline 2022. [online] Available from https://tbcindia.gov.in/showfile.php?lid=3668. [Last accessed February, 2023].
14. National Commission on Population, MOHFW. (2020). Population Projections for India and States (2011–2036). [online] Available from: https://main.mohfw.gov.in/sites/default/files/Population%20Projection%20Report%202011-2036%20-%20upload_compressed_0.pdf. [Last accessed February, 2023].

15. Office of Registrar General & Census Commissioner, (2022). Sample Registration System (SRS) Statistical Report 2019. [online] Available from https://censusindia.gov.in/nada/index.php/catalog/44375. [Last accessed February, 2023].
16. Sant'anna CC, Schmidt CM, March M de FBP, Pereira SM, Barreto ML. Tuberculosis among adolescents in two Brazilian State capitals. Cad Saude Publica. 2013;29(1):111-6.
17. Sawyer SM, Aroni RA. Sticky issue of adherence. J Paediatr Child Health. 2003;39(1):2-5.
18. Seddon JA, Chiang SS, Esmail H, Coussens AK. The Wonder Years: What Can Primary School Children Teach Us About Immunity to Mycobacterium tuberculosis? Front Immunol. 2018;9:2946.
19. Seddon JA, Thee S, Jacobs K, Ebrahim A, Hesseling AC, Schaaf HS. Hearing loss in children treated for multidrug-resistant tuberculosis. J Infect. 2013;66(4):320-9.
20. Simmons KB, Haddad LB, Nanda K, Curtis KM. Drug interactions between rifamycin antibiotics and hormonal contraception: a systematic review. BJOG. 2018;125(7):804-11.
21. Snow KJ, Cruz AT, Seddon JA, Ferrand RA, Chiang SS, Hughes JA, et al. Adolescent tuberculosis. Lancet Child Adolesc Health. 2020;4(1):68-79.
22. Snow KJ, Sismanidis C, Denholm J, Sawyer SM, Graham SM. The incidence of tuberculosis among adolescents and young adults: a global estimate. Eur Respir J. 2018;51(2):1702352.
23. United Nations. (2022). Sustainable Development Goals. [online] Available from https://sustainabledevelopment.un.org/topics/sustainabledevelopmentgoals. [Last accessed February, 2023].
24. Uppada DR, Selvam S, Jesuraj N, Lau EL, Doherty TM, Grewal HMS, et al. Incidence of tuberculosis among school-going adolescents in South India. BMC Public Health. 2016;16:641.
25. Volkmann T, Moonan PK, Miramontes R, Oeltmann JE. Tuberculosis and excess alcohol use in the United States, 1997-2012. Int J Tuberc Lung Dis. 2015;19(1):111-9.
26. World Health Organization. (2017). Moscow Declaration to End TB. [online] Available from https://www.who.int/publications/i/item/WHO-HTM-TB-2017.11. [Last accessed February, 2023].
27. World Health Organization. (2018). Roadmap Towards Ending TB in Children and Adolescents, Second Edition. [online] Available from: https://apps.who.int/iris/handle/10665/275422. [Last accessed February, 2023].
28. World Health Organization. (2019). Political Declaration of the UN General-Assembly High-Level Meeting on the Fight Against Tuberculosis. [online] Available from https://www.who.int/publications/m/item/political-declaration-of-the-un-general-assembly-high-level-meeting-on-the-fight-against-tuberculosis. [Last accessed February, 2023].
29. World Health Organization. (2021). Global Tuberculosis Report 2021. [online] Available from https://www.who.int/publications/i/item/9789240037021. [Last accessed February, 2023].
30. World Health Organization. (2022). Tuberculosis. [online] Available from https://www.who.int/news-room/fact-sheets/detail/tuberculosis. [Last accessed February, 2023].
31. Zvonareva O, Witte S, Kabanets N, Filinyuk O. Adolescents in a tuberculosis hospital: Qualitative study of how relationships with doctors, caregivers, and peers mediate their mental wellbeing. PLoS One. 2021;16(10):e0257379.

# 29 Asthma in Adolescents

*S Lakshmi Velmurugan, Utkarsh Sharma, S Kalpana*

## ■ EPIDEMIOLOGY

Asthma accounts for approximately 25% of all emergency room visits annually and ranks third in causes of hospitalization in children <15 years worldwide. Incidence and prevalence vary widely with geographic, ethnic, and socioeconomic factors. The prevalence of asthma has been increasing worldwide despite improvement in management and pharmacological advancements.

## ■ DEFINITION

Asthma is defined by two features:
1. Symptoms suggestive of airflow limitation like wheeze, breathlessness, cough, and chest tightness with variation in intensity over time.
2. Limitation in expiratory airflow that is variable.
   - Forced expiration volume in one second/forced vital capacity ($FEV_1$/FVC) ratio is below the lower limit at least once during diagnostic process.
   - Significant bronchodilator response of reversibility should be there.

There are three characteristic components of asthma:
1. Airway inflammation
2. Airway hyper-responsiveness
3. Reversible airway obstruction which may be absent during severe exacerbations or viral infections.

## ■ TRIGGERING FACTORS

Common triggers include infections, especially viral infections, dust mite, pollen, smoke, pollution, physical activity, drugs, e.g., aspirin, beta-blockers, food allergy, and chemical irritants.

## ■ RISK FACTORS
- Family history of atopy/asthma

- *Comorbid conditions:* Obesity/overweight, chronic rhinosinusitis, gastroesophageal reflux disease, and confirmed food allergy
- Tobacco smoke exposure
- Exposure to inhaled allergens (dust, mite, mold, and chemical irritants).

## ■ PATHOPHYSIOLOGY

Inflammatory cells such as mast cells and eosinophils have a significant role in the cellular inflammation that is associated with asthma. The allergic response starts with antigen (Ag) sensitization, in which an antigen is processed by an antigen presenting cell and is presented to a T cell. The T cell differentiates into a T helper 2 (Th2) cell which generated cytokines, such as: interleukin-4 (IL-4) which promotes immunoglobulin E (IgE) synthesis through the B cell; IL-5 that causes eosinophil maturation and activation; and IL-9 and IL-13, which promote goblet cell hyperplasia and mucous secretion. Triggered by the Ag–IgE cross-linking, the mast cells release mediators such as histamine, leukotrienes, and thromboxanes that cause smooth muscle contraction and airway edema. Airway injury is caused by eosinophil-derived granule proteins, proteases, and reactive oxygen species. Profibrotic cytokines such as transforming growth factor β promote fibroblast proliferation, generation, and deposition of extracellular matrix proteins, thus promoting subepithelial fibrosis and airway remodeling. A synopsis of the pathogenesis of asthma is given in **Flowchart 1**.

**Flowchart 1:** Pathogenesis of asthma.

```
Trigger factor
      ↓
Inflammatory mediators (IL-4, IL-5, IL-13, and chemokines)
      ↓
Airway inflammation
   ↙     ↓     ↘
Hyper-secretion   Airway smooth    Increased
of mucus          muscle constriction   reactivity
                  ↓
         Airway narrowing and obstruction
                  ↓
         • Cough
         • Wheezing
         • Shortness of breath
         • Tightness of chest
```

(IL: interleukin)

## CLINICAL FEATURES

Common chronic symptoms are dry cough, audible wheeze, and shortness of breath. Chest congestion and chest tightness are reported in older children. Symptoms vary with time and in intensity, being notably worse at night or in early morning. Physical activity during day often exacerbates the symptoms, especially in uncontrolled asthmatics. Laughter, cold air, and allergens can often trigger the event. If there is no significant improvement of symptoms with bronchodilator and regular corticosteroid therapy, consider asthma mimics in the differential diagnosis. Presence of risk factors including history of parental asthma helps in supporting the diagnosis. During acute exacerbations, auscultation will reveal expiratory wheeze and prolonged exhalation phase. Rhonchi and crackles may be appreciated. In severe exacerbations, signs of respiratory distress will be evident.

## DIAGNOSIS

Asthma is primarily a clinical diagnosis which is based on evidence of recurrent and reversible bronchoconstriction of variable intensity. A history of variable respiratory symptoms together with evidence of variable expiratory airflow limitation is the key to diagnosis.

Classification of asthma is also done in following categories:
- Severity classification (intermittent and persistent type)
- Control classification (well controlled/partly controlled/poorly controlled)
- Management type (easy to treat, difficult to treat, and refractory types).

## ASSESSING LEVEL OF SYMPTOM CONTROL

Assessing level of symptom control is shown in **Box 1**.

## DIFFERENTIAL DIAGNOSIS

- *Vocal cord dysfunction (VCD):* This is due to abnormal adduction of the vocal folds during inspiration that produces airflow obstruction at the

**BOX 1:** Level of symptom control.

| In the last 4 weeks, did the patient have: <br> 1. Daytime symptoms more than twice/week <br> 2. Any night waking due to asthma <br> 3. Short acting beta -2- agonist reliever needed more than twice/week <br> 4. Activity limitation due to asthma? | |
|---|---|
| Well controlled | None of the above |
| Partly controlled | 1 and 2 of the above |
| Uncontrolled | 3 and 4 of the above |

level of the larynx. The underlying pathophysiology of VCD involves a hyperfunctional and inappropriate laryngeal closure reflex. VCD frequently mimics asthma, as the adolescents present with frequent daytime wheezing. Flow volume loops in spirometry demonstrate inspiratory loop flattening due to decreased inspiratory flow during symptoms. Paradoxical adduction of the vocal cords can be seen during inspiration in laryngoscopy which usually confirms the diagnosis. The mainstay treatment of VCD is vocal cord relaxation techniques and breathing exercises.
- *Habit cough:* Habit cough or psychogenic cough can occur in adolescents. Typically, the cough is harsh, barking, and nonproductive. Characteristically, it disappears during sleep or distraction and is not exacerbated by physical exercise.
- Hypersensitivity pneumonitis (in adolescents living in farming communities and bird owners), pulmonary parasitic infestations, or tuberculosis may be common causes of chronic coughing and/or wheezing.
- Rare asthma masqueraders in adolescents may include retained airway foreign body and undiagnosed primary ciliary dyskinesia.

## ■ INVESTIGATIONS

- *Spirometry:*
  - It is recommended for adolescents for supporting the diagnosis of asthma, to identify patients at risk of asthma exacerbations, and also for consideration of alternative diagnosis, especially if there is a normal or near normal $FEV_1$ in a child with frequent respiratory symptoms (particularly when symptomatic)
  - $FEV_1/FVC$ ratio will be <80% in bronchial asthma.
  - Increase in $FEV_1$ by >12% (or >200 mL) of the prebronchodilator value indicates significant bronchodilator responsiveness.
- *Peak expiratory flowmetry:*
  - Less sensitive and less reliable as compared to spirometry
  - Simple and cost-effective tool for home-based measure of airflow
  - Excessive variability in twice daily peak expiratory flow (PEF) recorded over a period of 2 weeks suggests variability in lung function. Average daily diurnal variation in PEF of >10% indicates asthma.
- *Fractional concentration of exhaled nitric oxide (FeNO):* Not recommended for diagnosis of asthma as it can be elevated in nonasthma conditions and can be normal in some asthma phenotypes.
- *Chest X-ray:*
  - Chest X-ray is often normal in patients with asthma and hence has a limited role.

- May be useful to rule out differential diagnosis and also to look for complications.
- *Laboratory investigations:* Blood investigations have a limited role in the diagnosis of asthma.
- *Allergy test:*
  - These have supportive role in diagnosis of asthma.
  - Strong negative predictive value.
  - Contraindicated if high risk of anaphylaxis is anticipated.

## ■ MANAGEMENT

In the management of asthma, the long-term goals are to achieve good control of the symptoms and also to achieve reduction in deaths due to asthma, exacerbations, damage of airway, and adverse effects of medications.

### Risk Factors for Poor Asthma Outcome

In all children, in addition to assessing level of symptom control, risk factors for poor asthma outcomes including acute exacerbations, development of persistent airflow limitation, and medication side effects should also be determined. These are highlighted in **Box 2**.

Management involves assessment of treatment at regular intervals, adjustment of treatment as per need and review of response to treatment.

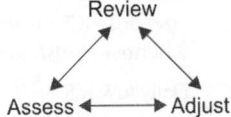

**BOX 2:** Assessing risk factors for poor asthma outcome.

---

**Risk factors for poor outcomes in asthma management**

*Risk factors for acute exacerbation:*
- High SABA use, inadequate ICS, poor adherence, incorrect technique
- Comorbid conditions
- Allergen and environmental smoke exposure
- Low FEV1 (<60% predicted)
- Past history of intubation or admitted in the intensive care for asthma

*Development of fixed airflow obstruction:*
- Prematurity, low birth weight, IUGR
- Eosinophilia in blood and sputum
- Hypersecretion of mucus
- Exposures to tobacco smoke and noxious chemicals

*Adverse effects of medicines:*
- *Systemic:* Oral corticosteroids used frequently, high dose of ICS
- *Local:* High dose potent side effects, poor inhaler technique

(FEV1: forced expiration volume in one second; ICS: inhaled corticosteroids; IUGR: intrauterine growth restriction; SABA: short-acting beta-2-agonist)

The Global Initiative for Asthma (GINA) (2021 guidelines) no longer recommend treatment of asthma in adolescents with short-acting beta-2-agonist (SABA) alone as reliever. Controllers in the form of inhaled corticosteroids (ICS) should be started as soon as the diagnosis of asthma is made.

## Personalized Management of Asthma in Children 6–11 Years of Age (Table 1)

- Inhaled corticosteroids are indicated in step 1 and 2 and SABA alone therapy has been discouraged. Early use of ICS has been associated with better lung function in future.
- SABA alone therapy does not protect patient against severe exacerbations. In fact, it increases the risk of exacerbations.

## Personalized Management of Asthma in Adolescents (Table 2)

- Low dose ICS-formoterol combination is the preferred ICS–long-acting beta-2-agonist (LABA) combination and when used as maintenance and

**TABLE 1:** Long-term management of children 6–11 years.

|  | Symptoms | Preferred controller | Alternate controller |
|---|---|---|---|
| Step 1 | Symptoms <2 times/month | Low dose ICS taken whenever SABA taken | Daily low dose ICS |
| Step 2 | Symptoms >2 times/month | Daily low ICS | Daily LTRA or low dose ICS taken whenever SABA taken |
| Step 3 | Symptoms most days or waking with asthma once a week or more | Low dose ICS-LABA or medium dose ICS or very low dose ICS-formoterol maintenance and reliever therapy (MART) | Low dose ICS + LTRA |
| Step 4 | Symptoms most days or waking with asthma once a week or more and low lung function | Medium dose ICS-LABA or low dose ICS-formoterol MART. Refer for expert advice | Add tiotropium or add LTRA |
| Step 5 | Short course oral corticosteroid may also be needed for patients presenting with severely uncontrolled asthma | Refer for phenotypic assessment + higher dose ICS-LABA or add on therapy, e.g., Anti-IgE | Add on anti-IL-5, or add on low dose OCS, but do consider side effects |

(ICS: inhaled corticosteroids; IgE: immunoglobulin E; IL-5: Interleukin-5; LABA: long-acting beta-2-agonist; LTRA: leukotriene receptor antagonist; OCS: oral corticosteroids; SABA: short-acting beta-2-agonist)

**TABLE 2:** Long-term management of asthma in adolescents.

| | Symptoms | Controller and preferred reliever | Controller and alternate reliever |
|---|---|---|---|
| Step 1 | Symptoms <2 days/month | As needed low dose ICS-formoterol | Low dose ICS whenever SABA is taken |
| Step 2 | Symptoms >2 days/month | As needed low dose ICS-formoterol | Daily low dose ICS plus as needed SABA |
| Step 3 | Symptoms most days or waking with asthma once a week or more | Low dose ICS-formoterol as maintenance and reliever therapy (MART) | Maintenance ICS–LABA plus as needed SABA |
| Step 4 | Daily symptoms or waking with asthma once a week or more and low lung function | Medium dose maintenance ICS-formoterol. | Add tiotropium (LAMA) or add LTRA |
| Step 5 | Persistent symptoms or exacerbations despite Step 4 treatment | Refer for phenotypic assessment + add on therapy including<br>• Combination high dose ICS–LABA<br>• Anti-IgE<br>• Anti-IL-5/5R<br>• Anti-IL-4Rα | |

(ICS: ICS: inhaled corticosteroids; IgE: immunoglobulin E; IL-5: Interleukin-5; LABA: long-acting beta-2-agonist; LTRA: leukotriene receptor antagonist; LAMA: long-acting muscarinic agent; SABA: short-acting beta-2-agonist)

reliever therapy (MART), the risk of severe exacerbations is considerably reduced.
- Preferably low dose ICS-formoterol in a single inhaler should be used.

## Step-down Treatment

Stepping down of treatment can be attempted once good control has been achieved and maintained for at least 3 months. Patient should be infection free, not traveling, or having any other associated condition like pregnancy. History of emergency visits along with exacerbations in the past is noted. Baseline status is to be documented. An action plan must be chalked out and follow-up must be planned. Reduction in the dose of ICS to the tune of 25–50% at 2–3-month interval while continuing ICS–LABA combination is initiated. Low dose ICS-formoterol is a step-down option in mild cases of asthma. Further, stepping down may be done with switching to as needed ICS–LABA or regular once daily ICS (budesonide, ciclesonide, and mometasone). Complete cessation of ICS increases the risk of severe exacerbation.

## Management of Asthma Exacerbations

### Assessment of Severity

Initial assessment of severity is the first step in managing children with acute asthma exacerbation. This will help in optimizing the choice of agent and also prioritizing care to children at risk of worsening. The GINA assessment of severity is presented in **Table 3**.

### Use of Rescue Therapy

Rescue medications are primarily taken to relieve the bronchospasm that occurs with asthma exacerbation. These include short-acting beta agonists (salbutamol and levosalbutamol), anticholinergic bronchodilators (e.g., ipratropium bromide), and short-term systemic glucocorticoids. In adolescents, ICS–LABA combination can also be used as reliever/recue medication. The maximum recommended dose of budesonide-formeterol in a single day is a total of 72μ of formoterol in out of hospital setting.

Monitor respiratory rate, heart rate, oxygen saturation, degree of alertness, accessory muscle use, and retractions.

Short-acting beta-2-agonists, such as salbutamol and levosalbutamol, remain a cornerstone of the treatment of asthma exacerbation in the hospital. Time to onset of action is approximately 5–10 minutes, peak effect beginning within approximately 50 minutes, and duration of action approximately 3–6 hours. Thus, as-needed, use of these drugs is the first-line therapy in patients with acute exacerbations.

Management will include the SABA at more frequent doses as described below, along with glucocorticoids. Again, SABA delivery by metered-dose inhaler (MDI) with spacer is most ideal. If the child is unfamiliar with MDI

**TABLE 3:** Assessing severity of asthma exacerbation.

| Mild or moderate | Severe |
|---|---|
| Assess presence of drowsiness, confusion, or silent chest at outset | |
| • Talks in phrases<br>• Prefers sitting to lying<br>• Not agitated<br>• Respiratory rate (RR) increased<br>• Accessory muscle not used<br>• Pulse rate (PR) 100–120 bpm<br>• Oxygen saturation (SaO$_2$) in room air 90–95%<br>• Peak expiratory flow (PEF) >50% predicted or best | • Talks in words<br>• Sits hunched forward<br>• Agitated<br>• RR >30/min<br>• Accessory muscle being used<br>• PR >120/min<br>• SaO$_2$ in room air <90%<br>• PEF <50% predicted or best |

**TABLE 4:** Drugs used in management of acute severe exacerbation of asthma.

| Salbutamol by metered-dose inhaler (MDI) | • 4–8 puffs every 20 minutes for three doses, then minimum 2 puff/dose<br>• Maximum 8 puffs/dose every 1–4 hours as needed |
|---|---|
| Levosalbutamol | ½ of recommended dose of salbutamol |
| Salbutamol by nebulizer | • 5 mg/dose<br>• Every 20 minutes for three doses, then switch to every 30 minutes to 4 hours |
| Ipratropium nebulizer solution (250 μg/mL)–add in moderate-to-severe exacerbation | • <20 kg—250 μg/dose<br>• >20 kg—500 μg/dose<br>• Every 20 minutes for three doses, thereafter 8th hourly if needed |
| Prednisolone | 1–2 mg/kg (maximum 40–50 mg) for first dose then 0.5–1 mg/kg twice for 3–10 days |
| Oxygen | Target saturation 93–95% |

**Flowchart 2:** Management of children with near-fatal asthma exacerbation.

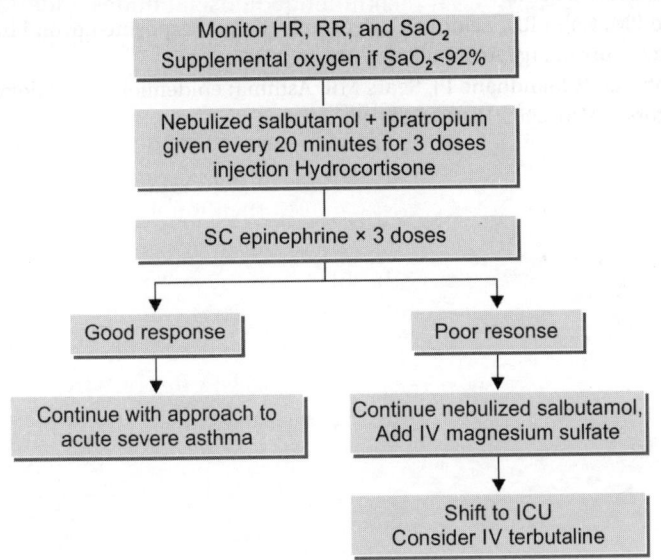

(HR: heart rate; ICU: intensive care unit; IV: intravenous; RR: respiratory rate; $SaO_2$: oxygen saturation; SC: subcutaneous)

usage or if MDI with spacer is not readily available, SABA can be delivered by nebulizer **(Table 4)**.

## Near-fatal Asthma

There is progressive respiratory failure, fatigue, and altered consciousness. The following algorithm **(Flowchart 2)** gives a general approach to management of children with near fatal exacerbations.

## SUGGESTED READING

1. Akinbami LJ, Moorman JE, Garbe PL, Sondik EJ. Status of childhood asthma in United States, 1980-2007. Pediatrics. 2009;123(Suppl 3):S131-45.
2. Bourdin A, Gras D, Vachier I, Chanez P. Upper airway 1: allergic rhinitis and asthma: united disease through epithelial cells. Thorax. 2009;64(11):999-1004.
3. Burke W, Fesinmeyer M, Reed K, Hampson L. Family history as a predictor of asthma risk. Am J Prev Med. 2003;24(2):160-9.
4. Global Initiative for Asthma (GINA). Guidelines for the management of childhood asthma 2021. Fontana, USA: Global Initiative for Asthma; 2021.
5. Lee J, McDonald C. Review: Immunotherapy improves some symptoms and reduces long-term medication use in mild to moderate asthma. Ann Intern Med. 2018;169(4):JC17.
6. Mims JW. Asthma: definitions and pathophysiology. Int Forum Allergy Rhinol. 2015;5(Suppl 1):S2-6.
7. National Asthma Education and Prevention Program. Expert Panel Report 3 (EPR-3): Guidelines for the Diagnosis and management of Asthma-Summary Report 2007. J Allergy Clin Immunol. 2007;120(5 Suppl):S94-138.
8. Pillai RA, Calhoun WJ. Introduction to asthma and phenotyping. Adv Exp Med Biol. 2014;795:5-15.
9. Salo PM, Cohn RD, Zeldin DC. Bedroom allergen exposure beyond house dust mites. Curr Allergy Asthma Rep. 2018;18(10):52.
10. Subbarao P, Mandhane PJ, Sears MR. Asthma: epidemiology, etiology and risk factors. CMAJ. 2009;181(9):E181-90.

# 30. Pneumonia in Adolescents

*V Poovazhagi, Kamal Kumar Singhal*

## ■ INTRODUCTION

Pneumonia in children and adolescents is a significant cause of hospital admissions. Pneumonia reportedly accounts for 15.1–22.7% of the patients who present at the emergency department with respiratory disease. Globally, pediatric community-acquired pneumonia (CAP) is associated with significant healthcare costs and impacts quality of life in many children and their caregivers. For the most part, physicians rely on an empirical diagnosis and therapy due to the difficulty in obtaining samples for laboratory diagnosis. Very less number of studies are available for adolescent pneumonia and the extrapolation has been done, based on studies in childhood pneumonia. Evidently, majority of the causes for adolescent pneumonia have been found to be of unidentified origin, followed by viruses, bacteria, and mycoplasma.

## ■ ETIOLOGICAL PROFILE OF ADOLESCENT PNEUMONIA

Adolescent pneumonias are of infectious etiology in majority and noninfectious pneumonias such as aspiration pneumonia and lipoidal pneumonia are less common. Apart from viruses, *Streptococcus pneumoniae*, *Mycoplasma pneumoniae*, and *Chlamydia pneumoniae* appear to be the most frequently encountered pathogens causing adolescent pneumonia. Less common are *Haemophilus influenzae* type b, *Staphylococcus aureus*, and group B *Streptococcus*. "Atypical pneumonia" refers to pneumonia not presenting with the usual clinical picture of pneumococcal infection (which includes high fever, productive cough, chills, and other "classic" features). The term is frequently used in adolescents with CAP. *Mycoplasma pneumoniae* is a major cause of CAP in school children and adolescents. Viral pneumonia is much more common in adolescents. By subtype, viral pneumonia includes influenza virus pneumonia, respiratory syncytial virus pneumonia, parainfluenza virus pneumonia, adenovirus pneumonia, and human metapneumovirus pneumonia. To complete the list are chickenpox virus (varicella), coronaviruses, aspiration, and tuberculosis.

Immunocompromised teens are more likely to get fungal pneumonia, such as aspergillosis and pneumocystis pneumonia.

## ■ RISK FACTORS FOR PNEUMONIA

Risk factors for pneumonia among teenagers include parental smoking, crowded living conditions, lung or airway issues, indoor air pollution, chronic diseases, such as cystic fibrosis, asthma, or sickle cell anemia, compromised immune system due to cancer, human immunodeficiency virus (HIV) infection, malnutrition, or other conditions.

## ■ CLINICAL PRESENTATION

Fever, cough, coryza, breathlessness, chest pain, anorexia, headache, and diarrhea are the common clinical presentations of adolescent pneumonia. Presence of lung crackles may be suggestive of pneumonia in an adolescent with fever without much symptoms. The signs may include chest retraction (intercostal, subcostal, sternal, and suprasternal), nasal flaring, grunting, groaning, and head bobbing. Auscultation may reveal rales, wheeze, and decreased breath sounds. These signs and symptoms have variable sensitivity and specificity in diagnosing pneumonia. Signs of severe illness such as cyanosis, grunting respiration, dehydration, and general danger signs like lethargy should be assessed in addition to vital signs and saturation.

Pneumonia following a short upper respiratory infection, with gradual onset of cough and fever, with wheeze, less toxic features and imaging showing bilateral involvement of lung will point toward a viral etiology. Predominant cough, chest pain, absence of wheeze in a not so sick looking adolescent with diffuse lung involvement will favor a diagnosis of atypical pneumonia. Presence of wheeze makes *M. pneumoniae* slightly less likely and the presence of crepitations (*i.e.,* crackles heard on listening to the chest) makes *M. pneumoniae* slightly more likely as the causative organism. Also mycoplasma infections are likely to have extrapulmonary features such as anemia, rashes, and neurological features. *Streptococcus pneumoniae* presents with high-grade fever, gastrointestinal symptoms with rapid progression to lobar pneumonia. Fever and respiratory symptoms such as cough and chest pain resolves early but tiredness and lethargy may persist for a few weeks. Complications include multiorgan failure due to sepsis, acute respiratory distress syndrome (ARDS), respiratory failure requiring ventilatory or breathing support, pleural effusion, and lung abscesses (pus-filled cavities in the lungs) that require surgical draining.

## ■ DIAGNOSIS

As current diagnostic tools lack accuracy and are unable to delineate different disease subtypes such as viral versus bacterial pediatric pneumonia, until today, the diagnosis is mainly based on simple diagnostic criteria such as tachypnea and fever. Diagnosis depends on the clues from history, clinical examination, complete blood counts, X-rays, and if appropriate, blood gases, viral studies, and inflammatory markers.

C-reactive protein (CRP), white cell counts [white blood cell (WBC)], and absolute neutrophil number in combination with fever, oxygen saturation, and absence of rhinorrhea still remain the most promising "biomarkers" to predict bacterial CAP. CRP may be used in adolescents to decide on withholding antibiotics and to assess response to therapy with antibiotics. Use of procalcitonin is not recommended to determine the need for antibacterial therapy. Multiplex polymerase chain reaction (PCR) assays using nasopharyngeal swabs, are particularly sensitive in diagnosing mycoplasma infections early, with sensitivity ranging from 80 to 100%. Induced sputum has been found to be useful in the diagnosis of CAP in children and adolescents. Routine culture of respiratory secretions and blood culture is not indicated in outpatients with pneumonia, unless they are categorized as severe pneumonia. Patients hospitalized for inpatient care in the preceding 90 days should be empirically treated for methicillin-resistant *Staphylococcus aureus* (MRSA) or pseudomonas infections.

When influenza is circulating in the community, testing is recommended using rapid influenza molecular assay over a rapid influenza antigen test. Urinary antigen tests for pneumococcal infection are not favored as the rate of colonization varies in different population and that will have an impact on the interpretation of the reports. Tuberculosis work-up is done in a subset of adolescents who are not very sick and toxic. Cartridge-based nucleic acid amplification test (CBNAAT) from sputum or induced sputum or gastric aspirates in hospitalized sick ventilated adolescents or tracheal or bronchial washings can be done. Viral studies do not give a high yield in case of infants and younger children with pneumonia. CT chest may be needed in severe patients or with complications. Other invasive procedures such as bronchoscopy and pleural fluid analysis need to be done in selected cases. Microbiological studies are not routinely recommended in mild pneumonias. Specific organisms like mycoplasma can produce pneumonia with hemolysis or aseptic meningitis and those subsets of patients need work-up for hemolysis and mycoplasma testing. Identification of mycoplasma infection is by culture separation, serological tests, and PCR. PCR is the most commonly used test as it is less time consuming and sensitive. Serological tests commonly used for the diagnosis are not very reliable in the acute presentation of *Mycoplasma pneumoniae* due to their persistence for longer periods. Loop-mediated isothermal amplification (LAMP) may be an alternative but needs to be studied in adolescent pneumonia. Cultures are time consuming and hence not favored.

## MANAGEMENT

Treatment includes supportive care and specific therapy with antimicrobials. Taking care of airway, breathing, and circulation; hydration; rest; and appropriate oxygen supplementation are the mainstay of treatment. Antibiotics and antivirals are required along with supportive therapy. Antivirals are not a routine in therapy for pneumonia in adolescents, other than in H1N1 pneumonia. Immunocompromised and those with malignancies may need antivirals much more than an immunocompetent patient. Viral pneumonia in adolescents will need oseltamivir, if suspected or identified to be H1N1, in an inpatient setting, irrespective of the duration of illness.

The World Health Organization recommends oseltamivir as first-line treatment for H1N1, with the use of zanamivir only for suspected or confirmed oseltamivir resistance.

Dosage of oseltamivir is given in **Table 1**.

Bacterial pneumonia can occur concurrently with influenza infection or later as worsening of symptoms; hence, antibacterial agents as recommended earlier have to be given with antivirals. They can be discontinued later, if there is no evidence of bacterial pathogen.

For bacterial pneumonia, initiation of antibiotics is decided based on clinical suspicion and radiological evidence among outpatients, the initial choice of empiric antibiotics will be amoxicillin or a macrolide. Hospitalized patients may need a combination of macrolide with beta lactam antibiotics such as amoxicillin/clavulanate or cephalosporin and/or monotherapy with fluoroquinolone. Patients with severe infection requiring admission to the intensive care unit or healthcare associated infection require dual antibiotic therapy, including a third-generation cephalosporin plus a macrolide in combination or a fluoroquinolone. Treatment options for patients with risk factors for *Pseudomonas* and MRSA species include administration of dual antibiotics, piperacillin or ceftazidime or cefepime with vancomycin or linezolid. It needs de-escalation if cultures are negative. There is no role for adding anaerobic coverage for suspected aspiration pneumonia unless there is a possibility of lung abscess or empyema. The duration of antibiotic

**TABLE 1:** Dosage of oseltamivir.

| Weight | Dosage (treatment) |
| --- | --- |
| Between 23 and 40 kg | 120 mg per day in two divided doses for 5 days |
| >40 kg | 150 mg per day in two divided doses for 5 days |
| Weight | Dosage (chemoprophylaxis) |
| Between 23 and 40 kg | 60 mg once daily for 10 days |
| >40 kg | 75 mg once daily for 10 days |

is guided by the clinical stability, as evidenced by resolution of vital sign abnormalities (heart rate, respiratory rate, blood pressure, oxygen saturation, and temperature), improvement of appetite and mentation. Antibiotic therapy should be continued until patient is stable and for not less than a total of 5 days. There are no recommendations for the use of corticosteroids in CAP except in patients with CAP and refractory septic shock.

For mycoplasma infections, ideally azithromycin, which is dosed at 10 mg/kg on day 1, with a maximum of 500 mg, followed by 5 mg/kg on days 2-5, with a maximum dose of 250 mg. It is unclear whether the utility of azithromycin in treating children with mycoplasma is due to its antimicrobial effects or its anti-inflammatory effects. Alternative regimens include clarithromycin at 15 mg/kg per day divided two times daily, with a maximum dose of 1 g, for 10 days; doxycycline 2-4 mg/kg either once or twice daily, with a maximum dose of 200 mg, for 10 days; or levofloxacin 10 mg/kg per dose daily, with a maximum dose of 750 mg, for 10 days. Erythromycin is less effective than clarithromycin as empiric treatment of CAP in adults and adolescents. Erythromycin, being less effective should not be used in CAP when azithromycin and clarithromycin are available. Linezolid use needs to be restricted as it is being used as a second-line antituberculous therapy.

## ■ PREVENTION

Vaccination, hygiene, handwashing, avoidance of smoking and overcrowding, wearing a mask, preventive medicines in immunocompromised, and oseltamivir prophylaxis for viral infections like H1N1 constitute the preventive measures. Vaccination has to be completed in adolescents including tetanus, diphtheria, and pertussis (Tdap), varicella, seasonal influenza, and coronavirus disease (COVID) vaccine.

## ■ SUGGESTED READING

1. Ashy N, Alharbi L, Alkhamisi R, Alradadi R, Eljaaly K. Efficacy of erythromycin compared to clarithromycin and azithromycin in adults or adolescents with community-acquired pneumonia: a Systematic Review and meta-analysis of randomized controlled trials. J Infect Chemother. 2022;28(8):1148-52.
2. Bhuiyan MU, Blyth CC, West R, Lang J, Rahman T, Granland C, et al. Combination of clinical symptoms and blood biomarkers can improve discrimination between bacterial or viral community-acquired pneumonia in children. BMC Pulm Med. 2019;19(1):71.
3. Cardoso MR, Nascimento-Carvalho CM, Ferrero F, Alves FM, Cousens SN. Adding fever to WHO criteria for diagnosing pneumonia enhances the ability to identify pneumonia cases among wheezing children. Arch Dis Child. 2011;96(1):58-61.
4. Gordon RC. Community-acquired pneumonia in adolescents. Adolesc Med. 2000;11(3):681-95.

5. Harris M, Clark J, Coote N, Fletcher P, Harnden A, McKean M, et al. British Thoracic Society guidelines for the management of community acquired pneumonia in children: update 2011. Thorax. 2011;66 Suppl2:ii1-23.
6. Jamieson B, Jain R, Carleton B, Goldman RD. Use of oseltamivir in children. Can Fam Physician. 2009;55(12):1199-201.
7. Kest H, Kaushik A, Shaheen S, Debruin W, Zaveri S, Colletti M, et al. Epidemiologic Characteristics of Adolescents with COVID-19 Disease with Acute Hypoxemic Respiratory Failure. Crit Care Res Pract. 2022;2022:7601185.
8. Krafft C, Christy C. Mycoplasma Pneumonia in Children and Adolescents. Pediatr Rev. 2020;41:12-9.
9. Lee CH, Won YK, Roh E-J, Suh DI, Chung EH. A nationwide study of children and adolescents with pneumonia who visited Emergency Department in South Korea in 2012. Korean J pediatr. 2016;59(3):132-8.
10. Matsuda C, Taketani T, Takeuchi S, Taniguchi Y, Nagira M, Moriyama H, et al. Usefulness of the Loopamp mycoplasma P detecting reagent kit developed based on the LAMP method. Rinsho Biseibutsuhu Jinsoku Shindan Kenkyukai Shi. 2013;23(2):53-9.
11. Metlay JP, Waterer GW, Long AC, Anzueto A, Brozek J, Crothers K, et al. Diagnosis and Treatment of Adults with Community-acquired Pneumonia An Official Clinical Practice Guideline of the American Thoracic Society and Infectious Diseases Society of America. Am J Respir Crit Care Med. 2009;200(7):e45-67.
12. Rueda ZV, Aguilar Y, Maya MA, López L, Restrepo A, Garcés C, et al. Etiology and the challenge of diagnostic testing of community-acquired pneumonia in children and adolescents. BMC Pediatrics. 2022;22(1):169.
13. Siemieniuk RA, Meade MO, Alonso-Coello P, Briel M, Evaniew N, Prasad M, et al. Corticosteroid therapy for patients hospitalized with community-acquired pneumonia: a systematic review and meta-analysis. Ann Intern Med. 2015;163(7):519-28.
14. Wang K, Gill P, Perera R, Thomson A, Mant D, Harnden A. Clinical symptoms and signs for the diagnosis of Mycoplasma pneumoniae in children and adolescents with community-acquired pneumonia. Cochrane Database Syst Rev. 2012;10(10):CD009175.
15. Wan YD, Sun TW, Liu ZQ, Zhang SG, Wang LX, Kan QC. Efficacy and safety of corticosteroids for community-acquired pneumonia: a systematic review and meta-analysis. Chest. 2016;149(1):209-19.
16. Wetzke M, Kopp MV, Seidenberg J, Vogelberg C, Ankermann T, Happle C, et al. PedCAPNETZ—prospective observational study on community acquired pneumonia in children and adolescents. BMC Pulm Med. 2019;19(1):238.

# CHAPTER 31

# Psychotic Disorders in Adolescents

*Megha Mahajan, Vinayak Koparde*

## ■ INTRODUCTION

Childhood and adolescence psychosis has always been surrounded by controversy due to lack of a uniform diagnostic criteria. Psychoses in children and adolescents have been diagnosed since the 1950s. In the 1960s, autism and childhood psychosis were together termed as "schizophrenia, childhood type". In 1980s, childhood schizophrenia and autism were seen as separate disorders. Autism or pervasive developmental disorder were more defined in subsequent editions of the Diagnostic and Statistical Manual of Mental Disorders (DSM) (i.e., DSM-III-R, DSM-IV, DSM-IV-TR, and DSM-5), and it helped to separate autism from childhood schizophrenia.

## ■ DEFINITION

Severe disruption of thought and behavior leading to the loss of reality testing is called psychosis. Varied definitions have been used to define psychosis in the past. Schizophrenia with onset at or after 18 years is adult onset and between 13 and 18 years is adolescent onset schizophrenia. Illness onset before 13 years is called childhood-onset schizophrenia and it carries a poorer prognosis.

## ■ PSYCHOTIC DISORDERS INCLUDED IN MAJOR CLASSIFICATORY SYSTEMS

Different types of psychotic disorders are seen in adolescents as shown in **Table 1**.

In adults, the most researched disorder among the above is schizophrenia. While schizophrenia is uncommon in childhood, its incidence increases during adolescence. Therefore, schizophrenia will be discussed in greater detail.

## ■ EARLY-ONSET SCHIZOPHRENIA

### Clinical Presentation

Diagnosis of this disorder (EOS) in children and youth is challenging. Misdiagnosis at the time of onset is not uncommon as psychotic symptoms

**TABLE 1:** International Classification of Diseases (ICD-11) and Diagnostic and Statistical Manual (DSM) psychotic disorders.

| ICD-11 | DSM-5 |
| --- | --- |
| Schizophrenia and other primary psychotic disorders | Schizophrenia spectrum and other psychotic disorders |
| 7A50 Schizophrenia | Schizophrenia |
| 7A51 Schizoaffective disorder | Schizoaffective disorder |
| 7A52 Schizotypal disorder | Schizotypal personality disorder |
| 7A53 Acute and transient psychotic disorder | Brief psychotic disorder |
| 7A54 Delusional disorder | Delusional disorder |
| 7A5Y Other specified schizophrenia and other primary psychotic disorders | Other specified schizophrenia spectrum and other psychotic disorders |
| 7A5Z Schizophrenia and other primary psychotic disorders, unspecified | Unspecified schizophrenia spectrum and other psychotic disorders |
| | Schizophreniform disorder |
| | Substance/medication-induced psychotic disorder |
| | Psychotic disorder due to another medical condition |
| | Catatonia associated with another mental disorder (catatonia specifier) |
| | Catatonic disorder due to another medical condition |
| | Unspecified catatonia |

*Source:* Sadock BJ, Sadock VA, Ruiz P. Kaplan and Sadock's synopsis of psychiatry: behavioral sciences/clinical psychiatry, 11th edition. Philadelphia: Lippincott Williams and Wilkins; 2014.

are often seen with other illnesses, including mood disorders, neurologic conditions, and acute intoxication. Usually, the illness is acute or insidious in onset, often starting with a prodrome having nonspecific symptoms such as sadness, anxiety, cognitive, and functional decline.

Individual are often seen to be socially withdrawn and have disruptive behaviors along with developmental delays and academic lag even before the onset of illness. Symptoms in adolescent onset schizophrenia **(Fig. 1)** (hallucinations, thought disorders, and flat affect) are almost similar to that in the adult except that systematic delusions and catatonic symptoms are uncommon here. Extreme anxiety, speech incoherence, self-absorbed behaviors, lack of concentration, and emotional dysregulation are commonly seen in adolescents. Assessment of delusions and hallucinations is often challenging in adolescents.

*Diagnostic issues and categories:* Diagnosis of early-onset schizophrenia (EOS) is made by using the criteria in adults **(Table 2)** defined in the DSM-5

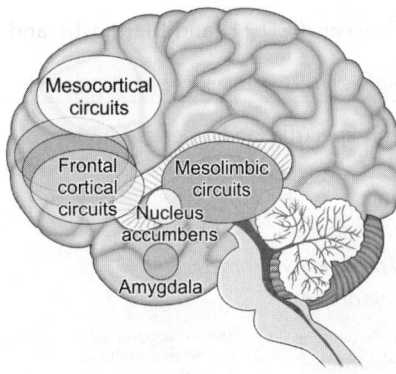

- Positive symptoms
  - Hallucinations
  - Delusions
  - Disorganized speech and behavior
- Negative symptoms
  - Blunted effect
  - Emotional withdrawal
  - Poor rapport
  - Passivity
- Cognitive symptoms
  Difficulties with:
  - Attention
  - Problem solving
  - Working memory
  - Speed of processing
- Affective symptoms
  - Depressed mood
  - Anxious mood
  - Guild
  - Tension
  - Irritability
  - Worry
- Aggressive symptoms
  - Verbal or physical abuse
  - Self-injurious behavior
  - Destructive behavior (arson, property damage)

**Fig. 1:** Symptom domains, clinical features, and neuroanatomy of schizophrenia.
*Source:* Stahl SM. Essential psychopharmacology: Neuroscientific basis and practical applications, 4th edition. UK: Cambridge University Press; 2000.

**TABLE 2:** International Classification of Diseases (ICD-11) and Diagnostic and Statistical Manual (DSM) symptom domains of schizophrenia.

| | |
|---|---|
| *Criterion A:* Two (or more) of the following, each present for a significant portion of time during a 1-month period (or less if successfully treated) | Symptoms must persist for at least 1-month in order for a diagnosis of schizophrenia to be assigned. |
| *Characteristic symptoms:* At least one of these must include 1, 2, or 3: <br>1. Delusions <br>2. Hallucinations <br>3. Disorganized speech <br>4. Grossly disorganized or catatonic behavior <br>5. Negative symptoms (i.e., diminished emotional expression or avolition) | *Core symptoms:* <br>1. Persistent delusions <br>2. Persistent hallucinations <br>3. Thought disorder <br>4. Experiences of influence, passivity or control <br>5. Psychomotor disturbances, including catatonia |
| *Criterion B:* Level of functioning (e.g., work, interpersonal relations, self care) markedly below the level prior to onset <br>*Criterion C:* Continuous signs of disturbance for at least 6 months (including the 1-month period covered under Criterion A) <br>*Criterion D-F:* Disturbance not attributable to other disorders with psychotic features or the effects of a substance | Additional detail (code) can be added to describe symptomatic manifestation (positive, negative, depressive, manic, psychomotor symptoms, cognitive) The symptoms are not a manifestation of another health condition (e.g., a brain tumor) and are not due to the effect of a substance or medication on the central nervous system (e.g., corticosteroids), including withdrawal (e.g., alcohol withdrawal). |

*Source:* Sadock BJ, Sadock VA, Ruiz P. Kaplan and Sadock's synopsis of psychiatry: behavioral sciences/clinical psychiatry, 11th edition. Philadelphia: Lippincott Williams and Wilkins; 2014.

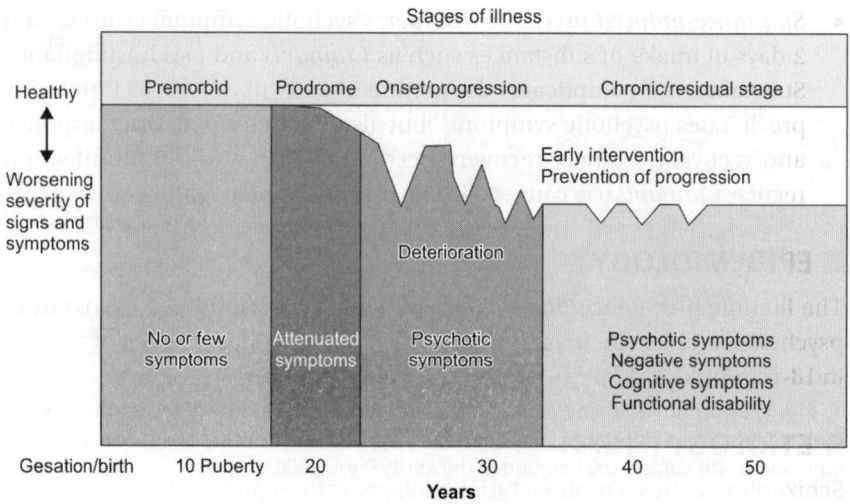

**Fig. 2:** Stages of illness: schizophrenia.
*Source:* Lieberman JA, Small SA, Girgis RR. Early detection and preventive intervention in schizophrenia: from fantasy to reality. Am J Psychiatry. 2019;176(10):794-810.

or International Classification of Diseases, 11 (ICD-11), which has good diagnostic reliability in adolescents unlike in children.

EOS is now seen as a phasic disorder **(Fig. 2)**.

*Prodromal phase:* Includes vague symptoms such as sadness, anxiety, cognitive, and functional decline.

*Acute phase:* This phase is dominated by positive psychotic symptoms with poor functioning.

*Recovery phase:* Improvement in active psychotic symptoms.

*Residual phase:* Predominantly negative symptoms seen here.

*Chronic impairment:* Persistent psychotic symptoms remain in few patients.

## OTHER PSYCHOTIC DISORDERS

- *Schizoaffective disorder* includes both psychotic and affective symptoms.
- *Schizophreniform disorder* has shorter duration (1–6 months) of psychotic symptoms.
- *Brief psychotic disorder* is not common in children.
- *Acute and transient psychotic disorders (ATPD)* have an acute onset of psychotic symptoms lasting transiently (few days to 3 months).
- *Reactive psychoses* are precipitated by a significant life stressor (death, trauma, war, abuse, etc.) with recovery within 2–3 months.
- *Delusional disorder* is uncommon in children and young adolescents.

# CHAPTER 31: Psychotic Disorders in Adolescents

- *Substance-induced psychotic disorder:* Psychotic symptoms start within 2 days of intake of substances such as *Cannabis* and psychostimulants. Substance use complicates the picture of early psychosis as it not only precipitates psychotic symptoms, but also interferes with drug response and recovery. Usually recovery occurs between 1 and 6 months, but regular *Cannabis* use causes chronic psychosis and cognitive worsening.

## EPIDEMIOLOGY

The lifetime prevalence of psychosis in adults is around 2–3%. All types of psychotic disorders increase during adolescence, with prevalence of 1 in 500 in 18-year-old.

## ETIOLOGY (FIG. 3)

Schizophrenia has a multifactorial etiology, with multiple genes interacting with various environmental factors leading to neuroplastic changes

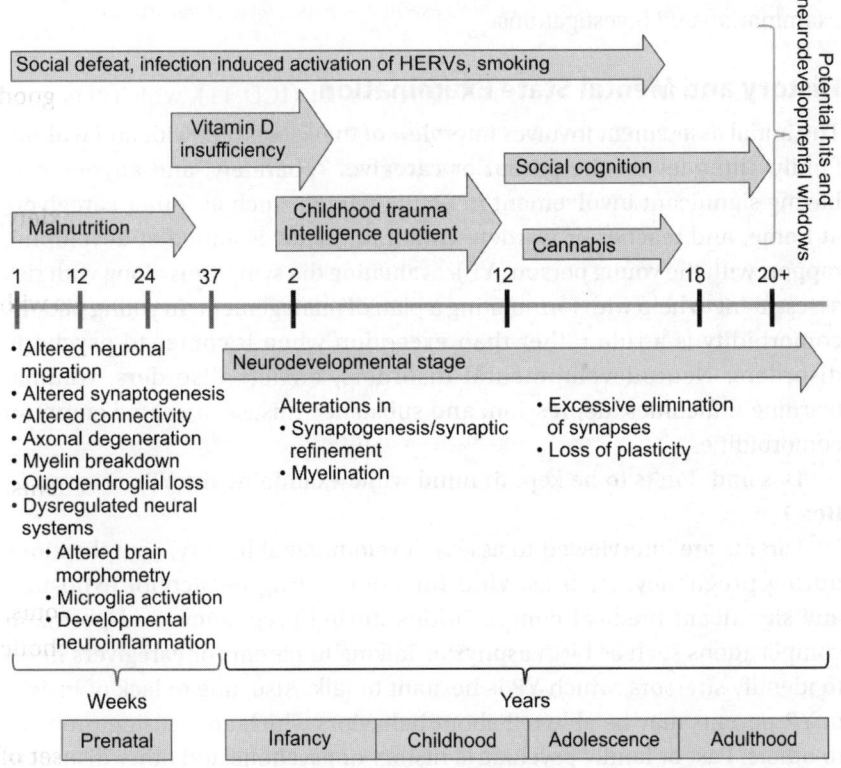

**Fig. 3:** Etiology of schizophrenia.
*Source:* Davis J, Eyre H, Jacka FN, Dodd S, Dean O, McEwen S, et al. A review of vulnerability and risks for schizophrenia: Beyond the two hit hypothesis. Neurosci Biobehav Rev. 2016;65:185-94.
(HERVs: human endogenous retroviruses)

during crucial developmental periods, hence causing disruptions in neurotransmitter regulated circuits and impaired connectivity especially in adolescence. Most genes are nonspecific, though some genes are also related to autism and bipolar disorders. The risk factors include family history of first-degree relatives with schizophrenia and personalities in the schizotypal, schizoid/paranoid spectrum. Factors that can precipitate the illness are organic factors, drug use, trauma, or any other psychological stress.

## ■ EVALUATION AND MANAGEMENT

## Assessment

Adolescents presenting with symptoms and signs of psychosis can have varied etiologies ranging from neurodevelopmental disorders, medical-neurological disorders, or psychiatric disorders as described in earlier sections. It is imperative to have a thorough assessment and investigation before a treatment plan is formulated. Assessment of the young person includes history taking, mental state examination, and physical examination and investigations.

## History and Mental State Examination

The initial assessment involves interview of the adolescent with and without family, interview of the parent or caregiver separately, and anyone else having significant involvement in young person, such as, other caregivers at home, and teacher or warden. Initial interview is aimed at developing rapport with the young person (YP), evaluating the symptoms along with risk assessment to help with formulating a plan of management. In young people, comorbidity is a rule rather than exception when it comes to psychotic disorders. Neurodevelopmental disorders, anxiety disorders, trauma, learning difficulties, depression, and substance misuse are some common comorbidities.

Dos and don'ts to be kept in mind while examining the YP are given in **Box 1**.

Parents are interviewed to assess developmental history, complications during pregnancy, such as, viral infections, drug or alcohol exposure, any significant medical complications during pregnancy, and perinatal complications such as birth asphyxia. Talking to parents or caregivers helps to identify stressors, which YP is hesitant to talk. Also, due to lack of insight in YP, parents may be able tell about behaviors which are causing problem to others. Past or family psychiatric history of psychotic and other disorders along with response to treatment, assessment of family dynamics, coping and explanatory models helps in management plan. Information from school and significant others is sought as psychotic symptoms may be present with only specific situation or people, such as declining grades in school,

**BOX 1:** Dos and don'ts to be kept in mind while examining the young person.

*Dos*
- Young person (YP) may prefer to be seen alone or with trusted adult to avoid embarrassment
- Discuss rules of privacy and confidentiality related to suicide and abuse
- See alone—substance history, suicide, and other risk assessment
- Start interview with neutral topics, such as, hobbies, likes, and friends to develop rapport
- Ask YP about specific concerns of anxiety, depression, bullying, and trauma. Also ask specifically about strange experiences to elicit hallucinations and other paranoid experiences

*Don'ts*
- Taking sides, blaming, not listening to YP, inadequate time, breaching confidentiality, and judging the YP without adequate discussion
- Antagonizing YP—can make a paranoid patient aggressive
- Starting treatment without adequate psychoeducation to YP and family or forcing YP to take treatment

peer problems, and substance misuse. Risk assessment for risk to self, risk to others and risk of neglect or abuse is done.

## Differential Diagnoses

Various medical, neurological, and psychiatric disorders can manifest with psychotic symptoms and first priority is to rule out organic causes of psychosis. Organic disorders can masquerade as psychotic disorders, hence it is important to first evaluate for thyroid disorders, vitamin $B_{12}$ deficiency, Wilson's disease, and inborn errors of metabolism. Common psychiatric differentials include substance intoxication or substance-induced psychosis, depression, anxiety disorders, autism spectrum disorder and post-traumatic stress disorders (PTSD). Auditory hallucinations experienced by a YP with depression may actually be their own thoughts (voices telling they are useless and good for nothing). Similarly, in anxiety disorders a YP may misinterpret shadows at night and believe that burglars have broken into the house.

Clinicians should be aware of common congenital disorders which may present with psychotic symptoms in the young. The most common ones are acute intermittent porphyria, glucose-6-phosphate dehydrogenase (G6PD) deficiency, Gilbert syndrome, Huntington disease, neurofibromatosis type 1, and XXX karyotype.

## Physical Examination and Investigations

Investigations are detailed in **Table 3** and need to be individualized. Investigations are done to evaluate any organic causes for psychosis in YP. They also help to monitor side effects of antipsychotic medication. Physical examination for dysmorphic features and signs of organic disorders

**TABLE 3:** Investigations for first episode of psychosis in adolescence.

| Test | Rationale |
|---|---|
| Complete blood count | Preexisting hematological disorders, anemia, clozapine-neutropenia |
| Creatinine, electrolytes, liver function | Preexisting disorders, polydipsia of psychosis, medication-induced hepatic impairment (Valproate) |
| Fasting glucose and lipid profile | Medication-induced insulin resistance and dyslipidemia. Biannual monitoring is required |
| Thyroid function | Psychosis due to thyroid disorders, lithium-induced hypothyroidism |
| Prolactin | Pituitary tumors, antipsychotic-induced hyperprolactinemia |
| Calcium | Low calcium rare cause of psychosis |
| CT or MRI | MRI brain preferable. Malignancy, injuries, deposition (Wilson's, NBIA) |
| EEG | Seizure disorder |
| Urine drug screen | Drug-induced psychosis (Cannabis, amphetamine, MDMA, cocaine, etc.) |

(CT: computed tomography; EEG: electroencephalogram; MDMA: methylenedioxymethamphetamine; MRI: magnetic resonance imaging; NBIA: neurodegeneration with brain iron accumulation)

(metabolic, thyroid, syndrome) is a must. Baseline and periodic monitoring of weight, height, and body mass index (BMI) help in identifying early signs of obesity/metabolic side effects. Blood pressure, pulse rate, and electrocardiogram (ECG) may be needed in some cases. Additional neurological, endocrine, or medical consultations may be required if the onset is acute and indicators for autoimmune pathology are present.

## Psychometric Testing

Psychometric testing of the YP using Thematic Apperception Test, Rorschach inkblot test, and Object Sorting Test can yield valuable information about rational and logical thinking, perceptual disturbances, defense mechanisms, and interpersonal stressors. This is especially important when the symptoms are developing, prodrome is suspected to guide treatment.

A summary of evaluation is presented in **Box 2**.

## Management

Early onset of psychotic disorders, especially schizophrenia requires a multidisciplinary treatment involving pharmacotherapy, psychotherapy, psychoeducation, family intervention, and liaison with the school. Treatment should be least coercive but admission to hospital may be needed if YP has

**BOX 2:** Evaluation summary.

*History*
- Nature and age of onset
- Developmental history
- Medical history
- Family history

*Psychological testing*
- Intelligence quotient (IQ)
- Psychometry-projective tests
- Academic and skills assessment

*Psychiatric examination*
- Conscious, orientation to r/o delirium
- Hallucinations, delusions, negative symptoms
- Risk assessment—suicide, harm to others

*Medical evaluation*
- Physical examination—thyroid, anemia, dysmorphic features
- Signs of substance misuse
- Neurological examination

**TABLE 4:** Second generation antipsychotics (SGAs).

| SGA antipsychotic | Dose range | Adverse effects |
|---|---|---|
| Risperidone | 2–6 mg/d | Extrapyramidal SE, metabolic |
| Olanzapine | 5–20 mg/d | Metabolic SE, weight gain |
| Quetiapine | 200–600 mg/d | QTc prolongation, sedation |
| Aripiprazole | 5–30 mg/d | Akathisia, insomnia |
| Paliperidone | 3–12 mg/d | Extrapyramidal SE, akathisia |
| Lurasidone | 40–80 mg/d | Somnolence, extrapyramidal SE |

high risk of violence, suicidal risk, risk of exploitation by other people, and inability of carers to manage at home. If YP lacks capacity to consent and has substantial risk if untreated, then admission may need to be involuntary or supported as per National Mental Health Care Act, 2017 of India which governs the rules for admission of minors for psychiatric treatment.

## Pharmacotherapy

Psychotic disorders, especially schizophrenia spectrum disorders, delusional disorder, and persistent psychotic disorders secondary to various causes are primarily treated with antipsychotic medication. Second generation antipsychotics (SGAs) are the preferred antipsychotics due to their favorable side effect profile. **Table 4** describes US FDA approved SGAs for use in adolescents for schizophrenia. First generation antipsychotics (FGAs), such as, haloperidol, loxapine, perphenazine, chlorpromazine are effective but associated with extrapyramidal side effects and tardive dyskinesia when used for long periods. In children and adolescents to minimize the risk of side effects "start low and go slow" is the mantra to be followed. Furthermore, it helps in improving compliance to long term treatment.

Behaviors which put the YP and others at risk of safety, such as, violence, destruction of property, and suicidal attempt require emergency sedation. If the YP is in a state to accept oral medication then rapidly acting tranquilizers should be given such as lorazepam 1 mg to start with and up to 4 mg if needed, risperidone 0.5 mg initially and 2 mg if required or olanzapine 2.5–5 mg. For uncooperative patients, intramuscular injection of lorazepam 1–2 mg or haloperidol for severely agitated patients 2.5 mg up to 5 mg are used.

Antipsychotic medication is continued for at least 12 months after remission of symptoms. This is to reduce the risk of relapse which is highest in the first year. When SGAs are used for longer duration, it is essential to monitor height, weight, and BMI by recording at the start of treatment. These are repeated after 1, 3, and 6 months of initiation and 6 monthly thereafter.

The evidence for treatment of schizoaffective disorder, psychotic depression, bipolar affective disorder (BPAD) with psychosis, and other psychotic disorders (substance induced) in adolescents is limited. There is scarcity of large and randomized controlled trials of pharmacological and nonpharmacological treatment methods. However, SGAs are commonly used for treating acute states and sometimes during maintenance period along with psychosocial interventions depending on the diagnosis.

## Psychosocial Interventions

*Psychoeducation*: The YP affected with psychotic disorder and their families are provided information about psychotic disorders, treatment options, and dos and don'ts in a structured way. Psychoeducation is done in an individual, family, or group for YPs or parent groups. Psychoeducation empowers families with right knowledge and in turn helps with treatment outcome by improving medication adherence, reducing blame/critical comments, recognizing behaviors which are maladaptive (substance misuse).

*Cognitive behavioral therapy (CBT):* The CBT is helpful in making the YP understand symptoms, teach coping strategies for psychotic experiences, and managing distressed emotions. CBT is most effective in the recovery phase of the illness, and helps in the management of symptoms of hallucinations, delusions, negative and cognitive symptoms persisting in spite of medication treatment. CBT helps patients in exploring ways of coping to manage hallucinations, challenge delusions, cope with negative emotions, and low mood.

## Working with Families

Families of YP are supported with learning effective ways of problem solving skills arising due to over expectations, poor understanding about the illness, and communication deficits. It helps families to deal with difficult situations effectively and reduce stress and risk of relapse.

## Recovery and Outcome

Psychotic disorders with onset in adolescence can have varied prognosis. Compared to adult onset, early onset of schizophrenia has worse outcome. YP with schizophrenia spectrum disorders are at risk of relapse, up to 90% in lifetime. YP may experience multiple episodes and about one third may continue to have symptoms and deficits. Negative symptoms (amotivation), cognitive deficits, or backlog of studies make it difficult for the YP to return to education. In such case, liaison with school for part time schedule, involvement of school counselors is helpful. Vocational training may be an option for significant academic difficulties. Other YP affected with psychotic disorder may require social skills training, cognitive remediation and rehabilitation to reintegrate with the community.

## ■ POINTS TO REMEMBER

- Psychotic disorders in adolescents are common and disabling if not treated at the earliest.
- Psychotic disorders in adolescents are characterized by delusions, hallucinations, disturbances in thought, motor function, cognition and negative symptoms.
- In the early stage many adolescents experience nonspecific symptoms, such as, low mood, anxiety, forgetfulness, falling grades, bizarre preoccupations and behaviors prior to developing overt psychotic symptoms.
- Evaluation involves mental state examination, risk assessment and investigations to rule out medical-neurological causes, substance-induced psychosis.
- Treatment is multidisciplinary and includes second generation antipsychotics, psychoeducation, cognitive behavior therapy, and family intervention.

## ■ SUGGESTED READING

1. Addington J, Piskulic D, Marshall C. Psychosocial treatments for schizophrenia. Curr Dir Psychol Sci. 2010;19(4):260-3.
2. Benjamin S, Lauterbach MD, Stanislawski AL. Congenital and acquired disorders presenting as psychosis in children and young adults. Child Adolesc Psychiatr Clin N Am. 2013;22(4):581-608.

3. Christian R, Saavedra L, Gaynes BN, Sheitman B, Wines RC, Jonas DE, et al. Future research needs for first- and second-generation antipsychotics for children and young adults. Rockville (MD): Agency for Healthcare Research and Quality (US); 2012.
4. Davis J, Eyre H, Jacka FN, Dodd S, Dean O, McEwen S, et al. A review of vulnerability and risks for schizophrenia: Beyond the two hit hypothesis. Neurosci Biobehav Rev. 2016;65:185-94.
5. Duffy RM, Kelly BD. India's Mental Healthcare Act, 2017. India's Mental Healthcare Act. Int J Law Psychiatry. 2019;62:169-78.
6. Edition F. Diagnostic and statistical manual of mental disorders. Am Psychiatric Assoc. 2013;21(21):591-643.
7. Gaebel W, Zielasek J, Cleveland HR. Psychotic disorders in ICD-11. Die Psychiatrie. 2013;10(01):11-7.
8. Kumperscak HG. Childhood and adolescent schizophrenia and other early-onset psychoses. In: Uehara T (Ed). Psychiatric Disorders–Trends and Developments. London: Intech Open; 2011.
9. Lieberman JA, Small SA, Girgis RR. Early detection and preventive intervention in schizophrenia: from fantasy to reality. Am J Psychiatry. 2019;176(10):794-810.
10. McClellan J, Stock S, American Academy of Child and Adolescent Psychiatry (AACAP) Committee on Quality Issues (CQI). Practice parameter for the assessment and treatment of children and adolescents with schizophrenia. J Am Acad Child Adolesc Psychiatry. 2013;52(9):976-90.
11. McDonell M, McClellan J. Early-onset schizophrenia. In: Mash E, Barkley R (Eds). Assessment of childhood disorders, 4th edition. New York: Guilford Press; 2007. pp. 526-50.
12. Palacio JD. IACAPAP Textbook of Child and Adolescent Mental Health. Virginia: United States American Psychiatric Association; 2017.
13. Poletti S, Anselmetti S, Bechi M, Ermoli E, Bosia M, Smeraldi E, et al. Computer-aided neurocognitive remediation in schizophrenia: durability of rehabilitation outcomes in a follow-up study. Neuropsychol Rehabil. 2010;20(5):659-74.
14. Remschmidt H, Martin M, Fleischhaker C, Theisen FM, Hennighausen K, Gutenbrunner C, et al. Forty-two-years later: the outcome of childhood-onset schizophrenia. J Neural Transm. 2007;114(4):505-12.
15. Sadock BJ, Sadock VA, Ruiz P. Kaplan and Sadock's Synopsis of Psychiatry: Behavioral Sciences/Clinical Psychiatry, 11th edition. Philadelphia: Lippincott Williams & Wilkins; 2014.
16. Stafford MR, Mayo-Wilson E, Loucas CE, James A, Hollis C, Birchwood M, et al. Efficacy and safety of pharmacological and psychological interventions for the treatment of psychosis and schizophrenia in children, adolescents and young adults: a systematic review and meta-analysis. PloS One. 2015;10(2):e0117166.
17. Stahl SM. Essential psychopharmacology: Neuroscientific Basis and Practical Applications, 4th edition. UK: Cambridge University Press; 2000.
18. Volkmar FR. Childhood and adolescent psychosis: a review of the past 10 years. J Am Acad Child Adolesc Psychiatr. 1996;35(7):843-51.
19. Xia J, Merinder LB, Belgamwar MR. Psychoeducation for schizophrenia. Cochrane Database Syst Rev. 2011;2011(6):CD002831.

# Index

Page numbers followed by *b* refer to box, *f* refer to figure, *fc* refer to flowchart, and *t* refer to table

## A

Abdomen, ultrasound of 184
Abnormal uterine bleeding 277-279, 287, 288
   causes of 279*t*
Abortive therapy 146
Acanthosis nigricans 210
Achondroplasia 94
Acid-fast bacilli 318
Acne 163
   adolescent 164*f*
   management of 164
   papulopustular 165*fc*
   scarring 164
   severe 166*fc*
   therapy 214
   vulgaris 163
Activated partial thromboplastin time 285
Acute psychotic disorders 352
Acute respiratory distress syndrome 344
Acyclovir 37, 38
Adolescent 85
   acne 164*f*
   anxiety 237
   assessment 33
   behavior develops 247
   biological framework of 217
   body image
      development of 20*fc*
      satisfaction scale 23
   brain 219
      development 9
   counseling 98
   development 220
   evaluation of 283*fc*
   friendly health clinic 116, 329
      role of 119
      services 116, 117
   growth spurt 269
   headache 139
   health academy 116
   hypotheses of 216, 217
   monitoring *physical growth* of 85
   obesity 190, 191
      etiologies of 194*t*
      management of 198
      pharmacotherapy for 202*t*
      overweight, prevalence of 190
   pneumonia, etiological profile of 343
   polycystic ovary syndrome 208
   pregnancy 34
      prevention of 271
   reproductive health 73, 76
   screening of 271
   sexual health 73, 76
   sexuality 30
      development 33*f*
   sleep problems 153
   substance abuse 308
   suicidal behavior 264*f*
      management of 256
   suicide 257
      biopsychosocial model of 257*fc*
      prevention of 265
   trajectories of 218
   vulvovaginitis 37
Aggressive behavior 229
Airway inflammation 333
Albendazole 272
Alcohol 309
Allergy test 337
Almotriptan 146, 147
Alpha-2 adrenergic agonists 130
Alstrom syndrome 191
Amenorrhea 277, 283, 286
   primary 278, 283*fc*
   secondary 278
American Academy of Neurology 146
Amitriptyline 148, 149
Amorolfine 169
Amphetamine 302
Anabolic steroids 302
Androgen insensitivity syndrome 278
Anemia
   correction 268, 288
   development of 269
   higher prevalence of 268
   programs 274
Anemia Mukt Bharat 272
Anger 155
Anna Freud's theory 31
Anthropometric indices, measurement of 87
Antiandrogens 214

Antidepressants 129
    tricyclic 149
Antiemetics 147
Antiepileptic drugs 191
Antifungals 169
Anti-müllerian hormone levels 209
Antipsychotic 129
    drugs 131
    medication 358
    second generation 357t
Antisocial personality disorder 248
Antitubercular treatment 319
Anxiety 155, 229, 232, 239, 243
    adolescent 237
    disorder 238, 240
    situational 240
Anxiolytic 131
Apocrine sweat glands 162
Aripiprazole 357
Arthritis 179
    juvenile idiopathic 143
Asthma 143, 156, 333
    acute severe exacerbation of 341t
    classification of 335
    exacerbation
        assessing severity of 340t
        management of 340
    global initiative for 338
    long-term management of 339t
    management of 337
    pathogenesis of 334fc
    personalized management of 338
Athlete's foot 168
Atomoxetine 130
Attention deficit hyperactivity disorder 54, 113, 126, 226, 231, 242, 247
    nonstimulant medication for 129
Audiometry 231
Aura 142
Autism 227, 349
    spectrum disorder 130
Autonomic nervous system 182
Autonomy 241
Axilla 169
Azithromycin 37, 38, 39, 347

### B

Bacilli, dissemination of 316
Back pain 178
Bardet-Biedl syndrome 191
Barrier contraceptives 35
*BEARS sleep screening* tool 157, 158
Behavior
    control 45

problems 52
    therapy 146, 253
Benzathine penicillin 38
Benzoyl peroxide 165, 166
Bichloroacetic acid 39
Bifidobacterium 180
Bile acid malabsorption 181
Biopsychosocial model 32, 275fc
Bipolar affective disorder 358
Bleeding disorders 279
Blood
    loss, gastrointestinal 179
    pressure 121, 123, 150, 197
    sugar 197
Body image
    assessment of 23
    development 18, 19
    disturbances, range of 18
    issues 6, 52, 269
        prevalence of 21
    questionnaire 23
Body mass index 26, 86, 88, 121, 123, 150, 190, 193f, 203
    assessment 191
    chart 91f, 93f
    formula 191
Bone age 86, 89
Boredom, negative spiral of 232
Bradycardia 25
Brain
    adolescent 219
    body-emotion-cognitive-changes 239
    development, culmination of 217
    gut interaction 179
    iron accumulation 356
Breast development 6
Breathing exercises 336
Breathlessness 344
Bristol stool form scale 176t
Bronchoalveolar lavage 320, 321
Buprenorphine 302
Butoconazole 40

### C

Calcium 287
Cannabis 353
Carotenemia 25
Cartridge-based nucleic acid amplification test 319, 345
Cefixime 37
Cefoxitin 38
Ceftriaxone 37-39
Celiac disease 179
Central nervous system 3

Cervicitis 37
Chancroid 38
Child's behavior 248
Childhood and adolescent migraine prevention 149
*Chlamydia*
    *pneumoniae* 343
    *trachomatis* 37, 38
Ciclopiroxolamine 166
Ciprofloxacin 38, 39
Clarithromycin 347
Clindamycin 37
Clonidine 130
Clotrimazole 40
Cocaine 302
Cognitive behavioral therapy 27, 54, 107, 146, 187, 265, 358
Cognitive defects 227, 228
Coliform bacteria 38
Combination pills 213
Comedonal acne, management of 165*fc*
Communication 119
Community programs 266
Comprehensive National Nutrition Survey 274
Computed tomography 194, 356
Conduct disorder 243, 247, 251
    treatment of 253
Confusion 239
Conners scale 250
Constipation 177
Contraception 34, 35
    postcoital 35
Contraceptive pill, oral 203, 288
Contrast-enhanced computed tomography 184, 320
Conventional therapy 145
Copper T 35
Core-learning disabilities 67
Coronavirus disease-2019 (COVID-19) 51, 238
    pandemic 51, 66, 104, 223
    vaccine 347
Corpus luteum secretes progesterone 276
Corticosteroids
    inhaled 337-339
    oral 338
    therapy 191
Corticotropin-releasing hormone 182
Coryza 344
Cosmetic procedures 214
Cosmetology 171
Cough 145, 336
    syrups 302

CRAFFT screening questionnaire 64*b*
C-reactive protein 345
Creatine phosphokinase 203
Criminal law (amendment) Act 41
Crisis care 265
Cryotherapy 39
Culture and drug susceptibility test 324
Cushing's disease 191
Cyber bullying 52, 257
Cyproheptadine 148
Cystic fibrosis 68
Cysts, ovarian 287

## D

Dating violence 34, 36
Day sleepiness 155
    excessive 156, 158
Dehydroepiandrosterone sulfate 284
Delayed sleep-wake phase disorder 155, 156
    treatment of 159*b*
Delinquency, juvenile 301
Delusional disorder 352
Dental erosion 25
Depression 52, 61, 76, 229, 232, 237, 241, 243
    persistent 243
    screening for 65*t*
Desvenlafaxine 130
Diabetes mellitus 68, 143, 155, 193, 194
Diarrhea 186
Dietary therapy 187
Digital media, benefits of 54*b*
Diphtheria 347
Disruptive behavior disorder 247, 248*b*, 251
    development of 247
    diagnosis of 248, 250
    early indicators of 249*t*
    treatment of 251
Disruptive mood dysregulation disorder 247
Dissocial disorders 247
Distant heart sounds 25
Dizygotic twins 178
Dizziness 239
d-lysergic acid diethylamide 302
Donovanosis 38
Down syndrome 94
Doxycycline 37, 38, 39
Drugs 63, 130
    abuse 229
Duloxetine 130
Dynamic psychotherapies 187

*Dysmenorrhea* 280, 285, 287, 288*t*
   primary 280, 282, 282*t*, 287
   secondary 282, 282*t*, 288
Dysphagia 179
Dysphoric disorder, premenstrual 280

### E

Ear, nose, and throat 150, 157
Eating disorders 25*b*
Eczema 167
Edema 25
Elbows 169
Electroencephalogram 157, 356
Electromyogram 157
Electronic
   cigarettes 301, 302
      nicotine delivery systems 302
Electrooculogram 157
Emotional disorders, childhood anxiety related 121, 230
Endocrine 279
   disorders 286
   regulation 4*f*
Endometrial regression 276
Endoscopy 184
Energy, loss of 242
Epididymitis, sexually acquired 39
Episodic syndromes 143
Erikson's theory 31
Erythromycin 38, 39, 347
*Escherichia coli* 177
Ethambutol 323
Exercise 61, 63, 63*b*, 200
Exhaled nitric oxide, fractional concentration of 336

### F

Facial petechiae 25
Famciclovir 37, 38
Fat, loss of 25
Fatigue 155, 341
Fecal calprotectin 184
Fecal test 184
Feet, hyperhidrosis of 170
Ferumoxytol 273
Fever 179
Figure rating scale 23*f*
Fluconazole 37, 40
Flunarizine 148
Fluoroquinolone 324, 325
Fluoxetine 243
Folic acid supplementation 272

Follicle-stimulating hormone 4*f*, 209, 276, 283, 284
Fragile X syndrome 229
   stigmata of 230
Frankfurt plane 87
Freud's psychoanalytic theory 31
Fungal infections 168

### G

Gastric aspirate 319, 320
Gender dysphoria 33
Generalized anxiety disorder 239
Genetic syndromes 191
Genital
   development 6
   ulcer disease 38
Genitalia 169
Glucagon-like peptide-1 203
Gonadotropin-releasing hormone 4*f*, 276, 283
Government Educational Schemes and Programs 233
Granuloma inguinale 38
Griseofulvin 169
Growth 85, 145
   charts 90, 121
   hormone 94
      deficiency 191
   monitoring 86, 87
      guidelines 191
      indices for 86
      process of 87
   physical 85
   velocity 89
Guanfacine 130
Guideline-driven care 119
Gut-brain interaction, disorders of 179
Gut-microbiota dysbiosis 180
Gynecomastia
   bilateral 87
   unilateral 87

### H

H1N1 pneumonia 346
*Haemophilus*
   *ducreyi* 38
   *influenzae* type B 343
Hair 171
   abnormalities 171
Hallucinogens 302
Harpenden calipers 89*f*
Head injuries 228

Headache 140f, 142, 150fc, 178
　adolescent 139
　characteristics of 142
　cluster 141
　disorders 139
　early morning 145
　frequency of 145
　medication overuse 141
　occipital 145
　primary 139, 144, 144t
　progressive 145
　secondary 144, 144t
　severe 145
　tension-type 139, 141b, 150
　thunderclap 145
Headspace modification 68
Healthcare
　accessibility of 118
　environment 118
　professionals, role of 48
　provider 75
Hearing impairment 228, 230
Heart rate 341, 347
HEEADSSS screening 143
Height 86, 87
　and weight chart 92f
　measurement of 195
Hemoglobin 288
Hemorrhage, subconjunctival 25
Hepatitis
　A 79
　B 79
Herpes simplex virus 37
Hirsutism 87, 171, 209
　progressive 210
Hormones 35
Human immunodeficiency virus 36, 73,
　　　77, 81, 83, 123, 166, 301, 320, 329
Human papillomavirus 36, 39, 79, 83, 170
Hydrogen breath tests 185
Hyperandrogenism 209, 210, 213
　biochemical evidence of 283
Hyperhidrosis, focal 169
Hyperinsulinemia 209
　compensatory 209
Hypersensitivity
　bisceral 179
　pneumonitis 336
Hypertension 140f, 145, 156
　persistent 198
Hypnotherapy, gut-directed 187
Hypochondroplasia 94
Hypotension 25
Hypothalamic dysfunction 191

Hypothalamic gonadotropin-releasing
　　　hormone 3
Hypothalamic-pituitary-adrenal axis 182
Hypothalamus, tumors of 278
Hypothermia 25
Hypothyroidism 191, 268

# I

Immune
　activation 180
　dysregulation 155
Immunoglobulin E 338, 339
Impulsive behavior 155, 219
Indian Academy of Pediatrics 57b, 94,
　　　116, 193f
Indian Penal Code 53
Infections 279
　gastrointestinal 177
　mycoplasma 347
　stage of 316
Infectious diseases 117
Inflammation, low-grade 180
Inflammatory bowel disease 179
Information and communication
　　　technology 154
Insomnia, psychophysiological 156
Insulin
　resistance 209
　sensitizers 213
Integrated health services delivery
　　　framework 328
Intellectual disability 130, 227
Intelligence quotient 228
Intensified-National Iron Plus Initiative 272t
Intensive care unit 341
Interferon gamma release assay 319, 329
Internet
　addiction 52
　gaming disorder 53
Intrauterine contraceptive devices 35
Intrauterine growth restriction 337
Iron
　deficiency 269
　　anemia 269, 271t
　parenteral 273
　requirement 273
　supplementation 272
Irritable bowel syndrome 175, 177, 186
　diagnosis of 182
　pathophysiology of 179
　post-infection 181
　practical management of 185
　subtypes of 175, 176t

Irritable mood 242
Isoniazid 322-324, 326, 329
   high-dose 325
Isothermal amplification,
       loop-mediated 345
Itraconazole 37, 169

## J

Jock itch 168

## K

Kallman syndrome 278
Keratosis pilaris 167
Ketoconazole 37, 166
*Klebsiella granulomatis* 38
Klinefelter syndrome 229, 231

## L

*Lactobacillus*
   *reuteri* 187
   *rhamnosus* 187
Latent tuberculosis infection 329
Learning disability 226
Leptin
   deficiency 191
   receptor defects 191
Leukotriene receptor antagonist 338, 339
Levofloxacin 39, 347
Life skills 26
   education 103
Linear growth
   deceleration of 179
   monitoring of 87
Lipoprotein
   high-density 197, 209
   low-density 203, 209
Lithium 129
Long-acting
   beta-2-agonist 338, 339
   muscarinic agent 339
Luliconazole 169
Lurasidone 357
Luteinizing hormone 4*f*, 209, 283, 284
   surge of 276
Lymph node 317

## M

Magnetic resonance imaging 284, 356
Major depressive disorder, symptoms of 242
*Malassezia* folliculitis 167

Mania 243
Manning's criteria 175
Measles, mumps, and rubella 79
Media
   adverse effects of 51
   benefits of 54
   education 26
   influence 76
   usage 50
   use
      guidelines 56*fc*
      health hazards of 52*b*
Medroxyprogesterone 284
   acetate 213
Melatonin 132
Menarche 276
   onset of 281
Meningitis 191
Menstrual abnormalities 282*b*
Menstrual bleeding
   chronic 279
   heavy 278
Menstrual calendar 290
Menstrual cycle 276, 281
   irregular 209
   normal 277*b*
Menstrual disorders 209, 210, 276, 280
   management of 286
Menstrual hygiene 290
Menstrual irregularity 87, 208
Menstrual losses 269
Mental
   disorders 228, 232
      diagnostic and statistical manual of 250, 251, 306*b*, 349, 350*t*
   distress 229
   health 238
      disorders, group of 238
      issues 76
      problems 244
      urgency of 261
   illness, treatment of 265
   state examination 354
Mescaline 302
Metabolic syndrome
   diagnosis of 197*t*
   prevention of 212
Metacarpophalangeal joints 25
Methicillin-resistant *staphylococcus aureus* 345
Methylenedioxymethamphetamine 356
Methylphenidate 129, 302
Metronidazole 37, 38
Miconazole 40, 169

Microorganic disorders 179
Micropenis 87
Midparental height 86, 88
Migraine 139, 140, 142, 143, 147*t*
    chronic 141
    criteria for 140*t*
    pediatric 142
    prophylaxis 148
    treatment modalities for 145*t*
Mild attention deficit hyperactivity disorder 227
Mood
    disorders 155, 244, 247
    stabilizers 131
Morning tiredness 155
Morphine 302
Motility studies 184
Motivational interviewing 106, 109
    treatment integrity 113
Moxifloxacin, high-dose 325
Multicomponent psychological therapy 187
Multisystemic therapy 253
Muscle relaxation, progressive 146
Myalgia 178
*Mycobacterium*
    growth indicator tube 321
    *tuberculosis* 315
*Mycoplasma*
    *genitalium* 37
    infections 347
    *pneumoniae* 343, 345
Myo-inositol
    administration of 213
    role of 213

## N

Naproxen 147
Narcolepsy 156
Narcotics 302
Nasha Mukt Bharat Abhiyaan 309
National Education Policy 233
National Family Health Survey 76, 117
National Iron Plus Initiative 272
National Tuberculosis Elimination Programme 315, 322
Near-fatal asthma 341
    exacerbation 341*fc*
Nebulized hypertonic saline 319
Negative body image, warning signs of 22*b*
*Neisseria gonorrhoeae* 37, 38
Neurodevelopmental disorder 132, 228
Neurohormonal dysregulation 182

Neuroleptic malignant syndrome 131
Neurotransmitters 181
Nicotine exposure 302
Nocturnal diarrhea 179
Nomophobia 52, 54
Nonalcoholic fatty liver disease 194
    symptoms of 198
Noncommunicable diseases 117
Nonepinephrine reuptake inhibitor 130
Nonsteroidal anti-inflammatory drugs 146, 150
    use of 287
Nonsuicidal self-injury 259, 261, 262
Norepinephrine reuptake inhibitors 130
Nucleic acid amplification test 321
Nystatin 40

## O

Obesity 52, 155, 156, 190, 210
    adolescent 190, 191
    comorbidities of 194*t*
    diagnosis of 193*f*
    etiology of 191
    pathological cause for 195
Obsessive-compulsive disorder 130, 239
Obstructive sleep apnea 156
    syndrome 194, 228
Odynophagia 179
Ofloxacin 39
Olanzapine 131, 357
Oppositional defiant disorder 247, 250
    treatment of 253
Oral contraceptive pill 203, 288
Organic disease 179*b*, 183
Orthostatic pulse 25
Oseltamivir, dosage of 346, 346*t*
Ovarian follicle 276
Ovulation, suppression of 35
Oxygen saturation 341

## P

Packed red cells, transfusion of 272
Pain 186
    chest 344
    chronic abdominal 178
    psychological 259
Paliperidone 357
Panic disorder 239
Papulopustular acne, mild-to-moderate 165*fc*
Parent child interaction therapy 252
Peak expiratory flowmetry 336

Pediatric
    intestinal pseudo-obstruction 183
    irritable bowel syndrome 175b
    migraine 142
        disability assessment
            questionnaire 143b
Pediatrician
    friendly growth charts 93
    role of 34, 54, 119, 303
    training of 266
Pelvic inflammatory disease 38
Peptic ulcer disease 179
Peptide receptor antagonists,
        calcitonin gene-related 147
Perirectal disease 179
Permethrin 169
Pertussis 347
Pervasive developmental disorder
        247, 349
Pethidine 302
Phantom vibration syndrome 54
Pharmacotherapy 146, 254
Pharynx, gonococcal infections of 39
Phasic disorder 352
Phenobarbitone 228
Phobic disorders 239
*Pityrosporum ovale* 166
Plus 79
Pneumonia 343, 344
    adolescent 343
    atypical 343
    bacterial 346
    risk factors for 344
Podofilox 39
Polycystic ovarian syndrome 194, 203, 208,
        211, 212, 277, 279, 284, 286
    adolescent 208
Polysomnography 157
Poor school performance 76, 225, 226,
        230t, 231
    causes of 226t
    prevalence of 225
Pornography 52
Post-traumatic stress disorder 240
Potassium hydroxide 169
Prader orchidometer 95f
Prader–Willi syndrome 94, 191
Pregnancy 34, 279
    adolescent 34
    medical termination of 41
    prevention 76
    teenage 73
Premenstrual syndrome 280, 289
Primary amenorrhea 278, 283fc
    etiologies of 278t

Primary headache 139, 144, 144t
    treatment of 145
Probiotics 187
Progesterone 213
    challenge test 284
Propranolol 148
Protection of Children from Sexual
        Offences (POCSO) Act 36, 53
Pseudohypoparathyroidism 191
Pseudomonas infections 345
Psilocybin 302
Psychiatric disorders 257, 303
Psychoactive substance 301
Psychoeducation 358
Psychological therapies 187
Psychometric testing 356
Psychomotor agitation 242
Psychosexual development, phases of 31t
Psychosis 243
    first episode of 356t
    lifetime prevalence of 353
    reactive 352
Psychosocial development, normal 7
Psychosomatic problems 229
Psychostimulants 129
Psychotherapy 100t, 243, 253
    role of 133
Psychotic disorder 349, 350t, 352, 357
    substance-induced 353
Psychotropic drugs 309
Puberty 3, 4f, 5, 145
    delayed 5, 87, 179
    monitoring of 5
    physiological processes of 218
    precocious 5
Pubic hair 6
Pyrazinamide 323

# Q

Quetiapine 131, 357

# R

Randomized controlled trials 149
Rapid diagnostic tests 319
Rashtriya Bal Swasthya Karyakram 328
Rashtriya Kishor Swasthya Karyakram 117
Red blood cell transfusion 273
Relaxation therapy 187
Reproductive health, adolescent 73, 76
Rescue therapy, use of 340
Respiratory failure 344
    progressive 341
Respiratory rate 341, 347
Restless leg syndrome 156

Retinal screening 198
Rifampicin 323
    sensitive tuberculosis 322*t*
Risperidone 191, 243, 357
Rizatriptan 146, 147
Road traffic accidents 155
Rotterdam criteria 208
Russell-Silver syndrome 94

## S

Sample safety plan 265*b*
*Sarcoptes scabiei var hominis* 169
Scabies 169
Schizoaffective disorder 352
Schizophrenia 349, 351*t*, 352*f*
    adolescent onset 350
    clinical features of 351*f*
    early-onset 349
    etiology of 353*f*
    neuroanatomy of 351*f*
SCOFF questionnaire 23, 24*b*
Seasonal influenza 347
Seborrheic dermatitis 165, 166
Secondary amenorrhea 278
    etiologies of 278*t*
Secondary headache 144, 144*t*
    red flag signs of 144, 145*b*
Sedatives 131
Seizures, coexistence of 145
Selective serotonin reuptake inhibitor 130, 265
Self-harm techniques 257
Sellar masses 278
Serotonin transporter 181
Sertaconazole 169
Serum glutamic pyruvic transaminase 194
    measurement of 198
Sexting 52, 53
Sexual abuse 34, 36, 76
Sexual activity 237
Sexual and reproductive health 73, 81
    assessment 73, 75*f*
Sexual behaviour
    high-risk 80
    promiscuous 301
Sexual development, adolescent 31, 32
Sexual exploitation 45
Sexual health
    adolescent 73, 76
    risk 78*f*
Sexual maturity
    monitoring of 94
    rating 5, 6*t*, 87, 195
Sexual orientation 30, 33

Sexual promiscuity 229
Sexual self-concept 32
Sexuality 30, 48, 61, 64, 64*b*
    adolescent 30
Sexually transmitted infections 35, 36, 37*t*, 73, 74, 76, 77, 79, 81, 83, 123, 170
Short-acting beta-2-agonist 337-339
Sialadenosis 25
Sinecatechins 39
Skin
    anatomy of 163*f*
    physiology of 163*f*
    test 318
Skinfold thickness 86
Sleep 153, 201
    diary 156
    disorders 155, 156*t*
    hygiene 159
        basic principles of 159*b*
    importance of 154
    problems 154
        adolescent 153
    walking 156
Slipped capital femoral epiphysis 194, 195
Social
    anxiety disorder 239
    influences 10
    isolation 229
    learning 32
    media usage 50*t*
Sociotherapy 254
Sodium valproate 149, 191
Somnambulism 156
Spasmo proxyvon 302
Special growth charts 94
Specific learning disability 228, 231
Spermatogenesis, suppression of 35
Spirituality 66, 66*b*
Spirometry 336
*Staphylococcus aureus* 343
Stimulants 302
*Streptococcus pneumoniae* 343
Streptomycin 323
Stress
    leads, perception of 221
    management 307*f*
Stressors 306
Striae distensae 167
Substance abuse 52, 76, 304*t*
    disorders 306*b*
    office management of 301
Substance use disorder 301, 304, 307
    screening for 303
Suicidal adolescent, office management of 258*b*

Suicidal behavior 155, 257, 262*fc*
  adolescent 264*f*
Suicidal ideation 241, 244
Suicidal risk, clinical assessment of 257
Suicide 52, 61, 65, 65*b*, 229, 256, 257
  adolescent 257
  screening for 65*t*
  warning signs of 260, 261*t*
Sulfamethoxazole 39
Sumatriptan 146, 147
Syphilis 38
Systemic disease 278
  symptoms of 145

### T

Tanner staging 94
Terbinafine 169
Terconazole 40
Testosterone 284
Tetanus 347
Thyroid 278
Tics 243
Tinea
  cruris 168
  pedis 168
Tinidazole 37
Tioconazole 40
Topiramate 148, 149
Tourette's syndrome 130
Transient psychotic disorders 352
*Treponema pallidum* 38
Triceps skinfold thickness 88
Trichloroacetic acid 39
*Trichomonas vaginalis* 37
Trimethoprim 39
Triptans 146
Tuberculin skin test 318
Tuberculosis 315, 317, 318, 329
  bacterium 316
  drug-resistant 320, 321, 324, 324*fc*, 325, 325*t*, 329
  drug-sensitive 320, 321, 324, 329
  drug-susceptible 323
  extrapulmonary 316, 320, 325
  infection 316
    pathophysiology of 317*fc*
  mono-resistance 326
  multidrug-resistant 321, 326, 326*b*
  mycobacterium 315
  poly-drug resistance 326
  pre-extensively drug-resistant 326
  psychosocial impact of 327
  pulmonary 320*fc*
  skeletal 318
  treatment of 321*fc*

Turner syndrome 94
Typical sleep dairy 157*b*

### U

Ultrasonography 283
United Nations Children's Fund 43, 103
United Nations Population Fund 43
*Ureaplasma urealyticum* 37
Urethritis 37
Urinary frequency 178
Uterine
  pathology 279
  problems 287

### V

Vaginosis, bacterial 37
Valaciclovir 37, 38
Valproate 148, 243
  sodium 243
Varicella 347
Venlafaxine 130
Verruca plantaris 170
Violence 155
Visual impairment 228
Vital sign abnormalities 347
Vitamin D supplementation 287
Vocal cord
  dysfunction 335
    treatment of 336
  relaxation techniques 336
Vomiting 145
Vulvovaginal candidiasis 40
Vulvovaginitis, adolescent 37

### W

Waist circumference 86, 88
Warts
  anogenital 39
  plantar 170
Weight 86, 87
  loss 179, 204
  measurement of 195
Wrist 169

### X

Xerosis 25

### Y

Young person's CORE 67

### Z

Zolmitriptan 146, 147